# THE WOMAN

FROM **PUBERTY** TO **MENOPAUSE**

# THE WOMAN

## FROM **PUBERTY** TO **MENOPAUSE**

Dr. Sola Akinniyi

DORRANCE PUBLISHING CO
EST. 1920
PITTSBURGH, PENNSYLVANIA 15238

The contents of this work including, but not limited to, the accuracy of events, people, and places depicted; opinions expressed; permission to use previously published materials included; and any advice given or actions advocated are solely the responsibility of the author, who assumes all liability for said work and indemnifies the publisher against any claims stemming from publication of the work.

All Rights Reserved

Copyright © 2020 by Dr. Sola Akinniyi

No part of this book may be reproduced or transmitted, downloaded, distributed, reverse engineered, or stored in or introduced into any information storage and retrieval system, in any form or by any means, including photocopying and recording, whether electronic or mechanical, now known or hereinafter invented without permission in writing from the publisher.

Dorrance Publishing Co
585 Alpha Drive, Suite 103
Pittsburgh, PA 15238
Visit our website at www.dorrancebookstore.com

ISBN: 978-1-4809-5750-3
eISBN: 978-1-4809-5773-2

## ACKNOWLEDGEMENTS

The realization of this book took time. Indeed, there were many times when reliance on the encouragement and inspiration from people around me were necessary to propel its progress.

My praise and deep appreciation go to the Almighty God for granting me the opportunity to bring this book to fulfillment. I am grateful to my darling wife, Mrs. Abimbola Akinniyi for her consistent provision of comfort, relentless effort and encouragement in ensuring the completion of this book; my lovely daughter, Oyinkansola Akinniyi deserves a special mention for her constructive criticisms and help where necessary.

My thanks also go to my great friend Mr. Akinkoye, Dr. and Mrs. Akinmolayan for their suggestions. I also sincerely thank my secretary, Edith, for doing a great job in typing out my clustered manuscript. I am most grateful to Mrs. Abimbola Oloyede, the veteran journalist for accepting to edit this book. Her expertise is evident in the diligent editing of the book.

Finally, I express sincere gratitude to Dorrance publishing company for ensuring the publication of this book.

This book is dedicated to the
GOOD HEALTH of millions of
adolescent girls and women
all over the world.

# CONTENTS

| | |
|---|---|
| ACKNOWLEDGMENTS.................................................... | v |
| Introduction................................................................... | xi |
| 1  -  Puberty and Adolescence......................................... | 3 |
| 2  -  Menstruation........................................................... | 27 |
| 3  -  Vaginal Discharge and Genital Infections............................ | 54 |
| 4  -  HIV and AIDS......................................................... | 69 |
| 5  -  Abortion................................................................. | 91 |
| 6  -  Family Planning...................................................... | 107 |
| 7  -  Uterine Fibroids...................................................... | 135 |
| 8  -  Polycystic Ovarian Syndrome (PCOS)..................... | 148 |
| 9  -  Endometriosis and Adenomyosis.............................. | 157 |
| 10 -  Infertility................................................................ | 169 |
| 11 -  Ectopic Pregnancy................................................. | 212 |
| 12 -  Pregnancy............................................................. | 219 |
| 13 -  Prenatal Care........................................................ | 261 |
| 14 -  Labor and Delivery................................................ | 292 |
| 15 -  Postnatal Care and Breastfeeding.......................... | 321 |
| 16 -  Cancers of the Cervix and Womb........................... | 342 |
| 17 -  Breast and Breast Cancer...................................... | 362 |
| 18 -  Ovary and Ovarian Cancer..................................... | 386 |
| 19 -  Weight Problems and Obesity................................. | 405 |
| 20 -  Menopause........................................................... | 414 |
| 21 -  Miscellaneous....................................................... | 437 |

# INTRODUCTION

Women are uniquely and specially endowed, both in body form and functions. In terms of anatomy and the complex tasks that women perform, they are different from men. Emotionally, women are also wired differently.

From the start of puberty, the female child experiences intricate and complex body and functional transformations, with the body becoming a battle ground for old and new hormones. At puberty, the pathway to adulthood, most of the bodily functions become progressive and automatic. The majority of the events are pleasant and physiological but a few are not so. Nevertheless, all must be learned and adapted to. Events change fairly rapidly, throwing up many questions that need answers. Therefore, from puberty up until menopause, every period in the life of a woman is unique, coming with its own measure of joy and challenges. To be able to understand the reasons for the various important occurrences and make necessary adjustments or adaptations, a reasonable amount of knowledge is essential. Knowledge empowers the woman to be able anticipate changes, adjust and adapt better to health and disease situations. Deliberate nutritional, habitual and lifestyles choices are pertinent for the furtherance of good health and the prevention of diseases.

This goal of this book is to provide answers to most of the important questions on the minds of adolescent girls and women. In the process of fulfilling this role, the book takes every opportunity to educate the reader on the essentials of her unique body form and functions. The deliberate question and answer arrangement of this book provides an accessible education for readers on the idiosyncrasies of the female body and functions. This style was deliberately chosen to make reading more enjoyable and engaging. As much as possible, medical jargons were avoided, so you don't need to have a medical dictionary by your side. While reading through, you will soon find out that the book talks; you will inevitably find yourself asking questions and hoping to find answers in the book. The answers have been presented in a friendly, easy to understand manner. Issues are discussed in a way that is frank and nonjudgmental. The pleasure of reading the book should make an average reader a resource person on the various topics discussed; You will probably become more useful to your friends, relations and community on feminine health issues.

The contents and topics covered in this book have also been carefully chosen, to cover the more important topical issues in feminine health, right from puberty to menopause. So, at various periods in a woman's life, the book comes- in handy, as a reservoir of information and help. If in the end, many girls and women find this book useful to themselves, relations and community, then, the purpose of writing would have been achieved.

Finally, the book is intended for the general public, especially women of all ages but healthcare personnel including nurses, and young doctors should find it useful in their practices. Enjoy your reading!

# THE WOMAN

FROM **PUBERTY** TO **MENOPAUSE**

# CHAPTER 1
# Puberty and Adolescence

*"It (puberty) is not that you lose control of your body so much as that you lose control over the way your body is interpreted. Your body becomes an alien body, a question rather than an answer."*
– CARINO CHOCANO

**1.    What does puberty mean?**
Simply put, puberty is the period in life when an adolescent is physically and physiologically mature to the point that reproduction is possible. It is a stage when a girl child can become pregnant while a boy child can impregnate a female. In other words, it is a transition period from childhood to adulthood. In terms of reproduction, the important thing is that the girl and her guardians should know that she has acquired the status of an adult and if she engages in sexual activity, she is in danger of conceiving an unwanted pregnancy.

**2.    What is the biological basis of puberty?**
At puberty, there are physiological, physical and emotional changes. The changes are initiated by the hypothalamus. The hypothalamus is an area in the brain which contains releasing hormones. The pituitary gland is a pea-shaped organ located at the base of the brain. The gland secretes and stores many hormones which perform different functions in the body. Both the hypothalamus and pituitary gland work together. When the pituitary receives the appropriate command from the hypothalamus, it releases two hormones – the luteinizing hormone (LH) and the follicle stimulating hormone (FSH). These two hormones stimulate the eggs in the ovaries which in turn produce the estrogen hormone. The estrogen hormone then stimulates secondary sexual characteristics, which includes the growth of female breasts, body hair in the private parts and armpits, as well as the occurrence of the first menstruation.

### 3. What are the features of puberty in females?

The hallmark of puberty is the appearance of secondary sexual characteristics; those physical features that suggest that an adolescent is becoming sexually mature. These include the appearances of female breasts, adult female-type body curves, armpit and pubic hairs. This period cumulates at the occurrence of the first menstruation.

### 4. What is the earliest sign of puberty?

Usually, the first sign is a growth spurt or a period during which a girl experiences accelerated growth in height. The accelerated tallness lasts for 1-2 years and should be quite noticeable by parents or keen observers, especially as this growth spurt is closely followed by the development of the breasts.

### 5. In what order do these physical changes occur in girls?

The appearances of the milestones of puberty overlap one another. Generally, they occur in the following order:

| Milestones | Average Age |
|---|---|
| Accelerated growth rate (rapid growth or tallness) | From 9 years |
| Breast development or budding (Thelache) | About 9 years |
| Pubic hair growth (Puderche) | 11 years |
| Armpit hair growth (Adrenache) | 11 years |
| First Menstruation (Menache) | 13 years or earlier |

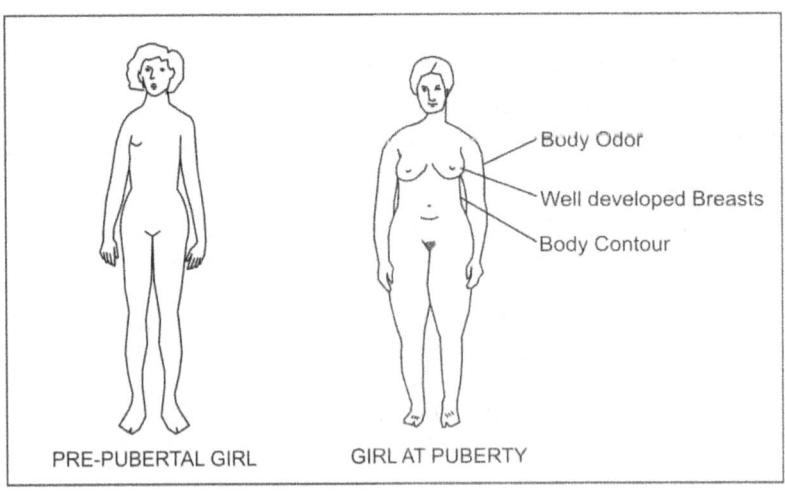

PRE-PUBERTAL GIRL   GIRL AT PUBERTY

## 6. At what age does puberty occur in girls globally?

Globally speaking, most girls attain puberty between the ages of 9-14 years. However, the age at puberty varies from one individual or community to another. The current global trend is that the average age at which girls attain puberty is decreasing.

## 7. What is responsible for the current reduction in the age of girls at puberty?

Globally, girls currently attain puberty at an earlier age than their counterparts in previous decades. There are suggestions that this trend may be largely due to changes in lifestyles, especially with the remarkable increase in the number of obese and overweight girls over the last few years. The influence of race is also important. Other reasons that have been suggested for the reducing age at puberty include:

- Diet and foods that enhance weight gain can increase the risk of obesity
- Increased consumption of meat
- Increased consumption of sugar-rich foods
- Increased consumption of dairy foods and beverages, which contribute to the accumulation of body fat and obesity
- Excessive stress
- Insulin resistance
- Increased use of hair products impregnated with hormones

Parents and girls should know how the current global trend in the use of hair attachments, affects young girls and women. The attachments are obtained from both human and artificial sources, many of which are laced with chemicals that contain the estrogen hormone. Although estrogen makes hair look natural, supple and shiny, the estrogen in such attachments penetrates the scalp, neck and upper back, where the attachments make contact with the skin. As earlier mentioned, Estrogen is the main hormone that promotes pubertal development, consequently early and prolonged exposure to this hormone, can facilitate early attainment of puberty in young girls.

## 8. So what is the average age of girls at puberty in the USA?

According to available data from the Center for Disease Control & Prevention (CDC), most girls in the USA attain puberty between the ages of 9 and 13 years. Of all the racial groups, African American girls attain puberty earlier than others. In very few cases, puberty may start in girls much earlier, around 8 years of age. However, the age at puberty varies from one racial group to another.

### 9. Is there any relationship between bodyweight and the timing of puberty?

Yes. A girl needs to gain sufficient weight for the onset of puberty to occur at the normal time. This is critical and especially true regarding the timing of the first menstruation, which most girls experience when they attain a critical body weight of 105.8 lbs (48kg). The range varies from 94.8 – 116.8lbs (43 - 53kg).

### 10. What about body fat content and timing of puberty?

The amount of fat in the body is also important for the initiation of puberty. It is believed that a girl must have about 17-22% body fat content for puberty to occur at the appropriate time. Therefore, girls that are excessively skinny may experience delayed puberty.

### 11. What are the common complaints at puberty?

At the onset of puberty, a girl child may experience some problems as a result of the various hormonal changes and their effects on her body. The changes include noticeable physical alterations. Some are bad, others are acceptable. The complaints and feelings are variable and depend on the individual girl. The common problems include:

- Acne or pimples on the face, chest and upper back; occurs in 85-90% of girls
- Weight gain, Changes in facial look and overall appearance
- Shyness and timidity
- Clumsiness
- Anxiety and mixed emotions
- Secrecy

### 12. What can be done to prevent excessive weight gain at puberty?

Weight gain is normal for most girls during the period of puberty. So, many things are changing in their bodies at this time during the process of transition from being a girl to a young woman. Women generally have more body fat than girls. However, you may be able to reduce the amount of weight gain by eating correct amounts of healthy food, taking food supplements and regular exercise. It is advisable that you discuss issues that may be bothering you at this period with your guardian, who should be willing to guide you through.

### 13. Why the shyness and timidity?

It is perfectly normal for a girl to feel shy and timid around puberty. This happens to many girls and the degree varies. To a large extent, this situation is as a result of the rapid changes in their physical outlooks, especially the appearances of robust breasts and adult body contours. Also, many of these girls have true profound emotional feelings towards males for the first time at this period. This may result in confusion and distancing from friends and associates, except the most trusted and intimate among them.

## 14. What are the 5 most common signs that parents should look out for that may signify that their daughter is attaining puberty?

There are 5 major physical features that are easily noticeable. They are:

- Growth spurt: Initial period of rapid growth or tallness. She can gain as much as 4 inches per year
- Breast development
- Hair growth in the armpits
- Rounding-up of body contours
- Unique Body Odor (BO): This happens at about age 11. This happens as a result of an increase in the activities of hormones and sweat glands. It is not foul smelling. It is unique to the girl. This is why it is possible for a mother to smell the clothes of her adolescent girl and correctly identify them

## 15. What is the current global trend in age for girls at their first menses?

Just like puberty, the age at which girls attain first menses (menache) is reducing globally. In many developed countries, puberty may occur as early as 8-9 years. In the less developed parts of the world, it is normal for girls to experience their first menses slightly later, commonly between 12 to 14 years of age.

## 16. When do girls commonly experience their first menses in the USA?

According to the statistics from the CDC, about 80% of girls experience their first menstruation at 11-13.75 years in the USA. The median age is 12.43 years. This is usually about 2 years after the beginning of breast development. Once again, there is disparity between the various racial groups. African American girls are more likely to experience menache earlier than girls from other racial groups.

## 17. What about those who attain puberty so early?

When a girl attains puberty before the age of 8 years, she is deemed to have precocious puberty. In some instances, precocious puberty may run in families for unknown reasons while in few cases, the reasons may be attributable.

## 18. What is the biological reason for precocious puberty?

More than 70% of cases of precocious puberty in girls happen for unknown reasons. However, there are two important areas in the brain, the hypothalamus and the pituitary gland, which are suspected to be biologically responsible for some cases of precocious puberty. Doctors believe that signals may occur from the hypothalamus and pituitary gland prematurely. These signals result in the release of hormones which accelerate physiological development in a girl at an earlier age, causing precocious puberty. Normally, signals for physiological and reproductive maturity do not occur until about the age of 10 years. Precocious puberty can also be caused by diseases such as:

- Brain tumors
- Tumors of the pineal gland
- Infection of the brain e.g. meningitis
- Hydrocephalus (abnormally large infant head)
- Head injury
- Drugs such as steroids, Oral Contraceptive Pills (OCP) etc. in childhood
- Liver diseases
- Endocrine disorders e.g. hypothyroidism

## 19. What are the factors that may increase the risk of precocious puberty in girls?

There are some conditions or factors that may predispose girls to precocious puberty. However, in over 70% of cases, precocious puberty occurs for unknown reasons. In some instances, it may occur in particular families, and it is possibly genetically inherited. Other factors include:

- Race: It is believed that being African or Black predisposes girls to precocity. Even in communities like the USA, Black or African American girls are more predisposed to precocious puberty than Whites
- Familial: In some families, precocious puberty may be more common than in other families in the same community for unknown reasons
- Affluence: children of wealthy people are more likely to experience precocious puberty more than other girls in the same community

- Obesity: Fat and obese girls are more likely to experience precocious puberty
- Effect of Equator and low altitude: Girls in communities located near the equator or low altitude are more likely to experience precocious puberty
- Radiation: girls who received radiation therapy of the central nervous system are more likely to experience the condition
- Exposure to sex hormones in childhood; especially estrogen

## 20. Is precocious puberty more common in girls than boys?

Yes, precocious puberty is more common and faster in girls than in boys. It is about 5 times more common in girls than boys. Therefore, it is very important for parents to diligently follow the pubertal process in their girls. This will enable them to guide and protect their children during this critical period of their lives.

## 21. What is the effect of precocious puberty on height?

The final height or tallness of an individual is partly determined by the length of the long bones of the limbs. When an adolescent girl matures early, the long bones also stop growing earlier than usual, thereby hindering the attainment of their maximum height. They therefore appear short, fat and more mature than their actual age.

## 22. How tall can a girl with precocious puberty be?

Most girls with precocious puberty are usually less than 5ft in height because, as explained above, the long bones of the body which are important determinants of final height, stop elongating prematurely.

## 23. What are the indicators that a child has precocious puberty?

Your attention may be drawn to the fact that the physical features of maturity like hip enlargement, breast enlargement, the appearances of pubic and armpit hairs and menstruation happen earlier than usual, when compared with other siblings or adolescents in your community. Also, because of hormonal transition from childhood to adult levels, the girl may experience early and unusual patterns of mood change, rapid growth or tallness. All these features will make her appear more mature than her age mates and many of these features are likely to appear before she is 8.

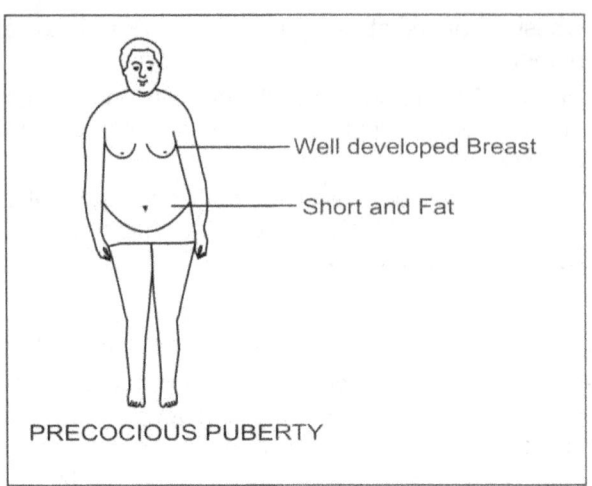

PRECOCIOUS PUBERTY

**24. What are the 3 most important worries of parents and girls with precocious puberty?**

The main problems are social and psychological. Firstly, the pre-pubertal girl may feel odd and out of sequence with her peers in the same community because although she is a young girl, she has mature adult features. However, despite her stature, she may not be able to cope with the social consequences. The second problem is the issue of premature closure of the long bones which limits her tallness and makes her short in stature. The third and most worrisome problem for parents is the fear that such girls may be taken advantage of by male sexual predators, with the ever present consequence of unwanted pregnancy.

**25. How does precocious puberty relate to intelligence?**

Despite the fact that girls with precocious puberty develop secondary sexual characteristics faster and appear more mature than their actual age, unfortunately, in terms of intelligence, their performance is on the average, the same as other girls of the same actual age. In other words, precocious girls do not enjoy any advantage over their peers in terms of intelligent quotient (IQ) or brilliance.

**26. What is the remedy for precocious puberty?**

It is important for girls with precocious puberty to be noticed by their parents as early as possible because the main remedy is to slow down the rapid development of sexual characteristics and features. This will also lead to improvement in the final tallness of the girls. This is achieved through the use of drugs under the supervision of a specialist gynecologist. Many of the drugs work by slowing down the development of secondary sexual features. Menstruation can then begin at the normal time and as a result, girls can attain their normal height. Such treatments are usually instituted for several years, up until the expected time of sexual maturity and that is why for optimal success, it is important for treatment to start as early as possible.

### 27. When should parents be worried about their child's development with respect to puberty?

When a girl attains 14 years and has shown no sign of breast development or any other secondary sexual characteristics, she should be taken to a doctor for assessment. If she has developed some sexual characteristic but has not menstruated, parents need to be patient and wait until she is 16 years. After the age of 16 years, she should be taken to the doctor for re-assessment. Though, the waiting period usually constitutes years of anxiety and worries for parents, most girls do attain puberty before the age of 16 years.

### 28. What is delayed puberty?

Delayed puberty is a situation where a girl is 14 years old and has not shown any sign of puberty or development of secondary sexual characteristics.

### 29. What is the most common cause of delayed puberty?

The most common cause of delayed puberty is a condition called Turner syndrome. This condition is due to some genetic abnormalities. The features include:

- Amenorrhea: This means inability to menstruate. Some of the girls lack functional ovaries
- Infertility: The girls are usually infertile. This is because they have miniature ovaries with scanty, abnormal eggs
- Short stature: They are usually short and stocky
- Webbed Neck: They have short, thick or wide necks
- Broad chest with small breasts: The breasts may be small and underdeveloped
- Abnormal curves of the upper limbs at the elbow joints: In medical parlance they are said to have high carrying angles.

This condition is usually brought to the attention of the doctor by parents when menstruation is delayed.

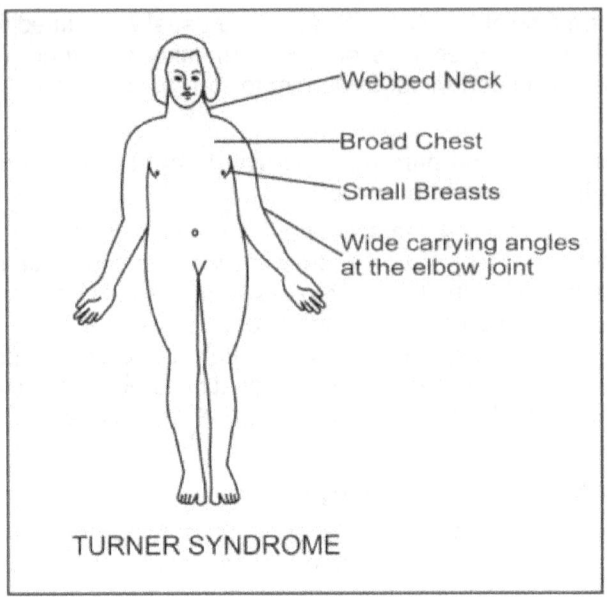
TURNER SYNDROME

### 30. What are the other conditions or situations that can result in delayed puberty?

In more than 30 % of cases, delayed puberty in girls occurs for unknown reasons. However, interviewing such girls or their mothers may reveal that some female siblings in the same family have this condition. This means that it runs in some families. Delayed puberty may also be caused by some chronic medical conditions in childhood. These conditions include:

- Malnutrition or starvation in childhood
- Tuberculosis infection, which is common in the developing countries
- Childhood Diabetes
- Chronic anemia, including Sickle cell anemia
- Endocrine disorders, including diseases of the thyroid gland
- Excessive stress in childhood
- Excessive exercise
- Severe obesity in childhood
- Failure to thrive in childhood

### 31. Can delayed puberty affect fertility?

Yes. Delayed puberty may occur together with delays in other developmental milestones in the adolescent period. Failure to attain puberty may translate into reduced ability for reproduction and therefore, some degree of infertility. Of course, as stated above, most girls with Turner's syndrome have very poorly developed ovaries and do not menstruate.

### 32. Why is it important for mothers to stay close to their girls at about the time of puberty?

The period of puberty is a turbulent one for adolescent girls. They have so many questions which must be answered. Their bodies are like battle grounds for the various hormones responsible for the changes in their physical appearances and emotions. At this time, they need to be mentored. They need people they are familiar with and to whom they can talk freely without much fear or intimidation. Mothers, guardians or some trusted 'big Aunties' can fit into this role so that only trusted people educate girls on all these issues to empower them to cope with the challenges as they arise.

Young girls therefore need education and guidance on issues like:

- Body change – Puberty comes with changes in appearance, including those of enlarging breasts and body curves. Faces also change and with stubborn pimples and ☐oily embarrassing skin, some may not like what they see in the mirror
- Weight gain - It is not unusual for girls to gain weight during the pubertal period, which may not be acceptable to those who are socially savvy or fashionistas
- Pubic hair – The appearance of pubic and armpit hair may not be totally acceptable to some girls who may hide such things or become unduly secretive in behavior. This is important for girls who share communal facilities like bathrooms in girls' hostels. In such situations, appearances of pubic hairs or enlarging breasts may be embarrassing and intimidating to them
- First menses - This is usually an embarrassing experience in the first instance or at the onset, even to those that have been tutored on how to handle the situation. It is the one phenomenon that may occur when least expected
- Sanitary Pads – Before the onset of menstruation, girls should be taught about the options and appropriate usage of sanitary pads, tampons, pant liners and other absorbents, with special reference to personal and environmental hygiene
- Premenstrual symptoms – Girls should also be aware of how to anticipate the onset of menses and what to do as soon as it appears
- Menstrual Cycle – It is equally important for girls to know how to estimate the approximate dates of their cyclical menses so they can prepare for it in advance

- Sexual education – At this time, it is most appropriate to introduce sexual education and discuss family planning. However hard it is, and many parents find it difficult, it is a necessary duty. Failure to do this, endangers young girls and they become gullible and vulnerable targets for more experienced boys and unscrupulous men

### 33. What is the general pattern of menstruation that occurs during the few years following puberty?

When a girl attains puberty, her first few monthly flows are more likely to be irregular in timing, cycle length and duration. In many cases, her menses may flow heavily for a long time or disappears for months without any cause. This may be a source of worry and creates anxiety for mothers. This is perfectly okay and will gradually become normalized as she gets older. Parents should know that this pattern may continue for 2-5 years.

### 34. Can a girl become pregnant even at this time?

Yes, she can become pregnant. It is true that their menstruation and ovulation are irregular at this time, however ovulation still happens occasionally and pregnancy is quite possible. Considering the fact that these girls are inexperienced, they may easily get into trouble from adolescent boys or the more matured male sexual predators. When girls become pregnant at this time, most of them will most probably seek to terminate it through an abortion. Many of such attempts have resulted in tragic incidents with short and long term complications, including death. This is another reason why it is important for parents and guardians to guide these girls through this critical period of their lives.

### 35. What should be done when girls feel sick and irritable before their period appears?

Many women have mood swings at this time. They are less cheerful, dull, irritable and more quarrelsome. Some girls experience lower abdominal discomfort, feel bloated, tired and clumsy. This is called premenstrual tension syndrome or PMS for short. It is common and not unusual. Girls can engage in regular exercise between or before menses. Reduced salt intake, avoiding caffeine and processed foods may help as well as avoiding heavy foods during such times. Light meals taken regularly in small quantities are more appropriate. Some women may benefit from vitamin supplements, especially vitamin B6 and primrose. However, you should visit your doctor for a more thorough appraisal and treatment.

### 36. How can pre-teens and young teenagers overcome the challenge and distress of pain during menstruation?

For many young girls who have just started menstruating, pain and severe discomfort are more frequent. The pain may be due to congestion but many of such cases cannot be traced to any cause. Generally, the pain should reduce and may even disappear completely as they grow up. Mild tone-up exercises between periods are helpful and other measures like hot baths and the use of simple pain killers or analgesics may help. In a few instances, the problem may be due to some identifiable causes which have definite remedies. In such cases, your doctor should be consulted for appropriate treatment.

### 37. If I had sexual intercourse with my boyfriend and he did not release semen inside me, can I become pregnant?

It is quite possible. During sexual intercourse and before the final ejaculation, there are multiple spurts of semen into the vagina. Even though the quantities released with each spurt are small, they may contain enough spermatozoa to fertilize your eggs and make you pregnant. So, it is unsafe to assume that you can only get pregnant when your partner releases the full measure of semen inside you at the time of orgasm.

### 38. Doctor, do you really think that it is appropriate to start family planning at the time of puberty?

Yes, in principle. All sexually mature or sexually active females who do not desire pregnancy should use family planning. The problem in many communities and cultures is that some parents consider sex education inappropriate for children. In some homes, it is regarded as immoral for parents to even talk about it in the presence of their children. So, sex education is not in agreement with many cultures and many believe that early exposure to sexual education may lead to promiscuity in young girls. Unfortunately, this attitude of rejection is partly responsible for the high rate of abortions and its complications, especially in developing countries. The truth is that after puberty, any mature girl that is sexually exposed and does not want to get pregnant must practice family planning.

### 39. Will starting family planning at this young age not result in infertility in future?

No. Rather, it will prevent unwanted pregnancy and the consequences of abortions which include infertility. Many types of family planning methods are suitable and convenient for young pubertal girls. The advice of a family planning giver or doctor comes in handy at this time.

**40. Who is an adolescent?**

Adolescence is the period in a child's life which starts from the beginning of puberty and ends at the time when the child has attained full physical maturity and development of secondary sexual characteristics. It is the beginning of being an adult. This period will commonly be about the age of 8-14 years. In the developed world like the United States of America, especially among African-Americans, puberty may begin earlier in girls and full sexual and physical development may be completed earlier than in other racial groups.

**41. What are the major problems of adolescents?**

The adolescent period is unique and turbulent for 3 main reasons:
- Adolescent girls are transiting in a situation that presents many new opportunities but a very short time for them to learn and adjust. In such a bewildering situation, young girls become very inquisitive, remarkably willing to take risks and try out new ideas, thoughts, objects, fantasies and even vices
- The girls experience physical, physiological, and emotional changes, all happening at the same time. Worse still, these changes are entirely new and relate with each other in a complex manner
- Adolescents are usually under peer group pressure and many of the things they do are influenced by what each member of the group has heard or seen from a distance. Consequently, instead of being taught or mentored by their mothers, guardians or aunties, they learn from one another and copy without questioning

Adolescents have many other challenges, the majority of which are social and psychological in nature. These problems include:
- Substance abuse
  - Alcohol and binge drinking
  - Smoking-tobacco
  - Marijuana
  - Other illicit or street drug use
  - Cocaine, Heroin, etc.
- Sex related concerns
  - Unwanted pregnancies
  - Increased request for abortions with the inherent risk of complications
- Challenges in Education
  - Truancy in school
  - Distraction during class

- Diminished ability to concentrate
- Social media vices
  - Pornography
  - Unwholesome associations with criminal gangs
  - Exposure to sexual predators
  - Internet addiction
- Psychological problems
  - Poor ability to communicate
  - Low self-esteem
  - Secrecy and introversion
  - Confrontation with representatives of authority

These are just a few of the important challenges related to adolescence, whose consequences have tremendous impact on what the young girls eventually become later in life.

### 42. What is the relationship between adolescence and puberty?

Puberty marks the onset of sexual maturity and starts at about the age of 9 years or beyond. Adolescence in some cases may precede puberty and last up to the early twenties. The adolescent period includes social and psychological growth, when the dependent child becomes a functionally independent child. It is a period when the girl is eager to explore herself and take more risks. She struggles for independence from her parents and other siblings. She is suspicious, inquisitive, aggressive and more individualistic. Puberty adds to these situations by causing more intense emotions.

### 43. In terms of behavior, what do puberty and adolescence represent?

At this time, children are rapidly maturing, both physically and physiologically. The girls experience many changes in their bodies. Guardians should therefore relate to their daughters more closely for the purpose of education, guidance and protection, otherwise, they may look for answers from other persons or resort to trial and error which may land them in trouble.

### 44. Why is conflict more common between adolescent girls and their parents?

Conflict is perfectly normal and natural at this time. This is partly due to the fact that many guardians try to avoid or suppress questioning by their daughters, instead of discussing issues with them. In fact, absence of such conflicts may suggest that a girl is hiding or suppressing her feelings or emotions. This is more harmful to the development and understanding of girls and may affect normal adult relationships in future.

### 45. What escalates the conflict?

Puberty and adolescence represent periods of intense hormonal and physiological changes. These changes translate into psychological, emotional and subtle changes in physical appearances in young girls. Many of these teenagers may not like the way they look as maturity sets in. Appearances of secondary sexual characteristics like breast enlargement may be embarrassing to them so they feel shy and uncomfortable with their first few menstruations, especially if they are the first or last among their peers to do so. They also generally feel clumsy, irritable, and insecure. These are potential causes of conflicts which demand understanding and empathy from guardians.

### 46. How can we resolve some of these adolescent problems?

Trying out new things and experiences are thrilling to adolescents so one effective way to redirect adolescent energy and focus is to carefully and strategically wean them from their peer groups. Adolescent problems are complex in nature. This is largely due to the adventurous nature of the young girls and the fact that most girls move in groups and are under peer pressure. Adolescents turn risky ventures to fun and think of fantasies as realities. Guardians need to be very patient with tactics and lots of motherly love. This may be tasking and demands perseverance from mothers who should help their daughters to see things from a different perspective because most adolescents believe that their parents are not only overbearing but also oblivious to their ideas and views. Sometimes, they think that guardians are old fashioned and unaware of current trends, so adolescent girls need the support and understanding of their guardians especially, mothers.

### 47. What is the solution to unwanted adolescent pregnancy?

Once a girl child attains puberty, the possibility of pregnancy is ever present. This danger must be recognized by guardians as a reality. This underlines the importance of sexual education for every girl at the attainment of puberty. There is no point in presuming that pregnancy is not a possibility because the girl was brought up to have high moral standards. Good moral standing is a great complement but it cannot objectively prevent unwanted pregnancy. Family planning is the best means of preventing unwanted pregnancy. This should always be kept in view and done as soon as possible, with the help and advice of the family physician.

### 48. How serious is the problem of unwanted pregnancy?

Most adolescents are not prepared for pregnancy. They become pregnant by "mistake" and are ill-equipped to deal with such situations. Some of such girls, in attempts to save their education, avoid public shame, scorn or even total rejection by their guardians, resort to abortion. In the absence of proper counseling and support, things can really go wrong. The alternative is to leave the pregnancy intact and risk the disruption of their education. Either way, the price is high!

## 49. What happens if I choose to keep the pregnancy?

It is not a good experience for a teenage student to become pregnant. There are both social and medical consequences, should you decide to keep the pregnancy. Firstly, the birth canal at such a tender age may not be mature or roomy enough to allow safe delivery through the vagina. This means that the choice of surgical operation becomes necessary. It is a known fact that teenagers also exhibit behaviors that make pregnancy a high risk venture. These behaviors vary from poor attendance in prenatal clinics to illicit drug use in pregnancy. Guardians of pregnant teenagers should give necessary and appropriate support, to ensure that their daughters get back to school as soon as possible, after a suitable period of parentage and care for their babies. With this type of experience, family planning should become an obvious necessity.

## 50. Who is a virgin?

A virgin is a girl who has never had sexual intercourse.

## 51. What does it mean to be a virgin in practical terms?

It means that the hymen, which is a thin membrane at the entrance to the vagina, is intact or has not been torn through sexual intercourse. In other words, a girl is said to be deflowered if her hymen has been torn through the act of sexual intercourse. Please, note that the hymen may be torn in many other ways. For examples, it may be accidentally torn during insertion of tampons or medications into the vagina or even during physical activities like jumping and riding bikes. These do not amount to loss of virginity because no sexual intercourse is involved.

## 52. What are the phases of the sexual act?

The sexual act in human beings is classified into 4 phases. These are:
- Excitement phase
- Plateau phase
- Phase of orgasm
- Resolution phase

## 53. What is the excitement phase?

The excitement phase, as the name implies, is when, due to stimulation or romance, the female becomes excited. Stimulation can be achieved by exhibiting romantic activities like whispering into the ears, body contact, cuddling, eye gestures and tactile stimulation in a conducive environment. In response, there is increased blood flow into all erectile tissues especially the clitoris which rises and becomes stronger. The clitoris behaves like the penis in men, because both of them are formed from a common embryologic origin. Stimulation results in copious secretion from the vestibular glands of the vagina. The cells of the vagina also produce copious fluid which helps to moisten the vagina and vulva, ensuring that the vagina and vulva become well lubricated. This facilitates easy penetration and thrusting of the penis during sexual intercourse.

### 54. What is the plateau phase?

This phase is next to the excitement phase. Here, there is an intense congestion of the blood vessels of the vulva and vagina. This means that the blood pipes fill up rapidly to full capacity and make the surrounding tissue more warm and tight. There are involuntary muscular contractions especially around the waist. The lower third of the vagina becomes engorged while the upper two third expands to accommodate and fit well into the robust and erect penis. The blood pressure and pulse begin to rise. Breathing also becomes more rapid at this time.

### 55. What is orgasm?

The plateau phase naturally progresses to orgasm. There are intense uncontrollable or involuntary contractions of the waist muscles and jerking of the body. The sensations in the vagina completely dominate the body at this time and all other sensory awareness seems not to matter at this moment of peak enjoyment. The whole body system is overwhelmed with pleasure. At this point, the vagina, the urethra, and the anus contract involuntarily and in some cases, fluid squirts from the urethra of the woman at the very peak of sexual pleasure. The blood pressure rises rapidly and may reach 180/120mmHg at the peak while the pulse and respiratory rates are doubled.

### 56. What is the significance of orgasm?

Orgasm is the phase of the sexual act that represents the very peak of sexual pleasure or enjoyment. It is a most desirable climax.

### 57. Is orgasm in a woman important for pregnancy to occur?

Though orgasm is the peak of sexual pleasure, it is not a condition for pregnancy to occur and failure to achieve orgasm does not cause infertility.

### 58. Do all women ejaculate?

No. Some women do not reach orgasm. Of those who do, some are capable of repeated or multiple orgasms. This is the type of orgasm in which urine squirts out of the urethra. This is called a 'squirt orgasm' and is the most fulfilling form of orgasm. Unfortunately, only a few women are capable of achieving this.

### 59. How can women achieve orgasm?

For some women, orgasm is achieved only after adequate sexual stimulation and foreplay, so failure to achieve orgasm may therefore represent inadequate sexual stimulation or the absence of stimulation. Failure to achieve orgasm does not mean that something is wrong or that the woman is sick so there is no need to feel guilty. For others, the ability to reach orgasm is a natural or in-born gift. Where causes of failure to achieve orgasm are identified, they should be discussed with your partner. Sometimes, a visit to your family physician, gynecologist or psychologist may be beneficial. Practical remedies include:

- Providing solutions to the problems that have been identified
- Confidence building activities
- Enhanced ability to express your feelings
- Sex education
- Adequate foreplay
- The right environment for sexual intercourse
- The right occasion
- The right partner
- Releasing yourself to your partner for mutual pleasure

### 60. What about the resolution phase?

At this phase, the body sensations return to normal. The pulse rate, respiratory rate and blood pressure all return to normal. The muscles relax once more and the clitoris is decongested over some minutes, eventually losing its erection. There may also be associated sweating which serves to cool the body.

### 61. What is the normal duration of sexual intercourse?

If we reckon that sexual intercourse starts from the first penetration of the penis into the vagina to the end of orgasm, the normal duration of sexual intercourse should be between 3 to 13 minutes. This duration does not include foreplay or romance. It has long been recognized that many men or couples would wish that the duration be as long as 30 minutes or more, just to prolong sexual pleasure. However, 30 minutes may be too long and may indicate sexual dysfunction or problems. It could also lead to exhaustion and other tragic consequences including heart attacks.

More emphasis should be placed on satisfaction rather than duration. Below is a guide to duration:

| Duration | Comment |
|---|---|
| 1 to 2 minutes | too quick |
| 3 to 7 minutes | adequate and normal |
| 7 to 13 minutes | desirable and normal |
| 14 to 30 minutes | too long and may be dangerous |

## 62. What is frigidity?

Frigidity more or less represents a complaint whereby the husband or partner does not derive the expected sexual satisfaction from the woman. Usually, this means that the woman does not respond to sexual stimulation or romance. She is not moved or seems indifferent. In other words, she provides little or no pleasure. Complaints like this may herald sexual disharmony so frigidity should be resolved from both sides. The woman should be able to discuss freely with her partner, explaining exactly how she feels about her interests, what turns her on and off and any deep seated problems on her mind. Sometimes, a husband's attitude may unconsciously contribute to the problem of frigidity, either directly or indirectly. Sexual harmony is an important obligation that keeps a marriage going, so problems like frigidity should be managed very promptly, in the most appropriate way, in the overall interest of the home.

The doctor and probably a psychologist should be informed as soon as possible.

## 63. What are the causes of failure of stimulation?

For profound sexual pleasure, both partners should be able to communicate and express their feelings without inhibition. The sexual response is mainly due to an autonomic nervous reflex. This means that as individuals, we cannot control it. It is not voluntary. However, the response may be enhanced or inhibited under certain conditions. In females, factors that may adversely affect response to sexual stimulation include:
- Illness including pelvic pain, pelvic infection etc
- Inappropriate environments or circumstances
- Fear, depression and anxiety
- Fear of pregnancy
- Grief

- Fatigue or exhaustion
- Systemic diseases - e.g. diabetes, hypertension
- Old age and menopause
- Socioeconomic issues such as lack of financial security
- Stress in marriage
- Social and religious taboos
- Bad experiences in previous relationships
- Addiction to Homosexuality
- Ugly incidences that haunt e.g. rape, abortion etc.

### 64. I am not circumcised; will this reduce my sexual enjoyment?

No. Circumcision does not reduce sexual pleasure; instead, it can lead to injuries to the external genitals and reduction in the degree of sexual stimulation. There are some cultures in the world where female circumcision is practiced. During circumcision, the clitoris, which is the most sensitive part of the female's external genitals, may be cut due to ignorance. The clitoris is the equivalent of the penis in the male. Just like the penis, the tip of the clitoris is very sensitive. When this tip is cut during circumcision, the cut heals with a scar. The remaining clitoris is shorter and far less sensitive to touch. This results in reduced response to stimulation during foreplay and sexual intercourse. In extreme situations where the whole clitoris has been removed during circumcision, sexual pleasure during romance is greatly reduced.

Female circumcision amounts to female genital mutilation and is one of the worst discriminatory practices against females. It has no medical benefits.

### 65. Does female circumcision reduce promiscuity in girls?

No, it does not. The notion of increased promiscuity in uncircumcised girls is widely held in some communities in Sub-Saharan Africa and other cultures. Unfortunately, this is why some guardians or tribes still allow it.

### 66. Does female circumcision prevent infertility?

No. Female circumcision or incisions on the vagina do not prevent infertility. Rather, they may cause sexual dysfunctions and injuries. When scarifications are made in the vagina, the resulting scars may partially narrow the vagina or cause pain during sexual intercourse.

### 67. What is the effect of premature ejaculation in a man on sexual harmony?

Premature ejaculation in the man means stimulation or sexual arousal in the female is halted halfway, most times, before the woman reaches her climax. If premature ejaculation is recurrent, the woman may perceive sexual intercourse as selfish and one sided; only for the man's enjoyment. If, she sees her partner as being selfish, she may eventually lose interest or commitment to sexual intercourse, unless the problem is corrected and her own fair share of enjoyment is guaranteed. The services of a gynecologist, urologist or psychologist may be useful and should be sought.

### 68. Is oral sex safe?
Oral sex is not completely safe. Apart from the fact that oral sex is dirty, the greatest danger is the ease of contracting and spreading infections. For example, with respect to transmission of the HIV infection, the potential effect of oral sex will be as bad as engaging in homosexuality, if not worse. Normal heterosexual vaginal intercourse is the most natural and socially acceptable coital practice globally. In most cultures around the world, oral sex is not socially acceptable. If people must indulge in oral sex, they must ensure that they are free from mouth ulcers and that their mouths are not bruised in the process. It is important to always remember the high risks and consequences of contracting many other sexually transmitted diseases.

### 69. What is masturbation?
Masturbation is a practice whereby a person stimulates his/her external genitals in order to derive sexual pleasure.

### 70. Is it abnormal to masturbate?
Masturbation is not as bad as many people think and has been practiced for a long time. It serves as a means of relieving sexual urges where there is no opportunity for normal sexual intercourse with a partner.

### 71. Does masturbation have any adverse effect on health?
Not quite. However, women who stimulate their genitals or clitoris with dirty fingers or objects may have increased risks of infection of the genitals, but this is not common. Infections can result in increased offensive vaginal discharge. Self-inflicted injuries due to sharp fingernails or other objects during self-stimulation are also not common.

### 72. Can masturbation cause infertility?
No, masturbation does not affect fertility in women. It does not affect ovulation or menstruation.

### 73. What are the 3 main advantages of masturbation?
Masturbation has several benefits but the 3 main advantages are:
- Self- release of sexual urge or tension

- Enjoyment of sexual pleasure at your own discretion
- No fear of unwanted pregnancy; therefore, no danger of abortion

## 74. What are the other advantages?

Perhaps the greatest advantage of masturbation is that it enables you to be in-charge of your own sexual life. You can derive normal sexual pleasure as long as you are not addicted to masturbation. Other advantages are that:

- It helps to relieve general and social stress
- It allows women to explore their bodies and know which parts give maximum sexual stimulation and pleasure. This may be an added advantage for women when they engage in normal sexual intercourse. They already know how and where they can be best stimulated by their sexual partners during foreplay and romance
- Masturbation guarantees sexual activity without a partner
- There is no risk of sexually transmitted infections

# DEAR DOCTOR:

## 75. I feel a sense of guilt and immorality after masturbation. Do others feel the same?

Some of the negative effects of masturbation include a sense of guilt and the feeling that masturbation is morally wrong and dirty. These feelings are more factual when you are just beginning to practice masturbation. Masturbation in secret worsens the sense of guilt and immorality. Unfortunately, the fact is that masturbation cannot be done openly, so here, there is no eating the cake and having it.

## 76. Is it right to use vibrators or genital stimulators?

It is normal to use vibrators or stimulators to derive sexual pleasure. However, the experience of the first few attempts may be disappointing. Once you can use the vibrator correctly, the amount and level of satisfaction will increase and you can build up confidence in your self-found sexuality.

## 77. If I masturbate with the aid of a vibrator, am I still a virgin?

Yes. You are a virgin as long as you have never had natural sexual intercourse with a male partner. Your hymen may be broken by the vibrator, but by definition, your virginity is still intact.

**78. I am addicted to masturbation; I think it is not just right. What should I do?**

This is a situation where a person feels a perpetual and an abnormal urge to masturbate as frequently as possible. In some cases, this is done many times in the same day. This is called compulsive masturbation. Many females who are addicted to masturbation withdraw to private places at odd times. It becomes an obsession and the only means of sexual pleasure. Once addiction happens, there is an aggravated sense of guilt and immoral feelings. There is a high probability that an addicted person would prefer to stay or be left alone to enjoy her privacy as much as possible. This is antisocial and at that level, help from a psychologist and your doctor is needed.

**79. What are the other problems of addiction to masturbation?**

An addicted person is more likely to be uncomfortably reserved as a person. She is also likely to have other problems and engage in antisocial activities. These include:
- Internet sex exposure especially pornography
- Solitude
- Anxiety
- Fear
- Depression

**80. So what is the solution to addiction to masturbation?**

It is a difficult and painstaking process. The addicted female must be weaned off in the first instance. This is followed by a period of abstinence from masturbation. This remedy requires determination, discipline and close supervision of a psychotherapist in order to achieve abstinence and be successfully re-integrated into a normal, natural partner-based sexual life.

# CHAPTER 2

# Menstruation

*"I mean if there was any justice in the world, you wouldn't even have to go to school during your period. You'd just stay home for five days and eat chocolate and cry."*
– ANDREA PORTES

**1.   At what age should a girl normally begin menstruation?**
Menstruation should start in a young girl between the ages of 11 and 14 years in most communities. The first menstruation is called Menarche (pronounced: me-nar-ke). The average age at first menstruation is about 12 years and 8 months. The age varies from one environment to another but it is earlier in the developed world. As a global trend, the age at first menstruation is decreasing.

**2.   What is the length of a normal menstrual cycle?**
In medical parlance, the first day that a woman sees her menstruation is counted as day 1, the second day is day 2 and so on. Using this method of counting, the length of a normal menstrual cycle is 21 to 35 days. Sometimes, 42 days may be regarded as normal in some individuals but the most commonly quoted number for a normal cycle is 28 days. In layman terms, this can be regarded as the number of days in between 2 consecutive menses.

**3.   What is the average duration of a normal menstruation?**
The duration of a normal menstrual flow is between 2 and 7 days. Menstruation of less than 2 days is short while bleeding beyond 7 days is too long.

### 4. What is the average blood loss during a normal menstruation?

The amount of blood loss by women during menses varies from one woman to another. Even in the same woman, the amount may be different from one cycle to another. Generally speaking, the average blood loss during menses is 35ml but doctors regard a menstrual loss of more than 80mls as excessive.

### 5. When is menstruation said to be irregular?

On the average, a woman is expected to menstruate once during her cycle length. Sometimes, she may bleed too early in a cycle when she does not expect to bleed, while at other times, the menses may be delayed, such that it occurs outside her normal cycle length. This means that the menses occurs in an unpredictable manner. In this type of situation, the menses is said to be irregular.

### 6. When is bleeding said to be abnormal?

Generally speaking, bleeding from the vagina at any other time except menstruation is regarded as abnormal. For example, prolonged or heavy bleeding, spotting and light flows outside menses are abnormal. However, a few women may experience spotting or scanty bleeding appearing once or twice on the same day during ovulation time, or implantation of the embryo. These are regarded as normal.

### 7. Is it normal to menstruate twice in the same month?

It is perfectly normal to menstruate twice in the same month, as long as there are at least 21 days in between each flow of blood. Menstruation should also last for 2 to 7 days.

### 8. What are the reasons why a young girl may experience menstruation earlier than usual?

There are many reasons but in about 50% of cases, the reasons are unknown. A girl's very first menstruation is called menarche. Early menarche is no doubt associated with precocious puberty. Apart from precocious puberty, early menstruation may occur in young girls for the following reasons:

- Girls in some families may menstruate earlier than other girls in the same community. It is familial or runs in the family
- Girls who live in low altitudes and cold climates
- Obesity is associated with accelerated sexual maturity and early menstruation

- Urban dwellers may experience early menarche more than rural girls
- High social - economic status of parents

9. **What is the relationship between menstruation and weight loss?**

Conditions that lead to extreme weight loss may also lead to stoppage of menstruation. When a woman's body weight falls below 25% of the ideal body weight, the functions of the hypothalamus in the brain may be disturbed. The hormones of the hypothalamus are not released to the pituitary gland. Hence, the follicle stimulating hormone (FSH) and the leutinizing hormone (LH) are not secreted. As a result, the growths of the follicles in the ovaries do not occur. In a normal situation, growing follicles produce estrogen hormone which in turn thickens the lining of the womb in preparation for pregnancy. So since there is no follicular growth, the womb is not physiologically prepared for menstruation, which is like a default state, if pregnancy does not take place in a given menstrual cycle.

10. **What is the relationship between strenuous exercise and menses?**

The leutinising hormone releasing hormone (LHRH) is a chemical produced by the hypothalamus in the brain. Its function is to release follicle stimulating hormone (FSH) and leutinizing hormone (LH) of the pituitary gland which are necessary for ovulation and subsequent menstruation. The hypothalamus is highly sensitive to physical and psychological stress and excessive exercise disturbs the production of LHRH. When FSH and LH are not secreted by the pituitary gland, ovulation and menstruation do not take place. This happens more often in competitive athletes, especially when they are training hard for competitions or tournaments.

11. **Is it possible for a woman to continue menstruating, even when pregnant?**

It is not possible to menstruate during pregnancy. However, a woman may bleed from the vagina in pregnancy. If such bleeding happens early during pregnancy or occurs at intervals, some women do confuse this type of bleeding with menstruation. The use of the word menstruation implies that you are not pregnant.

12. **Can women become pregnant if they have sexual intercourse during menstruation?**

Yes, it is quite possible even though the probability is very low. The first half of the menstrual cycle is called the proliferative phase. It lasts for about 14 days but varies in duration from one woman to another. The second half is called the Luteal phase and is fairly constant. It is the last 2 weeks of the cycle. Some females may ovulate early while others ovulate late in the cycle, depending on the lengths of the proliferative phase of their cycles. Since spermatozoa can survive in the female genital tract for some days, pregnancy is theoretically possible at any time. This means that there is no time that the possibility of pregnancy is zero. Therefore, have a family planning method in place or insist that your partner uses a condom!

### 13. Can women become pregnant if they engage in sexual intercourse during their safe periods?

There is never a time that a woman is 100% sure that she will not get pregnant. However, the least chance of becoming pregnant is from about 3 days after the estimated ovulation time and beyond. The female egg is only viable for about 12 hours after ovulation but it is possible for a woman to have multiple ovulations within the same cycle. For these reasons, engaging in sexual intercourse during the so called safe period may not be totally safe. Safe period refers to the time in your cycle when you are not likely to get pregnant if you engage in sexual intercourse without family planning. Please, note that unprotected sex is never safe. The safe period is not a recommended method of family planning. Family planning is cheaper and safer.

### 14. Is it appropriate to have sexual intercourse during menstruation?

Although it is normal, it is not to be recommended because menstrual blood is dirty and a good culture medium for harmful germs. Women should also be mindful of the fact that the vagina is tender at this time and could easily be bruised. If coitus does take place, in deference to hygiene and the higher possibility of contracting infection, partners should use condoms and be gentle in approach.

### 15. When is the menstrual flow said to be heavy?

Heavy menstrual loss is called menorrhagia (pronounced: me-no-ra-gia) in medical parlance. During menstruation, the quantity of blood loss may vary widely between 30 to 180 ml. In a more practical sense, the woman should use 3 to 5 sanitary pads per day. Using more than 5 pads per day, especially if they are fully soaked may suggest excessive menstrual loss. In many cases of heavy menstrual loss, blood clots are seen on the sanitary pads.

### 16. How common is a heavy menstrual flow?

It is fairly common. About 30% of women, between the age of 16 - 45 experience heavy menstrual flow.

### 17. What are the causes of heavy menstrual flow?

Heavy menstrual bleeding may occur for reasons that cannot be identified after thorough examinations. They are said to be idiopathic in such situations. However, there are many identifiable reasons why a woman may experience heavy bleeding. They include:

- Anovulation – that is the woman did not ovulate even though she menstruated
- Hormonal disorders – imbalances in the levels of hormones may result in anovulation as well as heavy flows at unexpected times
- Pregnancy - the woman may confuse bleeding in early pregnancy with menstruation if she is not aware that she is pregnant, so in a young woman with heavy bleeding, doctors normally take the possibility of pregnancy into consideration
- Infection – infection of the genital tracts may be associated with heavy and prolonged bleeding
- Drugs - some drugs may increase menstrual loss
- Masses in the womb like polyps, fibroids, adenomyosis and endometriosis cause heavy flows
- Ovarian tumors
- Coagulation disorders – women suffering from blood clotting disorders may bleed heavily for a prolonged time during menses
- Menarche – the first few menses on attainment of puberty in girls may be prolonged and heavy
- Excessive stress
- Excessive exercise

## 18. What are the effects of excessive menstrual bleeding?

Women who have heavy menstrual bleeding also suffer other adverse effects. The important ones among these include:

- Anemia - Anemia means shortage of blood in the body. This is perhaps the most important consequence. Women who lose more than 80mls of blood during menses are at risk of iron deficiency anemia. Anemia on its own adversely affects several other organs, systems and body functions. Thus, such women may become sick on and off from illnesses related to anemia
- Lack of ovulation - Women who bleed heavily for long durations in each cycle, spend a greater number of days of their cycles bleeding non-stop. In such a situation, ovulation becomes unpredictable. This reduces the chance of pregnancy and infertility may become an issue
- Social embarrassment - Imagine a woman who is afraid of venturing out of her home environment for fear of getting quickly soaked. Sometimes, simple functions like going to work, driving to the mall and going to the store for groceries may be problematic. Situations like these may be very frustrating for the woman and her family

### 19. When is menstruation said to be scanty?

This situation is called hypomenorrhea. This denotes menstruation with a reduced flow or one with a short duration. In extreme cases, the menses may come as a mild stain on the sanitary pad for a brief period or scanty flow for one day.

### 20. What are the causes of scanty menstruation?

Scanty menstruation is far less common than heavy bleeding and has fewer causes. Typically, the women complain of spotting or bleeding lightly for about one day. The causes include:

- Infection - Infection of the genital tract is one of the causes of scanty menstrual flow. The infection may involve the lining of the womb. When such an infection is neglected, it may become chronic and results in scar tissue formation in the womb, called adhesions. Adhesions can also be due to injury to the lining of the womb, such as when instruments are used during an abortion. The scar tissue replaces the normal endometrial tissue. Hence, there is much less normal endometrial tissue available for shedding, during menses. This manifests as scanty menstruation or no menstruation at all
- Anovulation - Women who do not ovulate regularly for various reasons are more likely to have scanty menstrual flow or complete absence of menstruation. Anovulatory cycles are common in young girls around puberty and in women around menopause
- Endocrine problems - Hormonal problems may also cause scanty menses. For example, polycystic ovarian syndrome causes anovulation and may result in irregular and scanty menses, while severe thyroid problems may lead to scanty menses or complete stoppage of menses
- Ovarian cyst - One of the effects of ovarian cysts is menstrual upset. This is more common with functional ovarian cysts because they secrete hormones. Many women with ovarian cysts may experience lack of menstruation for variable lengths of time
- Sheehans syndrome - This syndrome usually happens due to heavy bleeding following childbirth with adverse effects on the functions of the pituitary gland in the brain. In most cases, the menses stops completely
- Obstruction – The genital tract may be blocked due to conditions like narrowing of the cervical canal or imperforate hymen
- Oral contraceptives - Some family planning drugs usually lead to reduction of menses. In extreme cases, some women may experience scanty menses

- Medical illnesses - Chronic and severe medical conditions such as HIV/AIDS, tuberculosis, severe anemia and cancer can cause menstrual upsets
- Drugs and Herbs - Various drugs and herbs, especially when the correct amounts not used or when not prescribed, can result in scanty menses or complete cessation
- Extreme overweight and extreme underweight - In extremely obese and thin individuals, menstrual disturbances are common. These show up as cessation of menstruation in many cases, however, in some women, the menstrual flow may be scanty
- Extreme exercise - This may cause complete cessation of menses or scanty menses

## 21. What is the relationship between scanty menses and infertility?

A great percentage of women who have scanty menses do not ovulate regularly. They are said to have anovulatory cycles. Without ovulation, pregnancy is impossible. Also, some women experience scanty menses because of problems with the endocrine systems, especially of the pituitary – ovarian axis, this result in inability to ovulate. In developing countries, a remarkable number of women have damaged wombs as a result of severe or neglected infections of the inner lining of the womb. There can also be mechanical damage as a result of excessive scraping of the womb lining, especially during criminal abortions. When the lining of the womb is damaged, menstruation may stop completely or become scanty. In these situations, it becomes difficult to achieve pregnancy.

## 22. Are there any self-help measures?

Self-help measures are few. The main step is to see your doctor, in order to investigate the reason for the scanty menses. In many instances, once the underlying cause is corrected, menstrual flow improves. Change in life style such as reduction in weight in obese women and improvement in weight in extremely thin individuals, may also restore normal menstrual flow.

## 23. What is premenstrual syndrome (PMS)?

Many women experience some feelings or complaints regularly before their menstruation. The feelings may start just about 5 to 7 days before their menstruation or earlier but normally disappear once the menses starts or before it is over. The complaints vary from one individual to another. The common complaints include:

- Anxiety and depression
- Irritability
- Hostility

- Anger and aggression
- Fatigue and lethargy
- Poor concentration
- Tension and panic attacks
- Mood swings
- Breast pain and heaviness
- Changes in bowel habits, usually constipation
- Dizziness
- Headache
- Muscles pain or aches
- Palpitation
- Nausea and vomiting
- Bloating and Weight gain
- Acne or pimples

All these complaints or just a few may be experienced regularly before menses. As stated, in most cases, the symptoms and signs ease off once menstruation starts. They are called Pre-menstrual syndrome. Pre-menstrual syndrome (PMS) is not a disease. Rather, it is a combination of complaints noticed in such women.

## 24. What is the cause of pre-menstrual syndrome?

The cause of PMS is unknown, but there are suggestions. Majority of doctors suspect that PMS is due to the inappropriate interaction of hormones, especially estrogen and progesterone in the period of time leading to menstruation. This is because many of the complaints can be explained by the actions or effects of these two hormones. For example, progesterone is well known to cause constipation. It is possible that PMS is caused by many other factors apart from the effects of hormones.

## 25. What is the relationship between PMS and age?

The severity of most of the complaints in PMS reduces with age. Also, most women experience remarkable reductions in frequency and severity of symptoms once they begin child bearing.

## 26. Does the lack of vitamins cause PMS?

There are so many suggestions as to the causes of PMS and one of such suggestions includes vitamin deficiency. Others include low blood sugar, excess prolactin and aldosterone hormones. Doctors are still not certain as to what exactly is responsible for PMS.

## 27. What is the best treatment for PMS?

There is no 'best' treatment for PMS due to the poor knowledge doctors have as to what causes it. However, there are many remedies that may bring some

relief. Perhaps the most important aspect is a caring parent, husband or doctor whose support and empathy you can rely upon. Treatments that may be of benefit include:
- Vitamin B6 or pyridoxine
- Combined oral contraceptives for a period of time
- Progesterone vaginal pessaries
- Primrose oil
- Diuretics to relieve congestion
- Pain killers and antispasmodics
- Diet modification

## 28. What is Pre-menstrual Dysphoric Disorder (PMDD)?

Pre-menstrual dysphoric disorder (PMDD) could manifest as PMS. The main difference is that the complaints are more severe and associated with some sort of disability. For example, a woman may not be able to go to work or do her cooking.

## 29. Are there any self-help measures for PMDD?

Simple remedies may be applied according to the nature of the complaints. Complaints such as headaches usually respond to analgesics or pain killers. Exercise may reduce bloating while the use of oral contraceptive pills and bromocriptine may reduce breast pain. There are claims by some doctors that reduced consumption of caffeine or coffee is beneficial.

## 30. What are the instances when a woman may feel pain related to her reproductive life?

There are four major instances. These are:
- During menstruation
- Pre or post menstruation due to diseases of the genital tracts
- During ovulation
- During sexual intercourse

## 31. What is dysmenorrhea?

This is the medical term for painful menstruation. Many young girls and teenagers do experience pain in the first few years of menstruation, however, some older women do experience menstrual pain too. Dysmenorrhea may be primary or secondary. The third type, which is membraneous dysmenorrhoea is rare.

## 32. What is the difference between primary and secondary dysmenorrhea?

Dysmenorrhea is said to be primary when the cause cannot be identified. The pain of primary dysmenorrhea is typically described by women as spasmodic or gripping in nature. It is believed to be due to reduced blood supply to the womb. In secondary dysmenorrhea, the pain is due to congestion and as the name implies, it is usually as a result of some causes that can be identified. The pain is usually felt as a dull pain at the back, waist and lower abdomen.

## 33. How common is dysmenorrhea?

Pain during menstruation is common and occurs in 45 -72% of women. It is more common in adolescents and teenagers.

## 34. What is the difference between dysmenorrhea and PMS?

The main difference is in the pattern of pain. In dysmenorrhea, the pain starts at the beginning of menstruation and lasts for only a day or two. It may be associated with nausea and vomiting. Many women complain that the pain radiates down one or both legs. In contrast, the pain in PMS starts a few days before menstruation begins and stops before or at the end of the flow. So dysmenorhea starts at the beginning while PMS starts a few days before.

## 35. What is the medical treatment of primary dysmenorrhea?

There is no specific effective treatment for primary dysmenorrhea because the cause is unknown. Remedies that may be of help include:
- Non-steroid analgesics
- Combined oral contraceptives
- Synthetic progestogen
- Operative division of the nerve supply to the womb may be performed by doctors, if the pain is severe and does not respond to other common remedies

## 36. What are the causes of secondary dysmenorrhea?

The causes of secondary dysmenorrhea include:
- Pelvic inflammatory disease and other genital infections
- Pelvic tumors like uterine fibroids, polyps and ovarian cysts
- Endometriosis
- Presence of an IUCD or other foreign bodies in the womb

### 37. What is the treatment for secondary dysmenorrhea?

Unlike primary dysmenorrhea, doctors direct their efforts towards treating the cause of the problem. The first step is to see your doctor, who will examine you and carry out necessary investigations to find out the reason for the pain. Once the reason is identified, appropriate treatment can then be carried out. These may include antibiotics and analgesics for infections and pelvic inflammatory disease, surgical operations to remove fibroids or the removal of a troublesome IUCD, etc. Most of these treatments are beneficial and effective.

### 38. What is dyspareunia?

This is a medical term used to describe a situation where a woman feels pain during sexual intercourse. The pain may occur for unknown reasons but sometimes, such pains are caused by problems in the reproductive tract. Those caused without reasons are called primary dyspareunia, while those with identifiable causes are called secondary dyspareunia.

### 39. What are the causes of dyspareunia?

The causes include conditions like:
- Infections
  - Sexually transmitted diseases (STDs)
  - Pelvic inflammatory disease
- Endometriosis
- Erosion of the cervix
- Scars in the vulva, vagina and cervix
- Injury and ulceration of the genital tract
- Insertion of chemicals including herbs
- Vaginal dryness e.g. at Menopause
- Aggression during sexual intercourse
  - Rape
  - Drunken partner
  - Coitus under influence of drugs

### 40. What are the remedies?

The most important step is to see your doctor and find out the cause of the pain. The general remedy for pain during sexual intercourse is to treat the underlying cause. So, actual treatment will vary depending on the diagnosis made after a thorough examination by the doctor. Such treatments may include the use of appropriate drugs in cases of endometriosis, infections, pelvic inflammatory disease and corrective operations for scars and adhesions. For women who experience pain because of vaginal dryness due to menopause, estrogen creams and gels are useful vaginal lubricants that can reduce friction and pain remarkably. It is not advisable for you to indulge in the use of unprescribed analgesics solely for sexual intercourse. Rather, this points to a compelling need for you to see your doctor.

### 41. What are the other causes of lower abdominal pain that I should know?

Other important causes of pain include:
- Pelvic masses e.g. fibroids, ovarian cysts, abscesses
- IUCD – insertion of family planning coils
- Referred pain i.e. pain from other parts felt in the lower abdomen
- Ectopic pregnancy
- Physical injury
- Appendix problems: masses, infections, abscesses, stones
- Kidney problems: Stones, infections, cysts etc.
- Ureter: Stones and infections
- Infection and other problems of the Urinary bladder

### 42. What is an abnormal uterine bleeding?

A woman in the reproductive age group is supposed to bleed in the first few days marking the beginning of a new cycle, if the previous cycle has not resulted in pregnancy. Any other bleeding apart from menstruation is regarded as abnormal and the cause should be investigated. Important examples of abnormal bleeding are:
- Bleeding during or after sexual intercourse
- Bleeding in between menstruation
- Bleeding after attaining menopause
- Bleeding during pregnancy

Irregular, prolonged, or excessive menstruation is abnormal. All other cases of dysfunctional uterine bleeding (DUB) are also abnormal.

### 43. What is DUB?

DUB means dysfunctional uterine bleeding. This diagnosis is usually arrived at when the reason why a woman is having abnormal (heavy) menstrual bleeding is not known. This means that all probable causes of bleeding from the womb like fibroids, polyps and infections have been reasonably excluded through appropriate investigations. In developing countries, criminal, incomplete abortions are notorious causes of abnormal vaginal bleeding.

From experience, in some developing countries many young girls or women will attempt to have an abortion because of the implied shame and criminality.

### 44. How common is (DUB)?

Dysfunctional uterine bleeding (DUB) is common at the extremes of reproductive life, which is around puberty and before menopause. It is experienced by 20% of adolescents and 50% of women above the age of 45 years. Generally, more than 50% of all abnormal uterine bleeding are dysfunctional.

### 45. Does DUB cause infertility?

There is a relationship between DUB and infertility. About 10-20% of women with DUB do not ovulate regularly. This makes pregnancy more difficult to achieve.

### 46. What is the treatment for DUB?

The most important step is for the doctor to thoroughly investigate the cause of the bleeding. If no cause is found, then the diagnosis of DUB is justified. There are many modalities of treatment. The chosen treatment depends on the severity of bleeding and your doctor's opinion. Treatment modalities include:
- Dilatation and curettage (D&C) for the purpose of diagnosis and sometimes treatment
- Use of combined oral contraceptives
- Use of non - steroid analgesics
- Use of prostaglandin inhibitors
- Use of anti -fibrinolytics
- Use of Danazol

Also, there are some surgical procedures aimed at reducing or destroying parts of the inner lining of the womb. However, the most effective treatment for DUB is total surgical removal of the womb, called Hysterectomy. Hysterectomy is not a popular choice for many women although the benefits are numerous.

### 47. What is amenorrhea?

Amenorrhea is a medical term used to describe a situation where a woman of reproductive age has not menstruated for more than 6 months or more. It is also applicable to women who fail to menstruate for 3 consecutive cycles. Doctors and other health workers also often use the term in situations where there is absence of menstruation, even when the situation is temporary or menstruation is delayed. This term is also applicable to women who have not menstruated before or have missed their menses for whatever reasons. Amenorrhea is classified into primary and secondary.

### 48. What is primary amenorrhea?

This is when a girl of 14 years has not developed secondary sexual characteristics or failed to menstruate at 16 years. About 5% of all cases of amenorrhea are primary. In simple terms, a woman (more than 16 years old at least) is said to have primary amenorrhea if she has never menstruated before.

### 49. What are the causes of primary amenorrhea?

There are many reasons why a woman may not menstruate. Primary amenorrhea is far less common and the causes are few. Many of these causes are genetic. These include:

- Turner syndrome
- Mayer-Rokitansky syndrome
- Testicular feminization syndrome
- Kallmann syndrome
- Sywer syndrome
- Congenital defects of the female genital tract
  - Agenesis
  - Dysgenesis
  - Transverse vaginal septum
  - Imperforate hymen
- Hypothalamic dysfunctions
- Pituitary failure

### 50. What are syndromes?

In some health conditions, certain features or complaints commonly occur together to indicate that something is wrong. What they represent may not necessarily turn out to be a disease, but when one or more of the features are present, the others are more likely to be found too. So a syndrome is not necessarily a disease and the patient in some cases may look perfectly okay.

### 51. What is Turner syndrome?

Turner syndrome is a genetic disorder which is also called Trisomy-21.

In this condition, there is lack of formation or a disorganized formation of the reproductive tissues. Girls with Turner syndrome show the following features:

- Lack of menstruation

- Short stature
- Wide or webbed neck
- Wide chest with small breasts
- Wide carrying angles: this means that the angles at the elbow joint is wide such that the upper limbs appear bent at the elbow joints even when fully stretched. Also the upper limbs cannot be straightened completely as with other normal girls

Internally, the ovaries are either absent or miniatures and look more like streaks. The womb, vagina and vulva may be normal or poorly formed, for example the vagina may be shallow and inconvenient for sexual intercourse. In rare cases, a lady with Turner syndrome may menstruate, ovulate and possibly get pregnant after a long wait and therapy. However, most women with Turner syndrome have not menstruated before.

## 52. What is Mayer-Rokitansky syndrome?

The Mayer-Rokitansky syndrome is caused by the abnormal development of the reproductive organs very early when the baby is being formed in the womb. The ladies appear outwardly normal in physical appearance with well-developed feminine features such as breasts and body contours, but the main problem is primary amenorrhea due to absence of:
- The womb
- The vagina - sometimes a shallow vagina or dimple may be present

## 53. What is testicular feminization syndrome?

Testicular feminization syndrome is a condition in which the person appears externally as a full grown lady, usually tall with well-developed breasts, female body contours and all external appearances of a typical female, however, genetically speaking, the person is male. They actually have testes (instead of ovaries). The testes are usually located inside the abdomen. People with testicular feminization syndrome do not have wombs but a few women have shallow vaginas and many have normal vulvas. The presence of the vulva and vagina makes the situation more confusing. So in testicular feminization, the person is genetically male, does not have a womb, cannot ovulate or menstruate and therefore cannot be pregnant but due to the presence of a vulva and shallow vagina, such a person can have sexual intercourse. This condition is inherited and exists in some families.

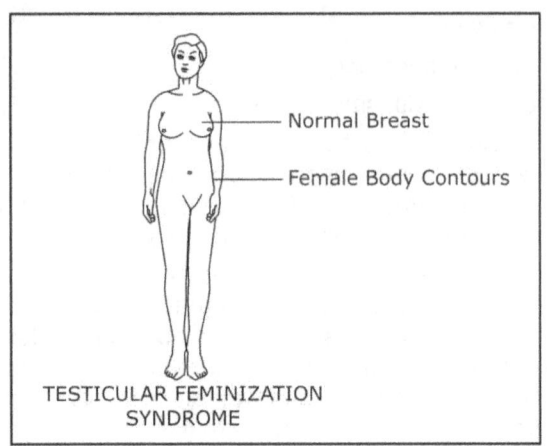

TESTICULAR FEMINIZATION SYNDROME

### 54. What about Kallmann syndrome?

Kallmann syndrome is a condition in which there is congenital lack of the Gonadotropin releasing hormone (GnRH) from the hypothalamus in the brain. Women with this syndrome have small, immature gonads and partial or total inability to perceive smell. Inability to perceive odor is called anosmia in medical palance. The secondary sexual characteristics leading to puberty are also lacking in such women. This means that they have poorly developed breasts, absence of pubic hairs, amenorrhea etc. Kallmann syndrome is one of the less common causes of primary amenorrhea.

### 55. What is Gonadal dysgenesis?

Estrogen is very important in the development of secondary sexual characteristics. In Gonadal dysgenesis, the ovaries which normally produce estrogen are poorly developed. This leads to estrogen deficiency which results in poor and disorganized development of the sexual organs. For example, in Turner syndrome, the ovaries are miniature as described above.

### 56. What is secondary amenorrhea?

This is when a woman of reproductive age who has menstruated before fails to menstruate for 6 months or more. 95% of all cases of amenorrhea are secondary. This definition excludes pregnancy, breastfeeding and menopause which are common reasons why women may not menstruate naturally.

### 57. What are the common causes of secondary amenorrhea?

A woman who has menstruated before may stop menstruating for several reasons. Perhaps the most common reason why a young woman may miss her menses is pregnancy. This is physiological because pregnancy is not a disease. Again, menstruation usually stops or becomes irregular for a variable length of time just before a woman finally attains menopause. This also happens during breast feeding. So the 4 main causes of physiological amenorrhea are:

- Pregnancy
- Lactation or breast feeding
- Pre Puberty and Adolescence
- Menopause

Apart from these, a woman may fail to menstruate due to diseases, illnesses, lifestyles and other factors. These reasons include:

- Problems of the Pituitary, hypothalamus and ovary such as:
  - Inappropriate breast milk secretion
  - Excessive prolactin
  - Consequence of severe, prolonged bleeding, usually during or after childbirth
  - Cancers of the pituitary that secrete prolactin
  - Problems of the ovary
    - Polycystic ovarian syndrome (PCOS)
    - Premature ovarian failure
    - Ovarian failure
    - Ovarian cysts
    - Irradiation damage
- Womb Problems
  - Destructive masses in the womb e.g. tuberculosis
  - Irradiation damage to the womb
  - Destruction of the inner lining of the womb e.g. following dilatation and curettage. This is common in developing countries, especially sub-Saharan Africa where criminal abortion is rampant
  - Adhesions and scars of the lining of the womb
  - Infections of the lining of the womb
- Major debilitating infections and illnesses e.g. Tuberculosis and AIDS
- Drugs such as:
  - Anti-hypertensive
  - Tranquilizers
  - Antidepressants
  - Anti-anxiety drugs
- Other causes include:
  - Overweight or obesity
  - Severe weight loss

- Severe exercise
- Severe stress
- Anorexia
- Contraceptives e.g. pills, the injectables
- Endocrine problems e.g. hypothyroidism

**58. At what times is amenorrhea regarded as normal?**

As mentioned above, a woman will naturally stop menstruating:
- During Pregnancy
- During Breast feeding
- On attaining menopause

In these situations, amenorrhea is regarded as normal.

**59. What are the diseases most commonly responsible for amenorrhea?**

The 4 most common causes of amenorrhea outside pregnancy, lactation, and menopause are:
- Polycystic ovarian syndrome (PCOS)
- Hypothalamic disorders
- Hyper-prolactinemia
- Ovarian failure

# DEAR DOCTOR:

**60. Can I become pregnant if I have sexual intercourse during menstruation?**

Yes, it is quite possible even though the probability is very low. The first half of the menstrual cycle is called the proliferative phase. It lasts for about 14 days but varies in duration from one woman to another. The second half is called the Luteal phase and is fairly constant. It is the last 2 weeks of the cycle. Some females may ovulate early while others ovulate late in the cycle, depending on the lengths of the proliferative phase of their cycles. Since spermatozoa can survive in the female genital tract for some days, pregnancy is theoretically possible at any time. This means that there is no time that the possibility of pregnancy is zero. Therefore, have a family planning method in place or insist that your partner uses a condom!

**61. Is it possible to continue to menstruate even when I am pregnant?**

It is not possible to menstruate during pregnancy. The use of the word menstruation implies that you are not pregnant. However, a woman may bleed from the vagina in pregnancy. If such bleeding happens early during pregnancy or occurs at intervals, some women do confuse this type of bleeding with menstruation.

**62. My girl is 13 years old and has not menstruated, what can I do?**

You need to observe her for signs of secondary sexual characteristics, that is, appearance of pubic hairs, hairs in the armpits, and breast enlargement. If these are not there, then she should be taken to see a gynecologist at the age of 14 or earlier, if you are worried. If the above secondary sexual characteristics are present, you may need to be patient and watch her till she is about 16 years old before taking her to the gynecologist. There is the possibility that your daughter may have delayed puberty or other important medical conditions.

**63. My first daughter is about 14 years old and has not menstruated. However, she complains of lower abdominal pain at monthly intervals. What do you advise?**

It is possible that she may actually be menstruating but the menstrual blood is blocked from coming out. One reason for this condition is an imperforate hymen. The hymen is a membrane-like structure which covers the entrance to the vagina. If there is no perforation or gap through which menstrual blood can drain, then menstrual blood may accumulate behind it, such that the vagina, womb and even the fallopian tubes all become filled with blood. This may result in progressive swelling or a bulge in the lower abdomen. On inspection, the hymen, which normally appears as a thin, pinkish membrane will appear bluish as a result of the accumulated blood. So, the periodic lower abdominal pain is as a result of the accumulated menstrual blood and it is cyclical because it is associated with her monthly periods. This condition is called hidden menstruation or cryptomenorrhea in medical parlance. Your daughter is actually menstruating, but the flow has accumulated behind the blockage. You need to take her to a gynecologist for confirmation and treatment.

**64. My daughter is 13 years old. She saw her first menstruation 5 months ago and up till now, she has not menstruated again. What is the problem?**

The first menses is called menarche. There are some hormones in the brain which should be produced in sufficient quantities and in regulated, frequent intervals. These hormones are responsible for stimulating the ovaries in order to produce eggs. The event results in ovulation. If pregnancy does not occur in that same month, eventually the inner lining of the womb, called endometrium, will be shed and menstruation will occur. In the first few years when young girls begin menstruating, because they are just becoming physiologically mature, the hormones may not be produced in sufficient quantities, so the ovaries are not adequately stimulated. The effect is that their menses may stop or become irregular. Even when they menstruate, many of such cycles are not preceded by ovulation. These are called anovulatory cycles. Anovulation, irregular menstruation or stoppage of menstruation for a variable period of time may last for 2 to 5 years. As a rule, menstruation gradually becomes regular and normalized with time, as the girl becomes more physiologically mature. It does not require treatment. However, it may be a source of worry and anxiety for you during the waiting period. You may need to see a doctor for further reassurance.

**65. I am 33 years old and I have 5 children. Unlike my friends, my menstruation comes regularly at about 40 days. Is this normal?**

Yes, I think it is normal for you, considering the fact that you have no other problems. Now as background information, the menstrual cycle is divided into 2 phases. The first half is called the proliferative or follicular phase. The second half is called the secretary or luteal phase. In the proliferative phase of each cycle, the woman recruits many follicles or eggs, some of these follicles mature but only one, the dominant or Graafian follicle will be ripe enough for ovulation. Ovulation happens at the end of the proliferative phase and marks the beginning of the luteal phase. The main activity in the luteal phase is the preparation of the inner lining of the womb for pregnancy. This preparation is done by the hormone called progesterone, which is produced by the corpus luteum in the ovary. While the proliferative phase varies in duration, the luteal phase is usually more constant at 14 days. Thus, most women can be categorized into early and late ovulators depending on the lengths of their cycles. In your own case, it is possible that your follicular phase is much longer, in this case, about 26 days (40 – 14 = 26). This simply means that you ovulate later than your friends at about day 26 of your cycle. This is an important clue to your fertile period and timing of sexual intercourse, if you still desire to get pregnant.

**66. I am 31 years old and I have had 3 kids. My menstruation is regular but most times, the flow is heavy and contains blood clots. Why do I have blood clots?**

A normal menstrual flow should not contain blood clots. In a normal situation, the womb contains some heparin-like substances which prevent clot formation. However, when the flow is heavy, the capacity of these substances to prevent clot formation is overwhelmed and becomes ineffective. Therefore, clots begin to appear in the sanitary pads. The immediate danger of heavy flow is the associated risk of iron deficiency anemia so you should see your doctor for proper evaluation and treatment.

67. **My menstruation is so heavy and during my periods, I feel so weak and incapacitated that I often don't go to the office. What should I do?**

You should see your doctor without further delay. There are many reasons why a woman may experience repeated heavy periods. Some of these have been listed above. Complaints of weakness, dizziness, fainting attacks and inability to function properly indicate the severity of blood loss. Apart from the issue of incapacitation and absence from work, the resulting anemia may also affect other bodily functions including your ability to menstruate in future. So, it is advisable that you see your doctor without delay for thorough investigations and treatment.

68. **I am 33 years old with 5 kids. I had a coil inserted about 6 months ago for family planning. Since then, I have been bleeding heavily during menstruation. Why is this so?**

One of the side effects of the coil is heavy menstrual bleeding. Other problems include lower abdominal cramps or pain and increased vaginal discharge. Coils may also migrate and disappear with the threads into the womb cavity. These problems are usually explained to women during the initial counseling for family planning. You need to see your doctor or healthcare provider to evaluate your situation. Depending on the severity of the bleeding as assessed by the doctor, you may need to discontinue the use of coil but I am confident that your doctor will assist you to choose another suitable and less troublesome family planning method. Please don't let this experience discourage you from using other forms of family planning.

69. **What is the best treatment for very heavy menses?**

When a woman has completed her family or stopped having children, the best treatment for troublesome, heavy menses is surgical removal of the womb. This solves the problem permanently. Some women do not like the idea that if their wombs are removed, they will not be able to menstruate again but this position is because of social beliefs and cultures. Conversely, in most developed countries like the USA, women are better educated and can make independent choices more freely. The most important function of the womb is to carry pregnancy and since the womb is different from the vagina, its removal does not stop enjoyment of sexual intercourse and should not cause any anxiety. Medically speaking, removal of the womb confers many other benefits. For example, a woman whose womb has been removed does not have to worry about the possibility of cancer of the womb anymore.

70. **What are the other treatments available for heavy bleeding?**

Other forms of treatment are available, but they are less effective. These include operations to remove identified causes such as fibroids or polyps - procedures that will burn off or reduce the inner lining of the womb from where the monthly bleeding normally comes. Various drug remedies including non-steroid anti-inflammatory drugs and family planning pills are also useful. The use of family planning pills or oral contraceptives may be particularly appealing to some women because they are familiar and also prevent unwanted pregnancy.

71. **When I complained of irregular and heavy menstruation to my doctor, I was surprised that he prescribed oral contraceptive pills Is this right? Will it not disturb me from getting pregnant in future?**

One of the benefits of oral contraceptives is the ability to correct irregular menstruation. It also reduces the amount of menstrual blood flow considerably by up to 50% in some cases. Its mode of action as a family planning method is to prevent ovulation when used as a daily pill. When a woman discontinues an oral contraceptive, its effects rapidly disappear because the daily pills do not accumulate in the body. Ovulation resumes immediately and in most cases, pregnancy can be achieved quickly. So, your doctor is perfectly right!

72. **I am 32 years old with a grown up kid. I have not menstruated for 7 months. My doctor said this is because I secrete excessive breast milk, despite the fact that I am not breastfeeding. Why is this so?**

In plain language, what your doctor means is that you have excess prolactin hormone in your blood. Excess levels of this hormone in the blood, is called hyperprolactinemia in medical parlance. In some cases, this is evident when there is inappropriate, copious discharge of milk on gentle squeezing of the breast. However, it is only in about 30% of such cases that the blood prolactin levels are truly raised. Hyperprolactinaemia prevents ovulation from taking place and menstruation may therefore not occur.

73. **So what are the causes of this type of inappropriate breast milk secretion?**

Causes of this condition include:
- Breast stimulation e.g. during romance
- Stress
- Anxiety
- Grief
- Drugs
- Tumors of the brain e.g. pituitary micro-adenoma
- Infections of the brain e.g. meningitis, encephalitis

### 74. I am a woman of 36 years of age. I noticed that for almost one year after the death of my husband, I did not menstruate, even though I was not pregnant. Please tell me why?

Loss of someone very dear, severe continuous emotional upset, mental anguish, depression, etc., will all disturb hypothalamic functions. The hypothalamus is an area in the brain that controls emotions and some important hormones that bring about ovulation and menstruation. When a woman is passing through severe emotional stress like you are doing, the hypothalamus may not be able to produce sufficient releasing hormones that are necessary for ovulation and menstruation. Again, in many cases of grief, there is weight loss which may also contribute to the problem. Time is a healer, says the adage and when the grief period is over and you are more stable emotionally, your menstruation should resume spontaneously. This is usually the case unless there are other underlying problems.

### 75. My doctor told me that some of the drugs that I take can stop me from menstruating. Which of the drugs?

I do not know the drugs that you are using now, but your doctor is right. Some drugs can stop your menstruation because of the way they work or due to their side effects. These drugs include:

- Anti-hypertensives
- Tranquillizers
- Oral contraceptives and the injectables e.g. Primolut - depo
- Cardiac drugs e.g. Digoxin
- Anti-cancer drugs
- Many herbal preparations with unknown active ingredients can also affect menstruation

That's why doctors always advise against self-medication. Please don't use drugs that are not prescribed by the doctor.

### 76. My menstruation has been irregular with occasional spotting of blood since I took the family planning injection prescribed by my doctor. Should I stop it?

Irregular vaginal bleeding, spotting of blood or "breakthrough" bleeding occurs in many women who are on contraceptive injections. These are some of the recognized side effects. If the spotting is so discomforting or embarrassing, you may need to change to another form of family planning. You should see your family planning provider or doctor for proper evaluation and guidance on a more suitable method.

77. **I had some problems during the delivery of my last baby. I bled severely because the placenta did not come out on time. I was given 5 pints of blood and discharged after 4 weeks. It is 2 years now and I am yet to menstruate. I am worried. Doctor, what is my problem?**

Sometimes, when a woman bleeds heavily, more often during or after child birth, the blood loss may be so severe that it sends her into a state of shock. In this situation, many organs in the body, including the brain, suffer the effects of the severe blood loss. The pituitary gland in the brain is partly responsible for the process that normally brings about ovulation and menstruation in women. In situations of severe blood loss like your own, when the pituitary gland also suffers from shock, its functions are badly affected and the result is that menstruation stops. In medical parlance, this is called Sheehan's syndrome. I strongly suspect that this may be the reason why you have not menstruated. You need to see a gynecologist who will evaluate your situation and give the necessary treatment.

78. **Doctor, why is it that women do not menstruate during breastfeeding?**

This is because during breastfeeding, the level of prolactin hormone is very high. High levels of prolactin suppress ovulation so menstruation may not occur for about 6 months or more, in women who are actively breastfeeding, especially if they practice exclusive breastfeeding.

79. **My daughter is 16 years old and has never menstruated. So, we took her to a scan center for an ultrasound scan of the womb. It was discovered that she had fluid in her womb, please what do you advise?**

It is possible that the fluid inside her womb is actually accumulated menstrual blood that was blocked from coming out. This blockage may be due to an abnormality of the vagina or a hymen that has not been torn, if she is a virgin. You should take her to a gynecologist for proper evaluation. The obstruction can be freed and the blood drained, so that your daughter can experience normal menstruation.

80. **Please doctor, can "washing of the womb" or D&C restore my menses?**

In some communities, washing and flushing of the womb are alternative names for dilatation and curettage (D&C). Doctors do not commonly do D&C in order to restore menstruation except when it is necessary to take samples of the lining of the womb for diagnostic purposes. Apart from the fact that this practice has no medical value whatsoever, it is harmful and can worsen the problem or lead to other complications.

This practice is rooted in the belief that failure to get pregnant or menstruate may be because the womb is dirty and hence needs to be washed and is common in many developing countries. In some women, aggressive scraping of the inner wall or lining of the womb during D&C many cause permanent stoppage of menstruation. Most of such obnoxious procedures are performed by quacks that use various tools to cause damage to the lining and walls of the womb, which may also result in infections, scar formation, and infertility.

### 81. If I menstruate regularly or monthly does it mean that I also ovulate regularly?

In most women, ovulation takes place and if pregnancy does not happen, menstruation should follow. So in normal circumstances, menstruation should be preceded by ovulation. However, this is not always so. Some women who do not ovulate can menstruate. Regular menstruation does not mean regular ovulation but the majority of those who menstruate regularly also ovulate regularly. Conversely, those who often miss their periods or do not menstruate regularly have higher probabilities of not ovulating regularly. They are said to have anovulatory cycles. For such reasons, it is necessary for doctors to conduct tests to determine why a woman fails to achieve pregnancy despite menstruating regularly.

### 82. So how do I know if I am ovulating?

The absolute evidence that you have ovulated is pregnancy. Most of the tests available are indirect evidences while a few are only suggestive of ovulation. Some of these include:

- Menstrual history: The majority of women who have regular menstruation are also likely to ovulate regularly especially if they do not have difficulty getting pregnant. So, doctors can have a fair insight into a woman's ovulation status from her menstrual history. In other words, regular menstruation may suggest regular ovulation
- BBT: This is basal body temperature. Soon after ovulation, the hormone progesterone is produced by the corpus luteum. The progesterone hormone is thermogenic because it produces heat, so the body feels hot around the time of ovulation. Consequently, due to the effect of progesterone, if ovulation has taken place, the temperature of the body, when taken every morning on waking up, would usually be about 33.8 – 35.6°F (1-2 °C) higher than usual. Thus, increase in basal body temperature is one of the indirect ways of knowing if ovulation has occurred. However, more superior and less cumbersome tests are currently available for the detection of ovulation
- Cervical mucus: At about the time of ovulation, there are profound changes in the mucus discharge from the cervix. It is usually copious, watery, and more elastic. At this time, most women feel wet. These

attributes are due to the effect of estrogen that is abundant in women around the time of ovulation. So, the appearance of this type of discharge may suggest ovulation

- Blood progesterone level: Doctors do blood estimation of progesterone, usually at about day 21 of the cycle, in order to make a judgment whether ovulation has occurred in the current cycle or not. Ovulation is deemed to have occurred if the blood level of progesterone measured is adjudged to be adequate
- Dip Stick testing of urine: Just before ovulation occurs, there is rapid increase in the Leutinizing Hormone (LH) level. This is called an LH surge. Currently, this surge is verified by plunging a dipstick into early morning urine, daily, for a few days close to the estimated day of ovulation. Ovulation is imminent if the strip changes color as indicated, after being dipped in the urine. This is a popular way of testing for ovulation worldwide
- Ultrasound Scan: The serial scan of the ovaries can also be done at about the time of ovulation to monitor the growth of follicles in the ovaries. This is called follicle tracking. Follicles can rupture once they attain a diameter of 18mm or more. The monitoring is done daily until the follicles rupture, thus confirming that ovulation has taken place

### 83. At about the middle of my cycle, I normally experience some low abdominal pain. Is this normal?

Ovulation could be likened to the process of plucking an orange fruit from the tree, which may involve twisting, pulling, etc. Similarly, the physiological process leading to the rupture of a follicle or ovulation is accompanied by pain. Some chemicals like prostaglandin which are involved in the normal process of ovulation are also known to cause pain. This type of pain is called ovulation pain. Many women experience this to various degrees. However, the pain is usually localized to the right or left, depending on which ovary is releasing the egg for the month. So in a way, this may be an indirect evidence of ovulation for you. If you experience it regularly during your cycle, it may assist you in the timing of sexual intercourse, in case you are planning to get pregnant. Please, note that it is not a recommended method of family planning.

### 84. My period is regular at 28 days, but sometimes I see a little blood for one day about the middle of my cycle. Why is this so?

This may be normal. This is because at the time of ovulation, when the follicle is being released, the estrogen hormone falls and the inner lining of the womb may be shed a little. This appears externally as spotting of blood. It is harmless and will not prevent you from getting pregnant.

**85. I have been unable to achieve pregnancy for about 6 years and have now been diagnosed as having PCOS. What does this mean?**

PCOS means polycystic ovarian syndrome. It is the most common type of hormonal imbalance in women. Women like you, who have PCOS, have numerous immature follicles in the ovaries. This makes the ovaries appear cystic and enlarged.

In this condition, there is excess and inappropriate Leutinizing Hormone (LH) production. The level of Follicle Stimulating Hormone (FSH) may be normal. The LH: FSH ratio, when calculated, is usually 2:1 or greater in women with PCOS. Furthermore, the levels of most androgens or male hormones such as testosterone, Dihydroepiandrosterone Sulphate (DHEAS) are high. In PCOS, there is also resistance to insulin hormone activity.

The result of all these is that even though you have many eggs, the eggs are in a male, instead of female dominated hormonal environment. The eggs are of very poor quality. Consequently, you may not ovulate or menstruate regularly. Other features of PCOS include obesity and excessive hair growth in areas like the face, upper chest, abdomen and limbs. It is not surprising therefore that you have difficulty in achieving pregnancy. Fortunately, there are a few ways to get around this problem, in the light of improved knowledge of the condition. You need to see a gynecologist who will evaluate your condition and treat you.

**86. I am 36 years old and I have had 4 children. Recently, each time I have sexual intercourse with my husband, he notices blood stains on his penis, what can be the reason for this?**

I do not know if you also bleed after coitus. If you do, this is called post coital bleeding (PCB). Post coital bleeding may also be associated with pain during sexual intercourse. The causes of such bleeding include:

- Problems of the cervix such as infections, erosion, polyp or cancer: The most important issue is the possibility of cervical cancer, which must be ruled out
- Problems of the vagina: such as infections including Candida or yeast infection, vaginal wounds, or bruises which may happen if your husband is not gentle during the act
- "Break-through" bleeding from the womb may happen occasionally, especially if you are on contraceptive pills

You need to see your doctor as soon as possible for examination and proper diagnosis. The doctor may order a Papanicolaou (PAP) smear or PAP test to screen for the possibility of cervical cancer. The ultimate treatment will depend on the cause identified.

## CHAPTER 3
# Vaginal Discharge and Genital Infections

*"I bet you're worried. I was worried. I was worried about vaginas. I was worried about what we think about vaginas and even more worried that we don't think about them"*
– EVE ENSLER

### 1. What is a normal vaginal discharge?

All girls and women have vaginal discharge at one time or the other, during their monthly cycles. Even women who have attained menopause have vaginal discharge. Therefore, it is perfectly ok to experience periods of normal, moderate discharge. The normal vaginal discharge is moderate in quantity, whitish in color and does not have an offensive odor. It is acidic and contains germs that are not harmful to the vagina.

### 2. What are the contents of a normal discharge?

The normal vaginal discharge has 5 main components. These are:
- Mucus or slimy secretions from the neck of the womb or cervix
- Fluids from cells lining the vagina
- Secretions from the Bartholin's glands
- Cells of the cervix and vagina that have peeled or fallen off
- Harmless vaginal germs, especially lactobacilli

**3. So, what is the typical smell of a normal vaginal secretion?**

Normal vaginal secretion does not have a specific odor. Certainly it is not foul smelling. It is also moderate in quantity depending on the time during the woman's menstrual cycle. At about the time of ovulation, the secretion may be increased, elastic and more watery. At other times, it should be moderate with a non-offensive odor.

**4. What is an abnormal vaginal discharge?**

It may be difficult to define an abnormal vaginal discharge, although it has some common features. These include:
- Offensive odor
- Copious quantity
- Discolored - yellowish, grayish, brownish etc
- May be blood stained
- Associated with other symptoms like waist pain, discomfort and fever

**5. What is leucorrhoea (pronounced: lu-ko-ria)?**

This may be regarded as a different form of the normal vaginal discharge. It is copious, watery, whitish but non–offensive. Leucorrhea contains shed vaginal cells, vaginal secretions, cervical mucus and harmless bacteria. Because it is usually excessive in quantity, it may be confused with abnormal vaginal discharge or vaginal infection. This innocent discharge may cause anxiety or worries for women.

**6. At what times could there be an increase in normal vaginal discharge?**

There are specific times when it is normal for a woman to experience an increase in vaginal discharge. These are at about the time of ovulation, when the woman feels wet, just before menstruation and during pregnancy. It may also increase in women who are on oral contraceptives or Family planning pills.

**7. Why does vaginal discharge increase during hot weather?**

Normally, the cells of the cervix or neck of the womb produce mucus secretion. The cells of the vaginal wall produce watery fluid while the Bartholin's glands make secretions. Other components include cells shed from the cervix and vagina along with bacteria or germs, especially lactobacilli, which are harmless. During hot weather, many women sweat a lot and with the under pants and clothing, the private part becomes more moist and hot. The protein materials in the vaginal discharge are broken down to produce ammonia salt which gets mixed with the sweat. This results in increased discharge with an unpleasant smell.

## 8. What is the main natural defense or protection of the vagina?

The main defense of the vagina is the acidic environment. The normal vaginal pH is 4 to 4.5. This acid is due to the harmless germs called lactobacilli, which are natural inhabitants of the vagina. Lactobacilli break down glycogen in the vagina to form lactic acid. This acidic environment promotes the growth of germs which are also harmless to the vagina, while making it difficult for harmful germs to survive. In this way, the harmless germs predominate in the vagina and continue to produce acid to protect the vaginal environment. This is a natural defense for the vagina. When there is an upset or reduced acidity in the vaginal environment, the risk of infection is increased.

## 9. Under what circumstances can this natural protection be weakened in a healthy woman?

When the acidic environment of the vagina is compromised, the population of harmful germs dominates that of the harmless germs. Consequently, there is increased foul smelling vaginal discharge. This may happen due to the use of oral contraceptives or family planning pills, antibiotics, and some vaginal preparations. Women who engage in frequent, regular douching or washing of the vagina may also have increased vaginal discharge. Other reasons include sexual intercourse with multiple sexual partners or change of sexual partners, as well as sexually transmitted diseases. When the immunity status or fitness level of a woman is depressed, she may have increased vaginal discharge because of the reduced protection against infections.

## 10. Can drugs cause an increase in vaginal discharge?

Yes. Some drugs may increase the quantity of vaginal discharge. Antibiotics, when not used appropriately, may kill off harmless germs in the vagina and encourage the growth of harmful ones leading to increased vaginal discharge. Other drugs including steroids and anti-cancer drugs may depress the body's immunity and allow harmful germs to multiply rapidly, resulting in genital infections. In such cases, vaginal discharge becomes copious.

## 11. Apart from the reasons given above, are there other causes of abnormal vaginal discharge?

Yes. Abnormal vaginal discharge can be caused by insertion of dirty foreign bodies into the vagina e.g. unclean tampons, dirty clothes, or tissue papers and newspaper waste during menstruation. This is a common practice by women in poor developing countries. Allergic reactions to drugs, chemicals, or other materials such as powders, soaps and spermicides can also result in increased vaginal discharge. Women who wear nylon pants or tight fitting under wears are also at increased risk of discharge.

## 12. What are the 4 most common germs responsible for copious vaginal discharge and infections in developing countries?

The most common germs are:
- Chlammydia germs
- Gonorrhea germs
- Trichomonas germs
- Vaginal yeast

It should also be added that staphylococcus, even though notorious in the African environment, is not as important or guilty as it is portrayed to be. This germ has assumed so much fame to the point that it is most probably the best known germ in the public domain.

## 13. Why are these germs very important to public health?

The infections caused by these germs are important for 2 main reasons. Firstly, the infections are all sexually transmitted with serious adverse consequences. Secondly, many women with infections by Chlamydia and sometimes, Trichomonas and gonorrhea may not experience pain, discharge or manifest worrisome symptoms. So in such situations, they may not go to hospital for treatment. This allows unintentional widespread transmission to their sexual partners.

## 14. What are the natural features of the external genital tract in women that make vaginal discharge more common?

The vagina connects with the womb through the cervix and opens to the outside of the body at the vulva. This makes it possible for germs to pass in and out easily. Secondly, the vulva lies very close to the anus and can be smeared with stool when cleaning up. Also, the urethra opens at the upper part of the vulva, so urine can easily stream down into the vagina when a woman urinates. All these factors make a woman naturally prone to repeated infections and vaginal discharge, because germs can pass easily from one area to another.

## 15. Is washing the vagina a method of reducing vaginal discharge?

No. In fact, this usually increases the severity of vaginal discharge. Whether the vagina is washed with clean water or chemicals, the effect is to remove harmless native vaginal germs, leaving behind the more harmful germs. With time, the vagina is overpopulated by harmful, disease producing germs. This results in the production of copious and offensive vaginal discharge. Washing of the vagina is called douching. It is not beneficial.

**16. Why do some old women experience vaginal discharge even though they are not sexually active?**

The estrogen hormone makes the normal vaginal skin strong and able to withstand infections. At old age, there is lack of estrogen, the vulva and vaginal skins become thin and dry and may be easily injured during sexual intercourse. Also, the vaginal environment is less acidic and therefore less protective than those of younger women because of reduced lactobacilli germs. This allows the growth of other harmful bacteria. Thus, the vulva and vagina in some old women may be prone to infections and can bleed easily.

**17. What are the causes of vaginal discharge in children?**

Vaginal discharge may occur in children naturally due to lack of estrogen hormone and poor hygiene, as a result of poor parental assistance or neglect. Some guardians leave their children to do the clean up after defecation; these children innocently smear the vulva with stool and urine. Also, children sometimes fiddle with their vulva with dirty hands and may insert foreign objects into the vagina. These are some of the common but avoidable causes of vaginal discharge in children.

**18. What is Pruritus (pronounced:Pru-ri-tus)?**

Pruritus is the sensation that causes an intense desire to scratch the body. This may be troublesome and felt around the vulva, anus, and other parts of the body. Sometimes, the sensation may be pleasurable which makes it more compelling to scratch the body even to the point of bruising the skin.

**19. What are the causes of itching in the vulva?**

Itching here means a sensation to scratch the private part, around the entrance to the vagina. This sensation is sometimes pleasant and because of this, some women are compelled to continue to scratch. The main causes are:

- Infections: In women, 3 conditions are mostly responsible. These are
  - Trichomonas germ infection
  - Yeast infection
  - Bacterial vaginosis

There are, of course, other less common reasons. These infections are all associated with vaginal discharges which are of different colors but all have offensive smells. Other reasons include:

- Infestations: Itching can be caused by infestations by Parasites like-
  - Scabies
  - Lice (Human pediculosis)

- Thread worms can also cause itching in the private parts like the vulva, anus etc. The itching here is irritating and troublesome, but the sensation is also pleasant
- Allergy: Some women are allergic to certain substances e.g.
  - Dye in clothes
  - Cotton clothes
  - Nylon pants
  - Family planning insertions into the vagina
  - Perfumes
  - Unclean water used on the skin for bathing
- Drugs such as Chloroquine and Penicillin also cause itching. Use of Chloroquine without an anti-itch drug can make life miserable
- Psychosomatic disorders:
  - Neurosis
  - Anxiety
  - Depression
  - Psychological and sexual problems may manifest as itching, though the origin may be unknown
- Poor hygiene: This is an important cause of itching in developing countries. Some women, for example, do not clean up at all or fail to clean up properly after defecation, urination, exercise or even sexual intercourse. The sweat generated is broken down to ammonia salt which is an irritant to the skin around the vulva and vagina. During menstruation, the use of non-sterile, dirty pieces of cloth or papers as sanitary pads, is also a source of itchy vaginal discharge.

It should be noted that warmth and wetness in the private part will encourage vaginal discharge and itching. So, it is always advisable to keep the pubic hair and private parts clean and dry.

### 20. Why are vaginal discharge and infections more common in developing countries?

This is because of poor genital hygiene, rampant sexually transmitted diseases and septic abortion, especially those procured through Dilatation and Curettage (D&C) by quacks.

### 21. What is vaginitis?

Vaginitis is the inflammation of the vagina. It is commonly caused by yeast infection. The discharge is whitish and thick. When this type of infection occurs in the entrance to the vagina called vulva, there may be associated irritation and an itching sensation.

## 22. What is bacterial vaginosis?

Bacterial vaginosis is a condition where there is overgrowth of harmful bacteria in the vagina. Consequently, there is heavy vaginal discharge which is extremely offensive in odor and leaves the underwear wet with discharge day and night. It is one of the most embarrassing situations that a woman may face, unless it is treated effectively. Bacterial vaginosis is caused by anaerobic bacteria, especially Gardnerella vaginalis and Mobillincus germs.

## 23. What are Sexually Transmitted Diseases (STDs)?

As the name implies, these are diseases that are mainly contracted through sexual intercourse. They include the following infections:

- Gonorrhea
- Syphilis
- Yeast infection
- Trichomonas
- Chlamydia infection
- Mycoplasma infection
- Granuloma inguinale
- Chancroid
- Scabies
- Hepatitis
- Herpes simplex infection
- HIV infection
- Human Papilloma Virus (HPV) infection

## 24. What is Gonorrhea infection?

Gonorrhea is a sexually transmitted disease caused by the bacteria called Nesseria gonorrhea. The disease shows up in 2 to 10 days after being contracted. Unlike men, most women who have gonorrhea infection may not have serious complaints, because women generally tolerate Gonorrhea infection better than men. In women with the severe disease, the complaints include copious, purulent, offensive vaginal discharge, increased frequency of urination, pain during urination and lower abdominal or waist pain. In some cases, there may be fever, weakness and other non-specific complaints. If not properly treated, acute gonorrhea becomes chronic and may result in damage to the fallopian tubes, inner wall of the womb and ovaries. In all cases, it is important to trace and effectively treat all sexual partners so as to prevent re-infection.

**25. What are the other consequences of gonorrhea infection apart from PID?**

Pelvic Inflammatory Disease (PID) is the most common disease caused by gonorrhea. However, gonorrhea may also cause inflammation or infection of the following parts:
- Joints (arthritis)
- Skin (dermatitis)
- Eyes (conjunctivitis)
- Blood

**26. What is Syphilis?**

Syphilis is also a sexually transmitted disease. It is most commonly caused by the germ called Treponema pallidum. It shows up at about 10 to 90 days after gaining entrance into the body. There are various stages of the disease. In the early stage, it commonly appears as a single, painless ulcer on the vulva, cervix, anus or lip. The tissues around the ulcer may become swollen. If not treated at this point, other skin ulcers, wounds, rashes and body swellings may appear. The woman may also suffer from headache, fever, poor appetite, mouth ulcers and multiple boils on her skin. At this stage, she is infectious and can pass the infection to other people. In the late stage, more serious skin infections and other health problems normally develop. The disease may practically affect all parts or organs of the body including nerves, womb, tubes, ovaries, eyes, brain, kidney, lung, heart etc, causing serious damage and disease. As in all cases of STDs, it is important to trace and treat the woman and all her sexual contacts early enough and adequately too.

**27. What is Trichomonas infection?**

This sexually transmitted disease is caused by the Trichomonas vaginalis germ. It has been suggested that this disease can also be contracted through the use of communal items like wet towels, dirty toilet seats etc. The disease shows up in 4 to 20 days after entering the body. It causes copious, yellow-green or grayish white, very offensive, vaginal discharge. There may be itching, frequent and painful urination, pain during sexual intercourse and vaginal bleeding or spotting after sexual intercourse. Unlike women, men can tolerate the disease without major complaints. Therefore, men can serve as carriers of the disease and continue to spread it among their female sexual partners.

**28. What is Chlamydia infection?**

This disease is caused by the germ Chlamydia trachomatis which is sexually transmitted. This disease is more common in patients with gonorrhea. It is a common cause of infection of the urethra, inner wall of the womb, cervix and fallopian tubes. The rate of sexual transmission is high and may be up to 50%.

It is responsible for many cases of tubal blockage in women, thus causing infertility. In Chlamydia infection, the vaginal discharge is a mixture of pus and mucus. Complaints like frequent, painful urination, low waist pain, pain during sexual intercourse and mild fever may be present. The consequences of untreated chlamydia infection include:
- Infertility due to tubal blockage
- Eye infection
- Post abortion infection
- Womb infection after delivery
- Premature rupture of the membranes during pregnancy
- Preterm labor
- Low birth weight babies

It is clear from the above that this disease must be adequately treated to avoid any of the numerous complications.

## 29. What about Candida infection?

This is a common infection in women in developing countries. It is also popularly called "toilet infection" by local women and men alike. It is sexually transmitted and commonly caused by the germ called Candida albicans or yeast. The discharge is usually whitish and thick. It may look like curds of spoilt milk or cottage cheese and may be associated with severe itching. Warm and wet environments encourage the growth of yeast. Improved hygiene, wearing of light underwear and keeping the private parts clean and dry may help to reduce yeast infection.

## 30. So why is it called toilet infection in some countries?

This is a local coinage in many rural African countries or communities that denote abnormal foul smelling vaginal discharge and itchy sensation. This is because many women think they contacted the infection as a result of using public toilets, hence the name toilet infection. In actual fact "Toilet infection" means sexually transmitted infections. The word "toilet infection" tends to make the disease more of a mere social condition which tends to reduce the stigma associated with the disease. In this way, women try to avoid the bad feelings, guilt and stigma associated with other sexually transmitted infections like gonorrhea and syphilis. Staphylococcus infection is the most popular "toilet infection" in women in developing countries.

## 31. What about HIV infection?

HIV means human immunodeficiency virus. Sexual intercourse is just one of the modes of transmission of this infection. Infection by this virus leads to the depletion of body immunity generally. Complications of HIV infection are numerous and affect virtually all parts and organs of the body. A chapter has been devoted to this condition due to its importance with regards to public health.

## 32. What is Genital herpes?

Genital herpes is a sexually transmitted disease caused by the Herpes simplex hominis type 2 Virus. The first infection may go unnoticed by the individual. The virus travels along nerve fibers to the skin of the genital tracts, especially the cervix and vulva in women. This produces local burning sensation and irritation. The infection causes numerous painful vesicles or blisters which burst to produce multiple painful ulcers on the vulva, vagina, cervix and skin. There is increased risk of this infection in situations where the body immunity is reduced such as HIV infection, use of immune suppressive drugs like steroids, sexual intercourse during menstruation and stress. Apart from the pain and severe illness that it causes, herpes infection is associated with spontaneous abortion, infection of the unborn baby, preterm labor and preterm delivery. Up to 50% of infected newborn babies die if the infection happens during pregnancy.

## 33. What are Genital warts?

Genital warts are fleshy tumors or growths. They are commonly found on the skin, vulva, vagina, cervix, urethra and anusamong others. Genital warts are caused by the Human Papilloma Virus (HPV). Human Papilloma Virus is transmitted during sexual intercourse or use of wet clothing of an infected person. An infected mother can also infect her baby during childbirth. Genital warts are associated with cancer of the cervix in women, cancer of the anus and external genital organs in both men and women. Genital warts also cause painful sexual intercourse, itching and burning sensation. Pregnancy, use of oral contraceptives and immune depleted states increase the risk of the disease.

## 34. What are the complications of STDs?

In women, the complications include chronic pelvic inflammatory disease (PID), infertility, menstrual disorders (excessive menses, painful menses, irregular menses etc.), pain during sexual intercourse, ectopic pregnancy, abortions and miscarriages. In infants, STDs can cause low birth weight, blindness and pneumonia in newborn babies.

## 35. How can STDs be avoided?

Most sexually transmitted diseases can be prevented, to a large extent by practicing safe sex. This means one man to one sexual partner who is free of STDs. Where casual sex is unavoidable, both partners must ensure adequate protection and safety. In most cases the man must use a condom. Women in particular must ensure good lower genital tract hygiene and avoid the use of communal items e.g. dirty public toilets, wet towels, etc. as much as possible.

### 36. What is Pelvic Inflammatory Disease (PID)?

PID means Pelvic Inflammatory Disease. It is a serious infection which involves the inner lining of the womb, fallopian tubes, ovaries and the tissue covering the inside wall of the pelvis. Most times, the germs usually spread upwards from the cervix. Doctors use the term PID to describe sexually transmitted infections (STI) in women in the reproductive age group, that is, from about the age of about 18 to 44 years.

### 37. How common is PID?

Pelvic inflammation disease (PID) occurs in 1% of women between the age of 15 to 35 years. It increases to 2% in younger girls and women between 15 to 24 years of age. This age range seems to be at the highest risk of PID. The age bracket also represents the period when women are highly sexually active and are more likely to have multiple sexual partners. PID is relatively more common in Africans than Caucasian women. Generally speaking, about 4% of women suffer from pelvic inflammatory disease.

### 38. Why is the occurrence of PID higher in developing countries?

The higher incidence of PID in developing countries is due to the fact that sexually transmitted infections are far more common than in developed countries. However, PID is one of the diseases that has been over diagnosed or misdiagnosed by quacks and other health workers, including some doctors.

### 39. What is the global trend in the incidence of PID?

Globally, the prevalence of PID is on the increase. In countries like the United Kingdom, there is up to 50% increase in PID in the 20- 24 year age group. This trend may be due to the global increase in sexually transmitted diseases and the fact that laboratories are now more equipped to diagnose STDs. There are also more sensitive and better tests for diagnosing PID, unlike in previous decades.

### 40. What are the common germs that cause PID?

The germs that cause PID in women may vary from one community to the other. Generally speaking, these germs are largely those that are also responsible for sexually transmitted infections in the same community. Most of the infections are called by the names of the germs that cause them. The common germs are:

- Neisseria Gonorrhea: The germ that causes gonorrhea

- Chlamydia: The germ that causes Chlamydia infections of the genital tract and other parts of the body
- Gram negative bacilli
- Trichomonas
- Haemophilus influenzae
- Group B and D streptococcus
- Mycobacteria hominis
- Bacteroides species
- Gram positive cocci

Mycobacterium tuberculosis, the germ that causes genital tuberculosis is still common in Africa and is one of the causes of infertility in developing countries. It is much less common in the USA. However, it may be a relevant health consideration in African American women.

## 41. What are the problems that may suggest PID?

The complaints in women with PID include the following:
- Pain: This is usually felt in the lower abdomen and around the waist. It varies from a deep and dull pain which may be constant, to the more severe and disenabling type. The pain may be increased by movement during walking and reduced by rest. It may also show up or be aggravated by menstruation and sexual intercourse. Occasionally, there may be associated pain during urination
- Fever: Hotness of the body may be a feature of PID depending on whether the disease is acute or chronic. For long standing PID, fever may be low grade or absent. The fever in PID is usually associated with nausea and vomiting, especially in acute cases when the temperature is high
- Vaginal discharge: Increased vaginal discharge may indeed be the most worrisome complaint by women suffering from PID. The discharge is copious and foul smelling. The color varies from light yellowish or milky to mixed muco-purulent. It may or may not be blood stained. More often, the woman experiences irritating, itchy sensations and the underwear is more likely to be wet and stained by the discharge
- Swelling: There may be small swellings on both side of the waist or groin. The swellings are usually painful and may be warm to touch. These are inguinal lymph node swellings. Lymph nodes are an important part of the natural body defenses against infection. They act like soldiers. In the process of fighting infection or defending the body, they become swollen, warm, and painful

- Irregular vaginal bleeding: PID may be associated with vaginal bleeding at unexpected times. It may also result in prolonged menstrual flow, which may stop and start unexpectedly

### 42. In developing countries, what typical events may be a pointer that a woman has PID?

In PID, it is normal to experience lower abdominal pain, fever and abnormal foul smelling vaginal discharge. The pain may be increased during menstruation, urination and sexual intercourse. These are the usual complaints, but in developing countries, when a woman or a young girl complains of having missed her period and presents with the complaints mentioned above, she is more likely to have procured criminal abortion or D & C. This is important because these ladies will not readily admit to having had an abortion until the situation becomes life threatening. Delay in diagnosis and treatment in this situation has resulted in many avoidable deaths.

### 43. What are the other conditions that may increase the risk of PID?

Those at increased risk of PID include women with multiple sexual partners and those who are sexually promiscuous. Women who have had surgical procedures with non-sterile instruments especially D & C, Hysterosalpingogram (HSG) etc, are at increased risk of PID. In developing countries, the insertion of herbal preparations into the vagina in a futile attempt to treat infertility is a serious issue. Naturally, women are prone to genital infections during and immediately after menstruation. So, engaging in sexual intercourse at this time may increase the risk of PID.

### 44. Why are STIs and other genital infections more common or aggravated just after menses?

During menstruation, and for the first few days after, infections are more common for 2 main reasons. Firstly, the menstrual blood is a rich medium where germs thrive more and can multiply rapidly leading to increased offensive vaginal discharge. Secondly, during menstruation, there Is a continuous communication from the cervix through the vagina to the outside, which means germs can pass freely into the womb. Outside menstruation time, there is usually a cervical plug of mucus that serves as a barrier to infection. The cervical plug is expelled at the beginning of menstruation, so infections at this time are more severe and common.

### 45. What are the 3 major consequences of PID in pregnancy?

Pelvic inflammation disease is not common in pregnancy but if it happens, it is associated with increased risks of abortion and preterm labor. Preterm labor implies that the babies are born prematurely, when they are not viable. Most times, such babies die shortly after birth. Pelvic inflammatory disease is also associated with post-delivery infection of the inner lining of the womb. This is called endometritis in medical parlance. This type of infection can lead to ill health in the mother in both short and long terms. It can damage the lining of the womb to the extent that the woman may find it difficult to conceive in future. So, abortion, endometritis and infertility are possible consequences.

### 46. What is the most important long term consequence of PID in women?

Infertility is the most important long term consequence as it leads to blockage of the Fallopian tubes. Tubal blockage is the most common cause of infertility in women in developing countries. After one episode of acute PID, the rate of infertility is 13%, after two episodes it is 36%. It is as high as 75% after the third episode. Therefore, all cases of PID must be adequately treated by a doctor, preferably a gynecologist.

### 47. Why is PID difficult to eradicate?

Perhaps one remarkable feature of PID is the fact that it recurs in 25% of all cases, which may be an indication of improper treatment of the first episode. Once the initial diagnosis is missed or the initial infection is poorly or incompletely treated, acute PID progresses slowly to chronic PID, which becomes deep seated and difficult to treat effectively. Like other diseases caused by sexually transmitted infections, re-infection is common and easy through sexual intercourse with defaulting partners.

## DEAR DOCTOR:

### 48. I have an offensive vaginal discharge, itching and an unbearable burning sensation. What should I do?

This type of complaint is typical of Trichomonas germ infection. This infection is caused by the trichomonas vaginalis germ. The infection is transmitted commonly through sexual intercourse. The discharge is usually copious, greenish, foul smelling and itchy with a typical burning sensation. You may experience lower waist pain and pain during sexual intercourse. In some women, this infection may cause pain when urinating. You need to see your doctor for further investigation and treatment. Your husband or partner must also be treated to prevent further spread and recurrence of the infection. If untreated or neglected, the infection may progress to pelvic inflammatory disease which may result in the blockage of your fallopian tubes.

**49. I am 27 years old and sexually active. I recently noticed that I spot blood after sexual intercourse. What is happening to me?**

There are many reasons why you may have this type of complaint at your age. The most important among these is infection of the lower genital tract, especially the cervix and vagina. This situation is typically associated with lower abdominal pain, pain during sexual intercourse and copious, foul smelling vaginal discharge. Chlamydia, Trichomonas, Gonorrhea, and staphylococcus infections are the main culprits. Other causes include wound-like lesions of the cervix which doctors call cervical erosion and trauma or bruises to the vagina. Bruises to the vagina may occur during forceful or aggressive intercourse and may have passed unnoticed initially. You are advised to see your doctor for proper evaluation and treatment.

**50. How would I know if I am suffering from an STD?**

You may be suffering from an STD if you have sudden onset of foul smelling vaginal discharge or unusual increase in offensive vaginal discharge, especially if you have been sexually active. The risk of STD is higher if you have multiple sexual partners or have had unprotected, casual sexual intercourse. Symptoms like fever, headache, weakness, and poor appetite as well as pain during urination may be pointers.

**51. So what should I do?**

You should see a doctor without delay for investigation and treatment. Remember that cutting corners or getting inadequate treatments may result in serious long term complications. In all cases, your sexual partners must be treated also. Otherwise, you may be re-infected or become carriers of STDs. Carriers of STDs are able to transmit and spread infections to other sexual contacts and the general public at large.

**52. Is it true that Intra-uterine contraceptive devices (IUCD) increase the risk of PID?**

Yes. Intra-uterine contraceptive devices (IUCDs) or coils are devices placed inside the womb cavity to prevent unwanted pregnancy. Pelvic inflammatory disease is more common in women using the IUCD family planning method. There are reasons why this may be so. The first is that IUCDs, even though sterile, are foreign bodies. Secondly, germs in the vagina may follow the thread through the cervix into the womb cavity. These two situations contribute to the ascendance of germs into the womb and affect other parts of the reproductive tract.

# CHAPTER 4
# HIV and AIDS

*"HIV does not make people dangerous to know, so you can shake their hands and give them a hug: Heaven knows they need it."*
– PRINCESS DIANA


1.  **What is HIV?**

HIV is an acronym for human immunodeficiency virus. Where

    H – stands for Human
    I – stands for Immune-deficiency
    V – stands for Virus

Viruses are infectious agents that are incapable of living independent lives except when inside other living cells. There are several groups. The human immunodeficiency virus is a retrovirus that can live in the human cell.

2.  **What is AIDS?**

It is an acronym for:

    A – Acquired
    I – Immune
    D – Deficiency
    S – Syndrome

It is one thing to be infected with the HIV and another thing to manifest the features of immune depletion or deficiency. AIDS refers to a situation where the infected person manifests clinical features and diseases associated with immune deficiency. The HIV can attack all parts of the body. Therefore, features of AIDS can manifest in any tissue, organ or system of the body. Hence, AIDs may manifest as diseases of the skin, lungs, gastro intestinal system, brain, bone, muscle, glands, etc. So, the sufferer may manifest myriads of clinical features and diseases of different organs, at different times or at the same time. Examples of such diseases are:

- Skin – rashes and Kaposi Sarcoma
- Lungs - opportunistic infections, chronic pneumonia
- Bowels - chronic diarrhea
- Connective tissue diseases
- Heart and blood - heart failure, anemia
- Kidneys - kidney failure
- Chronic weight loss

### 3. Where and how did HIV originate?

Scientists believe that HIV most probably originated from the Chimpanzee and that the virus had lived with these Apes as the Simian Immune Deficiency Virus (SIV) for a long time. It was transmitted to human beings who had contacts with the Apes. This was possible through hunting, where these animals were killed and consumed. In the process of transmission, the SIV changed into HIV in order to gain access and to live in human cells. The earliest records showed that this transmission happened around the 1920s, in the jungles of Kinshasa, in the Democratic Republic of Congo, Sub-Saharan Africa. Early cases of AIDS also happened in the Congo. So historically, HIV is widely regarded as having originated in the Congo.

### 4. When was AIDS discovered?

Acquired Immune Deficiency Syndrome (AIDS) was first discovered in 1983 in San Francisco, USA.

### 5. Where exactly was AIDS recognized first?

There was a period in California, when rare diseases such as cancer of the skin called Kaposi Sarcoma and some opportunistic infections suddenly became common. The World Health Organization (WHO), after in depth studies eventually traced the origin of the infections and Kaposi Sarcoma to prior HIV infection. AIDS was formally recognized and proclaimed by the WHO in September 1983.

### 6. What are the main types of HIV?

There are 2 main types of the Human immunodeficiency virus. They are the HIV type 1 and type 2 virus. One or both may be found at various locations or communities around the world. In most parts of the world, the HIV type I virus is more common.

## 7. How common is HIV?

The World Health Organization (WHO) has estimated that about 36.7million people were living with HIV globally as at end of 2016. This is a remarkable drop form the figure it was a decade ago. Globally, as at the end of 2016, the total number of people infected with the HIV virus stood at 70million.

## 8. What are the features of AIDS?

The features of AIDS are numerous because the virus is capable of infecting virtually all parts of the body system. Among the manifestations are infections that include the following:

- Tuberculosis
- Candida infections – mouth, bowels etc
- Pneumocystis carinii pneumonia
- Cytomegalovirus infection of the eyes
- Mycobacterium aviumintraculare complex infection
- AIDS dementia or forgetfulness
- Neurological
  - Toxoplasmosis of the brain
  - Streptococcal meningitis
- Chronic Diarrhea
- Weight loss
- Cancer
  - Kaposi Sarcoma of the skin, mouth cavity etc
  - Non-Hodgkins lymphoma
  - Hairy leukoplakia of the tongue – This is identified as white lines or ridges seen at the sides of the tongue. This lesion is almost unique to HIV infection. It suggests that immunity is much depressed

## 9. How does the HIV virus cause disease?

The HIV virus causes disease by depleting the immune system of the body, thereby increasing the risk of contracting other infections; viral, bacterial and parasitic. Apart from depleting the body's immunity, the virus also increases the risk of other diseases.

## 10. How does one get infected with the HIV virus?

There are various ways of contracting the HIV infection. However, the predominant method varies from one community to another. The main factor is hinged on the different cultures and sexual practices in the various communities. Generally speaking, the methods include:

- Sexual intercourse: HIV infection is most commonly transmitted through sexual intercourse. This may be heterosexual or homosexual intercourse with an infected partner. This is true in most developing countries like South Africa, China, India, etc. In the USA, the most common mode of transmission in men is through gay sexual practices, while heterosexual intercourse is the most common transmission mode among women generally
- Blood transfusion: Transfusion of infected blood or blood products is usually unintentional, and may be due to poor methods of screening of blood for transfusion. In remote health centers in developing countries, where there is lack of facilities for blood screening, blood may be transfused inappropriately without screening, in a desperate move to save lives, especially in cases of severe bleeding following child birth or road traffic accidents
- Use of unsterilized instruments: These include the communal use of syringes or needles among illicit drug users of cocaine, heroin etc. Currently, tattooing the skin with shared unsterile instruments in countries where tattooing is in vogue, may promote HIV transmission
- Mother to child: An infected mother can transmit HIV to her baby during pregnancy and child birth. This is one of the reasons why the infection should be adequately controlled during pregnancy and childbirth. Mother to child transmission is highest in West Africa
- Injuries: Infected material e.g. needle prick injuries in infected health workers can transmit HIV infection. However, the risk of contracting HIV infection through accidental needle prick is insignificant
- Sharing: Sharing of infected items like blades, nail cutters and barbing clippers are possible ways of transmitting HIV infection. This is common in developing countries where awareness of HIV is low and it is difficult to possess personal or disposable clippers and other instruments

**11. What are the signs or complaints that may suggest that someone has contracted HIV infection?**

HIV infection may be contracted without much illness to signpost it. The transmission may mimic other infections, with symptoms like:
- Fever
- Headache
- Body aches
- Poor appetite
- Weakness or easy tiredness
- General ill health

These complaints may be experienced for a few days or happen intermittently for weeks at a mild to moderate level. The complaints may also not be significant. The period of febrile illness usually gives way to the window period when tests for HIV infection may be negative or inconclusive. However, the tests for HIV should be repeated at intervals in suspected cases.

## 12. What are the stages of HIV infection?

Generally speaking, HIV infection usually progresses through 3 main stages. These are:

- Stage 1 - Stage of primary infection:

When someone contracts HIV infection, in a matter of days or weeks, the person produces antibodies to the HIV. At this time, most people feel well and the infection may not be noticed at all. In some cases, those infected may have fever or exhibit symptoms of common cold. These symptoms include:

- Headache
- Weakness
- Muscle pain and body pain
- Fever
- Sore throat
- Lymph node enlargements

At this stage, seroconversion is taking place. Seroconversion means that the viruses are present in the blood stream and the infected person continues to produce antibodies against the virus at this time. This production of antibodies is a means of self-defense as the body attempts to fight back the infection. It may be difficult for doctors to suspect HIV infection at this early stage, because people suffering from other febrile diseases like enteric fever, pneumonia, malaria, and even cold can have all these complaints

- Stage 2 -The asymptomatic stage:

With seroconversion and the production of antibodies, the HIV infected person may not show any sign of illness for weeks or several years. However, the immune system becomes depleted gradually as the disease gains ground and spreads around the body. The victim may feel well for several years, sometimes up to 15 years, while immune depletion continues. If blood tests or other tests for HIV are performed at this stage, the test should be positive because seroconversion has already taken place

- Stage 3 - The symptomatic stage:

If not treated, over time, the immune system becomes very depleted or compromised. This leaves the person at the risk of opportunistic infections including yeast, tuberculosis, other symptoms and diseases such as chronic fever, diarrhea and weight loss

### 13. How is HIV diagnosed?

The first step is voluntary counseling by the laboratory scientist or other healthcare providers, followed by the HIV screening test. Whether the screening test is positive or negative, post screening counseling is also done. If the screening test is positive, a confirmatory test is mandatory. An HIV screening test is conducted by performing blood tests using HIV rapid test kits, which detect the antibodies to the virus.

### 14. What is the difference between screening and confirmatory tests?

When the body is infected, it produces antibodies which are defensive proteins in an attempt to fight the virus. Screening tests are performed to detect these antibodies. Sometimes, antibodies to different diseases may be similar or only slightly different from one another. This makes it difficult for screening tests to correctly identify the specific antibodies each time. For this reason, a screening test cannot give a yes or no answer, like a confirmatory test. Confirmatory tests like the western blot are performed to identify the actual viral particles or antigens. Since confirmatory tests are definite and ensure validity, it is mandatory to perform confirmatory tests whenever screening tests are positive.

### 15. Which conditions are associated with increased risk of HIV infection?

The risks of contracting HIV infection are increased in situations where repeated transfusions of blood or blood components are used for routine treatments. These situations include:

- Hemophiliacs
- Sickle cell anemia
- Heroin and cocaine intravenous drug users
- Homosexuals

Other disease situations are:

- Immune compromised states
- Tuberculosis
- Cancers e.g. Cancer of the cervix

### 16. How is HIV infection monitored?

HIV is monitored by measuring the level of CD4 lymphocytes in the peripheral blood. The normal value of CD4 is greater than 0.5/l. Reducing levels of Blood CD4 indicate progression of the HIV/ AIDS. Currently, it is also possible to measure the viral load.

### 17. What is viral load?

This is a term used by doctors and other health care providers to denote the amount of virus in the body. This term indicates the level or severity of the burden or health status of a person suffering from a viral infection like HIV. The viral load is measured as the number of viral particles per ml of blood. Viral particles are also called copies. When the viral load is high, the disease burden is likely to be serious too. In people with HIV, when the viral load is more than 100,000 copies per ml of blood, it is said to be high.

### 18. When is the viral load said to be undetectable?

Sometimes, it is possible to effectively treat viral infections like HIV to an extent that the viral load in the blood cannot be detected by conventional tests. This is one of the desirable goals of HIV treatment. When the viral load becomes undetectable, the HIV patient is most probably in the best state of health, with a good immunity status, as far as the infection is concerned.

### 19. What is the pattern of increase in viral load during viral infections?

Viral load is usually very high few weeks after a recent infection. After this period, it reduces and may be low for several months or years. A high viral load at other times suggests more serious evidence of disease.

### 20. What is the importance of checking the viral load?

If a person is already infected with a virus e.g. the HIV, doctors may sometimes order the viral load estimation at intervals. At the same time, the CD4 lymphocytes count may be requested. These are used for 2 main reasons:

- To estimate the extent and severity of the viral infection
- To know how effective a particular drug combination is. If the drugs are effective, the measurement of viral loads at intervals should show reduction in levels. Rising viral load levels suggest that the disease is getting worse. This may indicate the need for increased drug dosage or a change of prescription.

### 21. What parts of the body can be tested for HIV?

The most common practice is to test the blood for HIV. However, HIV infects all parts of the body without exemption. Scientists and doctors find it easier to test body fluids for HIV infection but apart from blood, other body fluids can be tested for HIV. These fluids include:

- Saliva
- Tears
- Fluid from wounds

- Urine
- Sweat
- Nasal discharge etc

## 22. Please, explain the meaning of window period?

Window period is a quiet period of apparent good health when an already infected person tests negative for the HIV. The person does not show any feature that may suggest HIV infection. The duration starts from the time of infection to the time that the person eventually tests positive for the virus. During the window period, most of the virus would have left the blood stream and are busy invading the various body tissues and organs. This explains why blood tests at this time are negative.

## 23. When are HIV test results said to be indeterminate?

Sometimes, a laboratory scientist may not be sure of the outcome of an HIV test he has performed because the color indicator is ambiguous i.e. neither here nor there. So, it is difficult to interpret the result as positive or negative. Such reports create a dilemma for doctors as well as the person being tested. In this situation, the test should be repeated after a period of time. If the result remains the same, other superior methods like PCR testing for actual DNA detection can be deployed. This will reduce the patient's anxiety. PCR is an acronym for polymerase chain reaction, which is an enzymatic method of amplifying DNA and investigating and identifying its structure.

This situation presents a hard nut for doctors to crack especially where clinical features suggest that the patient is more likely to have HIV infection. When results are of doubtful value and cannot be confirmed as positive or negative, they are said to be indeterminate.

## 24. What is the relationship between viral load, CD4 lymphocytes count, and immunity?

Increasing or high viral load means that the viral infection is getting worse or more severe. This causes the CD4 lymphocytes count and the level of immunity to fall. So, increased viral load brings about reduced CD4 count. The values of these two important parameters therefore run in opposite directions: viral load rises while the CD4 count falls with increasing disease.

## 25. What other associated infections may occur in women with HIV?

In HIV patients, the main effect is immune depletion, which increases the risk of infections by other germs. Most of the infections are opportunistic in nature. These include:

- Increased incidence and severity of Human Papilloma Virus (HPV) causing genital warts
- Vulva intraepithelial neoplasia or pre-cancer lesions of the vulva
- Persistent severe Pelvic Inflammatory Disease (PID)
- Persistent post-partum endometritis
- Herpes simplex infection
- Tuberculosis – common in developing countries
- Extensive yeast infection
- Pneumocystis carinii Infection

## 26. How does the practice of oral sex encourage transmission of HIV infection?

Oral sex means licking the penis of a man by a woman or licking the vulva of a woman by a man. HIV infection can be transmitted if infected semen or vaginal fluid comes in contact with the mouth, especially if the mouth, gum, vulva or penis have ulcers or are inflamed.

## 27. Can deep or open mouth kissing cause HIV infection?

The risk is extremely low, because saliva does not contain significant amounts of HIV germs. However, it is best to avoid this saliva-to-mouth contact. Prevention is better than cure!

## 28. Can "fingering" during romance cause HIV infection?

Yes. If there is exposure to infected blood through a cut in the finger, nail bed, or vagina. The risk is extremely low, but it is not worth taking.

## 29. Can someone contract HIV while visiting the doctor or dentist?

Yes, even in doctor's clinics, if poorly sterilized or infected instruments are used. Be careful and insist on well sterilized or "one-use-only" instruments and disposables. It is your right to be served well in a manner that guarantees your safety.

## 30. Can HIV infection be contracted through human bites?

Yes, but once again, the threat is minimal. If, however the bite results in an open, bleeding wound, as in all cases of human bites, the site should be immediately cleaned with water and the injuries properly treated by a doctor or qualified healthcare provider. Remember that other infections like tetanus can be transmitted in this way, so an anti-tetanus injection may be needed.

### 31. Can mosquitoes transmit HIV?

No. When a mosquito bites, it does not inject blood from previous bites. It only injects saliva, which acts as a lubricant to facilitate feeding. Fortunately, mosquitoes are not known to transmit HIV infection, for if that were the case, the devastation of AIDS would be too horrible to contemplate, especially in malaria endemic regions like West Africa.

### 32. Does HIV infection mean a death sentence?

HIV infection should not necessarily result in death if effective treatment is commenced early. This means that people should know their HIV status as early as possible. They must also disclose and commit themselves to their treatment regimens, including drugs, instructions, and appointments. As often happens, it is a big mistake to assume that one is free from the disease simply because of adequate weight gain and improvement in general well-being. The infection is currently incurable and treatment is lifelong. People living with HIV should have appropriate lifestyle modifications to enable them live a healthy, stress free life, free of vices. With early detection and strict adherence to treatment instructions, HIV infection should not mean a death sentence.

### 33. What is the current trend in monitoring the progress of treatment in HIV/AIDS?

There are two options available to the doctor for monitoring the progress of HIV/AIDS. These are through estimating the patient's CD4 lymphocyte counts and viral load. Currently, doctors believe that viral load estimation is more cost effective and superior to CD4 Count.

### 34. Since it is a viral infection, is there no vaccine that can prevent HIV?

There is no doubt that progress is being made by researchers in different parts of the world to find a lasting cure or vaccine against HIV infection but for now, there is no such vaccine. Some vaccines are at different stages of testing and hopefully, a few of these will be ready for use in human beings in the near future.

### 35. Are there no drugs that can cure HIV or AIDS?

As at now, there are no drugs that can cure HIV. Many claims by some people, especially herbalists and other alternative medical practitioners, have turned out to be false after investigations. However, with early detection and proper treatment, the amount of virus in the body or viral load can be kept at the minimum. In some instances, the viral load may be pushed down so low, that the virus becomes undetectable. This is a desirable goal of treatment, but it does not amount to a cure.

### 36. Why is HIV infection not curable?

When an infected person is on an anti-retroviral drug regimen or combination, the drugs suppress the replication of the virus, pushing the viral load down. However, if the drugs are stopped, because the virus also infects long-lived memory cells, the virus can begin to replicate from these memory cells and re-infect the body. This makes a cure impossible for now, consequently people living with HIV must continue to use their drugs for as long as they are alive.

### 37. When is a patient said to have a severely compromised immunity?

A person with AIDS is said to have a severely compromised immunity when the CD4 count is less than 0.5/l. The level of compromise is useful to doctors in planning drug treatment, in the management of AIDS patients.

### 38. How is HIV treated?

HIV is treated with anti-retroviral drugs. Two or more drugs are usually combined in order to make them more effective and to prevent resistance of the virus to the drugs. Some drugs in common use include Zidovudine, Didanosine and Nevirapine.

Treatment of other underlying diseases like opportunistic infections, tuberculosis and other systemic illnesses are also necessary to maintain a stable health.

### 39. What are the aims of treatment?

The aims of treatment are to:
- Reduce viral load to 'zero'
- Keep viral load down perpetually
- Prevent HIV from progressing to AIDS
- Curtail opportunistic infections
- Prevent further transmission of infection through counseling and education

### 40. Why is it important to start treatment early?

Not everybody infected with the HIV will develop AIDS. With early treatment, many people lead normal lives, however, if treatment is not started quickly, most people infected with HIV will progress to AIDS within 10 years. For the few who develop AIDS despite early treatment, the time between HIV infection and the development of AIDS is much longer than the mean time of 10 years. These patients probably have additional underlying illnesses and compromised immunity. The patients who begin treatment late or who default in their treatments, also progress to AIDS faster.

## 41. How is AIDS monitored?

AIDS is pretty much monitored in the same way as HIV infection but more regular CD4 and viral load quantifications are done at shorter intervals. Tests to monitor and treat complications from other AIDS related diseases are also necessary.

## 42. What are the common factors that can aggravate HIV/AIDS?

Briefly these include:
- Smoking
- Too much alcohol
- Stress – physical, emotional
- Drug abuse –heroin, cocaine
- Use of un-prescribed drugs especially steroids
- Inter-current Infections:
  - Tuberculosis
  - Pneumonia
  - Yeast infection of the mouth and bowels
- Systemic Diseases
  - Uncontrolled diabetes
  - Malnutrition, Starvation

## 43. Why is AIDS such a devastating disease?

HIV/AIDS has one of the most devastating impacts on public health because of:
- Transmission through sexual intercourse which makes transmission more rapid and difficult to control
- Mother to child transmission during pregnancy and childbirth
- Death of one or both parents and the economic and social consequences of millions of orphans worldwide
- Preponderance among the youths: The most sexually active group in any population is the youth. They are also the group at the highest risk of having multiple sexual partners. So, HIV is most devastating among the youth

## 44. What are the complaints that may suggest depressed immunity?

People with reduced immunity suffer more frequent illnesses with recurrences at shorter intervals. Such illnesses include:
- Recurrent attacks of bacterial infections
- Recurrent herpes zoster (shingles) infections
- Genital herpes
- Vaginal and oral candidiasis or yeast infections
- Presence of hairy leukoplakia
- Skin lesions:
  - Recurrent dermatitis or skin inflammation
  - Tinea infections (Tinea pedis)
  - Folliculitis or occurrence of multiple boils at different parts of the body

## 45. Where is HIV infection most prevalent?

HIV infection is more common in developing countries than in developed countries. There is no doubt that the infection is most prevalent in West Africa. This may be related to the degree of poverty, low education, the poor level of awareness and poor health infrastructural development which are typical of developing countries. Another reason is the added fact that tuberculosis and sexually transmitted infections (STIs) are rampant in many communities in West Africa. The high prevalence of tuberculosis and STIs correlates with that of HIV infections and AIDS.

## 46. What is the pattern of the spread of HIV among the racial groups in the USA?

The estimated numbers of new HIV infections in 2010 for the most affected sub-populations and racial groups in the USA are as shown in the table below:

| Racial Group | Number Affected |
|---|---|
| White gay | 11,200 |
| Black gay | 10,600 |
| Hispanic Latinos | 6,700 |
| Black Heterosexual Women | 5,300 |
| Black Heterosexual Men | 2,700 |
| White Heterosexual Men | 1,300 |
| Hispanic/Latino Heterosexual Women | 1,200 |
| Black Male intravenous drug users | 1,100 |

Source: CDC estimated incidence among adults and adolescents in the USA, 2007 – 2010 HIV.

**47. What is the trend of HIV infection in the USA?**

For some time now, the occurrence of new HIV infections appears to have plateaued or become fairly constant at 50,000 per year. Currently, HIV infection in gay men is the single most important contributor to new HIV infections in the USA and since 2010, new HIV infections among gay men have been on the increase. Despite the smaller percentage of the population of African Americans in the USA, the majority of new HIV infections are among young African Americans.

**48. What are the differences in the mode of transmission of HIV between developed and developing countries?**

In the developed countries like the USA, UK, Australia, etc. the main routes of transmission of the virus is through homosexual intercourse and the use of intravenous drugs. In developing countries, HIV is acquired mostly through vaginal intercourse, as a sexually transmitted infection. The problem of homosexuality, especially men-sex-men (MSM), is much less rampant in the poor developing countries.

**49. Which groups of people are more likely to contract HIV infection?**

The risk of HIV infection is higher in sexually promiscuous individuals with multiple partners, those who engage in casual sex, commercial sex workers, homosexuals and illicit intra venous drug users.

**50. What is the death burden of HIV?**

Globally, the rate of infection is reducing, thanks to wide spread campaigns, public education, wider coverage, treatments with highly effective drugs and increased voluntary testing. Correspondingly, the deaths due to HIV and related illnesses have reduced remarkably. In 2015, about 1.1 million people died of the disease. This represents about 45% reduction from the figure in 2005.

# DEAR DOCTOR:

**51. Can I contract HIV infection through activities like hand shake or swimming in the same pool with an infected person?**

No. Ordinary life activities like these are not usual ways of contracting the HIV infection.

**52. What about sharing cutlery and eating together?**

No. HIV is not transmitted through food. Also, HIV cannot survive on its own, outside the body for a long time. Therefore, one cannot contract the infection by merely sharing cutlery or eating together with an infected person. This is an important issue in the care of persons living with HIV or AIDS in our various communities. Eating with them does not cause HIV. They do not need to be stigmatized or isolated. Rather, they need to be encouraged through love, empathy and care.

**53. Can I contract HIV if I live in the same house with a person living with AIDS?**

No. HIV is not an airborne infection and cannot be contracted by cohabiting with somebody living with HIV/AIDS. You cannot contract the infection through ordinary life interactions like shaking the hands of an infected person.

**54. Is it true that HIV does not survive outside the body?**

Yes. The virus can only survive for a short time outside the body. It cannot live an independent life of its own. It can only survive inside the cell of another animal like monkeys or human beings. It dies quickly when exposed to air or an environment outside the cell. For this reason, leaving infected body fluids like expressed breast milk in a cup for several minutes on a table should kill the virus. However, this is not a widely used method of sterilizing breast milk. It is not recommended for nursing mothers with HIV infection.

### 55. My screening test is negative. Does it mean that I am forever free from HIV infection?

No. If you have tested negative, congratulations! However, a negative test has two meanings. It is either you are not infected or you are in the window period of infection. To rule out the window period scenario, you should repeat the test in another 6 months. If you are truly negative, then you are encouraged to live a safe life. Keep to a single uninfected sexual partner. If you unavoidably have to engage in casual sexual intercourse, please ensure that you play safe also. Wear a condom. Abstain from sharing communal things like needles, barbing clippers and insist that only sterile instruments should be used on you. The issue of tattooing is worrisome. It is becoming more popular among the youth, people in the entertainment industry as well as sports men and women. Please, if you must be tattooed, then ensure the instruments are sterile or disposable. Finally, a negative test warrants that you check your HIV status at regular intervals, at least once a year.

### 56. What is the role of voluntary counseling?

The objective of counseling is to inform and educate you on important aspects of the disease and ensure that you are able to take appropriate decisions. Information is power and you will also be encouraged to express yourself and cast away timidity. During counseling, the benefits of knowing your HIV status and the dangers of doing otherwise will be explained to you. What your attitude should be to a positive or negative test result, will also be discussed. If you test positive, you will be advised on the need for a confirmatory test, immediate commencement of treatment, and other dos and don'ts going forward. If you test negative, the need to repeat the test in 6 months will be discussed. More importantly, the need to lead a safe life will be stressed. It is better to have information than to grope in the dark. So, if you are yet to know your HIV status, please step out and be tested now!

### 57. I have just tested positive for HIV. What do you advise doctor?

At this time, it is better to remain as calm as possible while you follow the steps of recovery outlined below:

- Accept the situation. This is a verdict and rejection does not alter the result
- Ask other questions that may come to your mind and clarify doubts from the counselor or doctor

- Ask the doctor when, where and how to start treatment
- Ask for information on the cost of drugs and where to get them. Some Non-governmental organizations (NGO) offer free and potent drugs, while some subsidized drugs are also available
- Ask for the nearest support center where clubs or associations of people living with HIV/AIDS do support and encourage each other
- Tell your confidants and beloved ones the truth about your situation. They are more likely to support than reject you
- Do not spend much time thinking about stigmatization and other negative attitudes because that will not help you
- Try and get as much information as you can on living well with HIV
- Focus on starting therapy on time in order to prevent the infection from progressing to AIDS
- Discuss with your counselor or doctor what changes in lifestyle are needed in order to lead a healthy life. These include:
  - How to get sufficient rest at all times
  - How to ensure good nutrition
  - Taking your drugs exactly as prescribed
  - How to ensure safe sexual practice
  - Quitting alcohol, smoking, and the use of hard drugs
- Be convinced that if you keep to your treatment, you can lead a normal life. Think positive that death is not an option

## 58. Now that I have tested positive, how do I save my face and what will I say to my family and friends?

Your feelings are typical of the shock and emotions that people feel when they have just tested positive for HIV. Many All these problems and more will come like a flash and flood your emotions. This is one important reason why all tests for HIV should be preceded by voluntary counseling. Voluntary counseling should also be repeated after the test, to advise on some of the challenges in the immediate period after testing positive. These include:

- Shock
- Initial rejection
- Emotional upset
- Confusion over what to do
- How to handle the reactions of parents, siblings, friends and others
- Who to talk to
- How to get care
- Possibility of stigmatization
- Fear of the ultimate consequences, including death

In all these situations, remain calm and open minded. Share your thoughts with your care giver. It is important to let your parents, friends and confidants know about your condition as early as possible. They are most likely to give you the support you need and reduce your burden.

**59. How long does it take for the disease to show?**

The duration varies from a few weeks to months, sometimes up to few years before the features of the disease begin to manifest in the body. However, there are individual differences. Also, HIV infection and AIDS manifest faster in the presence of other pre–existing debilitating conditions and systemic illnesses like tuberculosis, un-controlled diabetes, or sickle cell anemia.

**60. If my HIV screening test is negative, can the confirmatory test be positive?**

Yes. It is possible for your screening test to be negative whereas you are actually positive. This is possible if your screening test was performed during the window period. Again, there are situations when the body cannot react immunologically because of severely depleted immunity due to other chronic severe diseases. In such a situation, the individual is said to be in a state of anergy. In some instances, blood samples might have been labeled wrongly or exchanged for someone else's sample unintentionally, which may lead to false results. The confirmatory test or RNA testing should be done because they test directly for HIV viral particles and not antibodies as in the case of screening tests.

**61. I tested positive for HIV a few months ago. It was a surprise to me because I was not sick at all. Could the report be wrong?**

The report could be absolutely true. Most times, people who test positive are not sick and may not know that they are already infected with the virus. This is because the Initial infection may not cause any unusual ill health or be remarkable enough to warrant suspicion. Such is the nature of HIV infection. You are advised to go to the hospital quickly. There are designated treatment centers in the community and you should be able to find one that is near and convenient for you. Treatment is free at most of the centers, so cost should not be a barrier. Please, do not spend valuable time hiding your condition or doubting the result. If you are not convinced, you may repeat the test in another laboratory rather than staying away from treatment. Remember that if the infection is ongoing, you need to attack it right away!

**62. What if I am infected and desire to get pregnant, what do I need to do?**

It is advisable that your health be optimal if pregnancy is being contemplated. The outcome of pregnancy is better when:

- General health is optimal
- Viral load is lowest
- CD4 count is high
- Opportunistic infections or other complications are absent
- You are on an effective anti-retroviral combination therapy or Highly Active Anti-Retroviral Therapy (HAART). Pregnancy poses two challenges. First, pregnancy reduces the level of immunity in women generally. So, this is a physiological stress which may be too much to bear, if you are not fit enough. Secondly, the risk of transmitting the HIV virus to your baby is higher when your viral load is high. Therefore, women living with HIV should use additional family planning apart from condoms. Pregnancy should be planned when health parameters are optimal, as advised by the doctor

### 63. If I am HIV positive, can I become pregnant?

Yes, you can become pregnant as easily as any other woman. However, if the HIV infection has progressed to AIDS, then your fertility potential may be reduced. In such a situation, it is advisable that the pregnancy is well planned. Your health should be optimal and your viral load at its lowest. Therefore, it is necessary for your doctor to plan along with you. You will need to be closely treated and supervised throughout pregnancy, labor, and delivery.

### 64. Why do I still need family planning if I am already infected with HIV?

If you are lucky to have completed your family, it is better to practice family planning and totally stay out of pregnancy. It is a known fact that pregnancy can reduce your immunity further if you are living with HIV/AIDS.

### 65. If my infected partner does not ejaculate inside me during sexual intercourse, can HIV infection still occur?

Yes, but the pre-ejaculated semen usually contains very little quantities of the HIV. This makes the risk of contracting HIV infection in this way lower than after ejaculation. However, it is better to practice safe sex than take such a dangerous gamble. Please insist that your partner uses a condom. Also, remember that your partner may not be able to fulfill his promise not to ejaculate into the vagina or withdraw the penis from the vagina just before ejaculation.

### 66. If my sexual partner is not infected with HIV, can I be infected?

You cannot be infected by having sex with him since he is not infected. Both of you should have your HIV tests done at regular intervals, not fewer than once a year. This could be during your annual medical checkups. You should also be aware of other ways by which this infection is transmitted.

### 67. What are the precautions that I need to take to stay healthy, in view of my positive HIV status?

Here are some helpful tips to stay healthy:
- Get as much information as you can and stay on top of fresh developments on HIV infection. Information is power
- Keep all clinic appointments with your doctor or care giver
- Adhere strictly to your drugs and treatment instructions. When you take ill, get treated without delay
- Keep good overall hygiene
- Eat nutritious foods with enough protein and fruits. Take sufficient vitamin supplements. Eat right!
- Rest well and live a stress-free life
- Regular light exercises are beneficial
- Stop all social vices like smoking, alcohol abuse, illicit drug use, too much sex, etc. Moderation should be your virtue
- Report any change in your health or well-being to your doctor immediately
- If you do all of these, you should be able to lead a normal life

### 68. Why is it important to have my HIV test done even when I am healthy?

The important thing to note is that a person who has been infected with the HIV virus may look normal without any sign of ill health for a variable length of time. In the established disease or AIDS, the ill-health of the sufferer will be clear and noticeable. This is why it should never be assumed that a person is free of HIV/AIDS until the test to determine her status has been done. As the slogan goes "HIV does not show on the face". Only tests, not looks can confirm or refute whether somebody has HIV infection or not.

### 69. Is it true that some people are resistant to HIV infection?

Yes. There is evidence to show that some people have natural immunity or resistance to HIV infection. For example, some commercial sex workers in some parts of the world have shown that despite being constantly exposed to the virus, the prevalence of HIV infection among such groups are unexpectedly low. It is also known that about 1% of Caucasians has mutation in CD4 receptors. This seems to give them some relative protection or immunity to HIV infection. However, this is never a license for people to be reckless, regarding HIV.

**70. If I suspect that I have been accidentally exposed to HIV, what should I do?**

You should have emergency treatment to attempt to prevent HIV infection. It is called post exposure prophylaxis (PEP). This entails starting anti-retroviral drugs within 72 hours of such an exposure. The drugs should be continued for 4 weeks. The doctor must be informed immediately. In case of a wound such as needle pricks, the wound should be immediately washed thoroughly with running water as the first step while awaiting the arrival of drugs. When you are accidentally exposed to someone with HIV or AIDS, you may be overwhelmed with anxiety. It is normal to be worried about whether you will contract HIV or not. From the time of the exposure until the next 3 – 6 months when you run the HIV test on your blood sample, you may live in fear and confusion. The best thing is to get PEP as fast as you can and hope that it is sufficient to prevent the transmission of HIV. At this period and while waiting to be re-tested, it is beneficial to discuss your questions and worries with your doctor. In many countries, there are designated centers where PEP, HIV counseling and support are available. The good news is that PEP is effective in preventing HIV infection.

**71. How do I cope with the cost of my care, especially since my drugs are meant to be taken for life?**

The huge financial costs of drugs and appropriate nutrition in the face of reduced productivity in persons living with HIV are enormous. The most important aspect is to ensure that your drugs are procured and used as prescribed without fail. In most advanced countries, there are many centers that provide ready help and support for people living with HIV/AIDS. Such help includes on-going counseling, emotional support, cost of living subsidy and free or heavily subsidized potent drugs. There are also special centers, where in addition, information can be provided round the clock. In developing countries where the greatest burden of HIV/AIDS is felt, the situation is different. In such communities, there are no support centers or subsidies for drugs. Worst of all, drug supplies are irregular and may not be available for several weeks at a time. This means that people living with HIV/AIDS cannot even get these drugs to buy. Non-availability of basic drugs seems to be the greatest problem confronting people living with HIV/AIDS in the developing world, especially sub-Saharan Africa. The situation is gradually changing, thanks to the help and support of donor nations like the USA, UK and Non-government organizations (NGOs).

**72. Can HIV/AIDS cause cancer?**

HIV infection does not cause cancer. In many instances, HIV infection may be detected too late so that treatment is also started late. Therefore, some cases of HIV infection eventually progress to AIDS. There are no reasons to suggest that AIDS causes cancer, but it is capable of affecting any part of the body. However, it is well known that some types of cancers are closely

associated with AIDS. This means that they are more common in people living with AIDS than people without AIDS. Such cancers include:
- Kaposi Sarcoma
- Non-Hodgkins Lymphoma
- Primary Lymphoma of the brain
- Cancer of the Cervix

# CHAPTER 5
# Abortion

*"Abortion should not only be safe and legal, it should be rare"*
— BILL CLINTON

### 1. When does life start?
One way to look at this issue is by recognizing the beliefs of the various religions which have different views about when life starts in the womb. The common view is that all religions believe in the sanctity of life which must be respected. However, the preponderance of current medical opinion is that life starts when the fetus has grown to a stage when it is capable of independent life or viability. Here, independent life means that the fetus is able to survive on its own outside the mother's womb. As expected, the age at which survival starts, varies from one country to another, depending on the level of facility and support available to the fetus outside the womb.

### 2. What is abortion?
Abortion is the termination of pregnancy before the age of viability of the fetus. The age of viability in the developed countries like the USA is 20 weeks, at this time the fetus weighs about 500g. So abortion can also be defined as the expulsion of the fetus from the womb before 20 weeks or expulsion of a baby that weighs less than 500g. After, 20 weeks and up until 37 weeks, such an expulsion is termed premature birth; not an abortion. In most developing countries, 28 weeks is the age at which pregnancy is deemed to be viable, so abortion is said to occur when pregnancy is terminated before 28 weeks. Therefore, the definition of abortion with regards to the cut off age differs between developing and developed countries.

### 3. What does the word abortion connote?
When people mention the word abortion, what readily comes to mind is the criminal intent. This is because induced or criminally procured abortion is rampant in some communities, especially in developing countries. In many

developed countries, abortions are allowed, subject to legal indications. However, abortions can occur unintentionally or spontaneously due to various reasons.

### 4. Who is an abortionist?

An abortionist is a doctor or somebody that performs abortions on women. In developing countries, going by current usage, the word abortionist connotes a criminal intention or quackery.

### 5. When is abortion said to be illegal?

As the name implies, illegal abortions are those performed without valid license or authority and against the law governing abortion in a particular society or country. In most cases, such abortions are performed because of unwanted pregnancy. These abortions are mostly requested by women, girls or couples for social reasons. Illegal abortions are mostly done in secret with the attendant high risk of complications.

### 6. What is the difference between an abortion and a miscarriage?

A miscarriage is an unintended or spontaneous abortion, whereas an abortion can be spontaneous or induced. Most miscarriages happen between 4-6 weeks of pregnancy.

### 7. What is spontaneous abortion and how common is it?

Spontaneous abortions are those that occur of their own accord. In other words, they are unintentional. The occurrence of spontaneous abortion is believed to be higher than the often quoted figure of 15%. It is estimated that about 50% of all pregnancies are aborted spontaneously early in pregnancy. Many of such abortions happen because the pregnancies are not compatible with life, due to genetic problems. A remarkable percentage of these spontaneous abortions happen even before the woman misses her period and may therefore go unnoticed. Spontaneous abortion is more common in older women.

### 8. What are the different types of abortion?

There are different ways to classify abortion. When abortion occurs naturally, it is said to be spontaneous or a miscarriage. On the other hand, abortion may be intentionally procured or induced. The importance of this classification is that procured abortions connote criminal intentions. There are also safe and unsafe abortions; this consideration places emphasis on the safety of the process, expertise and authority of the abortionist. Is the person a doctor or a trained healthcare provider? Is there any genuine medical reason to perform the abortion? Will the method and environment guarantee safety? The most

common classification is to consider abortion according to features. Going by this consideration, abortion is classified into:
- Threatened abortion
- Inevitable abortion
- Incomplete abortion
- Complete abortion
- Spontaneous abortion
- Induced abortion
- Missed abortion
- Legal abortion
- Illegal abortion
- Therapeutic abortion
- Recurrent or habitual abortion
- Medical and surgical abortions

Using the criterion of infection, abortion can also be grouped into septic and aseptic abortions. Most septic abortions have criminal intentions.

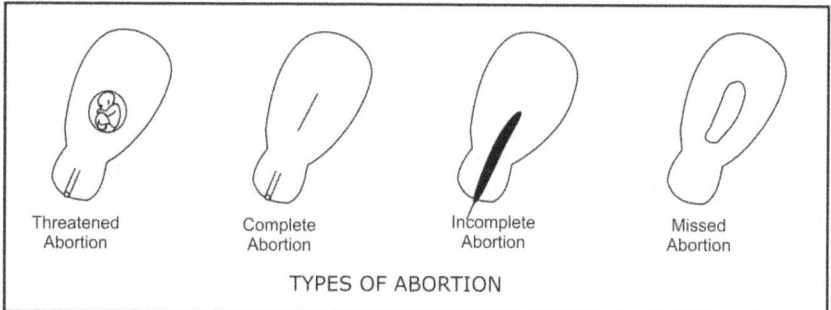

TYPES OF ABORTION

## 9. What is induced abortion?

Though abortions can happen spontaneously, they can also be initiated by the doctor, health care providers or abortionists for various reasons. In some cases, abortions may be induced by qualified healthcare givers, if the pregnancy constitutes a risk to the mother, the fetus is deformed or for other reasons. Depending on the law regulating abortion in a country or state, such abortions may be legal or illegal. The majority of induced abortions are legal in the USA and other developed countries.

## 10. What is threatened abortion?

This term is applied when a pregnant woman spontaneously experiences cramp-like pains with or without vaginal bleeding that may be followed by the spontaneous expulsion of the fetus, during the first 20 weeks of pregnancy. In threatened abortion, the baby is alive and the womb is closed. These are hallmarks of threatened abortion. Despite the fact that the woman may be worried when abortion is threatened, about 75% of such women still carry their pregnancies to term. In threatened abortion, the bleeding may be brief or intermittent. When a woman bleeds in pregnancy for any reason, she should see her doctor as early as possible.

### 11. What is inevitable abortion?

In this case, the baby may be alive or dead but unlike threatened abortion, the womb is open. It denotes that the pregnancy is on its way out and abortion is sure to happen. It is inevitable.

### 12. What is incomplete abortion?

In this case, some of the products of conception have been expelled through the dilated cervix, leaving some remnants inside the womb. There may be pain. Vaginal bleeding is present, but it may happen on and off. Because of the remnants in the womb and the continuous loss of blood, the woman is in danger of infection and anemia. In developing countries, infection of the womb and anemia are major killers of women during abortion.

### 13. What is complete abortion?

This means that abortion has taken place and all the products of conception have been expelled completely. The womb is usually closed. If abortion is complete, pain should stop. Bleeding should also stop completely. Sometimes, there may be scanty bleeding for a short duration.

### 14. What is missed abortion?

This is when the fetus or baby is dead but the products of conception are retained inside the womb. The cervix is closed. In most cases, the fact that the pregnancy is no longer viable is known to the woman. The woman may not even bleed. The woman may however stop having the feeling that she is pregnant, as some of the pregnancy symptoms like nausea, vomiting, breast fullness and pain have disappeared. The tummy is also lighter. In a few instances, this situation may persist and remain unnoticed for several months. In developing countries, due to ignorance, some women may move from one quack to another, seeking to deliver their long-overdue pregnancies.

### 15. What is recurrent pregnancy wastage?

By definition, this term is used by doctors when a woman has lost 3 or more pregnancies in a row. However, many doctors now believe that instead of waiting for women to lose 3 pregnancies, investigation and treatment should begin after a woman has lost two consecutive pregnancies, or even one. In the former, investigation and treatment should begin within the first 3 months of pregnancy, while in the latter, between the 4th – 6th months of pregnancy.

### 16. What is septic abortion?

In this type of abortion, the retained products of conception have been invaded by harmful germs in the womb. In developing countries, abortion is mostly illegal and further criminalized by moral, cultural, and religious beliefs. Most septic abortions result from such criminal acts. Septic abortion is responsible for most deaths due to abortion in developing countries. It is a major cause of maternal deaths in pregnancy. In many cases, the woman bleeds continuously or intermittently and soon becomes anemic and then runs into shock. The degree of shock may be out of proportion to the amount of blood loss. She appears pale or "white" with cold hands and feet and low volume pulse. This is the classical picture presented by those who will eventually die if help does not arrive quickly. It is important for parents to recognize this classical appearance in their adolescent girls and call for help on time. Due to the criminal nature of such abortions, young girls usually deny having procured abortions until they are at the point of death, when it may be too late to save their lives.

### 17. How dangerous are septic abortions?

In septic abortions, severe vaginal bleeding, lower abdominal pain, fever, chills, weakness and other complaints of serious ill health are common. This is a killer situation in many developing countries and has resulted in the deaths of many young girls and women. The typical story is that of a teenager or unmarried woman who has already had dilatation and curettage (D&C) in a quack medical practice downtown and ends up as an emergency case in the clinic a few days later. She is usually in a moribund state of health due to severe infection, dehydration, vaginal bleeding, anemia and shock. On a few occasions, the womb may be perforated with associated injuries to the intestines. This scenario is common in many developing countries.

### 18. What is unsafe abortion?

Unsafe abortions are those performed by unskilled personnel in a dirty environment. This means abortions performed by quacks, lacking in skills in a medically unsafe manner and dirty environment. Most times, unsafe abortions lead to severe complications and sometimes death.

### 19. Why is it attractive for women to procure abortion rather than prevent pregnancy?

There are two reasons that make abortion more of a solution to unwanted pregnancy for some women. These include:

- Ignorance: In some parts of the world, women grossly lack knowledge of family planning. This ignorance is more prevalent in developing countries. Family planning may be out of reach in some communities
- Many women who seek abortion do so because, in their own perception, pregnancy can be removed swiftly and safely through abortion. They see abortion as a readily available correction for an unwanted pregnancy. They assume that abortion is completely safe, whereas it is wiser and much cheaper to practice family planning, prevent unwanted pregnancy and avoid the complications inherent in abortion

### 20. What is a medical abortion?

The term medical abortion is applied when drugs are used to cause abortion. Such drugs include mifepristone (RU486) which is anti-progesterone. This drug is usually used in combination with another drug called prostaglandin. Medical abortions are done for early pregnancies and should be supervised by a doctor.

### 21. What is surgical abortion?

Surgical abortion is an abortion performed through surgical methods and can be done in two ways. The contents of the womb can be sucked out using a suction device like the Karman's syringe or vacuum evacuator. Usually, this is done for pregnancies of 9 weeks or less. For older pregnancies, the cervix or neck of the womb may be surgically dilated, prior to evacuation of the contents. Final evacuation may be achieved by causing the womb to contract in order to expel its contents. Womb contraction is achieved through the use of drugs. Evacuation may also be achieved through mechanical removal, such as curettage.

### 22. When is an abortion said to be therapeutic?

There are situations when it is not advisable for a woman to continue with pregnancy. In most cases, for medical reasons, continuation of pregnancy may lead to dangerous complications and cause harm to the woman. In some cases, the baby in the womb may be so abnormal that it is better to terminate the pregnancy as early as possible. In all such instances, abortion can be considered as a form of treatment, in order to prevent problems or complications. This type of abortion is called therapeutic abortion because it is perceived by health care givers, as a form of treatment.

### 23. What are the causes of spontaneous or unintended abortions?

Abortions may occur spontaneously without any identifiable cause. However, well known causes of spontaneous abortions include:

- Chromosome abnormalities - These account for more than 50% of cases of unintended abortions. The genetic problems may be inherited from the mother, father or both parents. Genetic abnormalities usually manifest in physical deformities, mental and behavioral problems. The timing of abortion depends on the severity of the abnormal genetic inheritance. Some abnormalities may result in early abortions while others may allow the baby to survive for some months before being aborted
- Cervical incompetence – An inherent weakness or damage to the cervix may cause it to give way or open up when pressure is exerted on it by the contents of the womb during pregnancy. In such a situation, the cervix is said to be incompetent. This usually happens from the 13th week of pregnancy. It is a major cause of recurrent abortion
- Abnormalities of the womb – Some wombs are deformed from inside. This makes implantation of pregnancy difficult. Masses such as fibroids or polyps also cause abortions when located right inside the womb cavity. They act like sitting tenants in the womb and soon "force the baby out." This results in pregnancy wastage
- Infections and infestations – This is a major cause in the developing world, mainly because of poor hygiene. Infection of the inner lining of the womb and scar formation, make normal implantation and pregnancy difficult. This is usually as a result of badly managed PID and septic abortions. Also, many viral infections, especially Toxoplasmosis, Rubella, Cytomegalovirus and Herpes (acronym: (TORCH), viral infections, cause various congenital abnormalities, many of which result in abortions. Abortions may also be caused by parasites and bacteria. Examples include malaria, typhoid fever and sexually transmitted infections
- Systemic diseases - When systemic diseases like hypertension or diabetes are not properly treated or controlled, they are associated with the increased risk of abortion
- Thyroid disease and other endocrine problems – The probability of pregnancy and its outcome depend to a great extent on a very intricate balancing of some hormones in the body. Hormonal problems lead to menstrual disorders, inability to achieve pregnancy and abortion. The most common hormone imbalance in women is polycystic ovarian syndrome (PCOS). Abortion is common in these women. Severe thyroid diseases usually result in infertility. If the disease is not treated effectively and the woman manages to get pregnant, it is more likely to trigger an abortion
- Systematic lupus erythematosus – This is a disease that may involve many body systems at the same time. The rate of pregnancy loss is high; up to 40% in some cases. Other diseases such as Tuberculosis and sickle cell anemia are associated with increased risks of abortion

- Smoking – Heavy smokers not only risk placental problems, premature labor and low birth weight babies but also higher rates of abortion and pregnancy wastages
- Alcohol and drugs – Female alcoholics, pregnant women who drink heavily or use illicit drugs are more prone to abortion
- Immunological – A woman may have unfavorable immune response to her husband's tissue antigens. Therefore, her body recognizes the pregnancy as a foreign body and eventually rejects it. Such unions almost always result in pregnancy wastage.

**24. What are the other factors that may increase the risk of abortion?**

Apart from diseases, others with higher risk are:
- Age – women who are younger than 20 and those older than 35 years of age
- Multiple pregnancy – Women who are pregnant with twins or more are more disposed to abortion. In this regard, the more the number of babies in the womb, the higher the likelihood of abortion
- Pregnancy spacing – The interval between successive pregnancies is also important. Inappropriate spacing between pregnancies of less than 6 months (short) and more than 3 years (long) are associated with higher abortion rates. The recommended interval between consecutive pregnancies is between 1-3 years

**25. What are the signs that a normal pregnancy may be aborting?**

The warning sign may start with lower abdominal discomfort or heaviness, which increases in intensity with time. Sometimes, bleeding may be noticed first and become progressively more severe. Lower abdominal pain and bleeding are the most common complaints. With more intense pain, the neck of the womb opens up and at this point, abortion becomes inevitable. In a more advanced pregnancy, loss of birth water or liquor from the vagina may happen early. Once any of these signs happen and become progressive, you should go to hospital where attempts will be made first to salvage the situation or prevent complications, if abortion becomes inevitable.

**26. How can abortion be prevented?**

Once you are sexually active, the surest way to avoid abortion is to prevent unwanted pregnancy through the use of appropriate family planning measures. However, in many developing countries, despite the preventive role of family planning, less than 20% of sexually active women utilize family planning. Consequently, abortion replaces family planning in these societies.

### 27. When is abortion most dangerous for a pregnant woman?

Abortion is never safe, but illegal abortion is more dangerous. The risk of complications increases in situations where:
- Pregnancy is advanced
- There is more than one fetus
- Very young girls and old women are involved
- The woman is sick
- Infection is more likely or already present
- The age of pregnancy cannot be determined with accuracy
- The procedure is not performed or supervised by a doctor or other healthcare providers with enough experience
- Wrong methods are used
- Abortions are performed in secret

### 28. What are the methods used to procure abortions legally?

Abortions can be performed through medical or surgical methods. Generally, for pregnancies of about 9 weeks or earlier, medical abortion or suction termination is used. For pregnancies of 9 – 14 weeks, suction termination is done. Beyond this age, when pregnancies are more advanced, careful medical abortion or dilation and evacuation may be performed. Abortions in advanced pregnancies are more dangerous and should be performed by healthcare providers that have the required skill.

### 29. What is recurrent pregnancy wastage?

By definition, this term is used by doctors when a woman has lost 3 or more pregnancies in a row. However, many doctors now believe that instead of waiting for a woman to lose 3 pregnancies, investigation and treatment should begin after she has lost one or two consecutive pregnancies. Investigation and treatment should begin within the first 3 months of pregnancy.

### 30. Are there abortion laws in developing countries?

Yes. Many developing countries have abortion laws, but they are largely restrictive. For example, in Nigeria, these are prescribed under the Penal Code in Northern Nigeria and the Criminal Code in Southern Nigeria. The Law prescribes a jail term of up to 14 years for an abortionist and up to 7 years for the woman who aborts. Essentially, it only allows abortion to be performed in order to preserve the mother's life and not for social or non-medical reasons. Some developing countries do not have abortion laws.

**31. What is the difference between the abortion laws in developing and developed countries?**

The big difference is that most developed countries like the USA and UK have well defined abortion laws that stipulate the conditions under which abortions can be legally procured. In countries where there are no abortion laws or where the laws are restrictive, death and complications due to abortions are usually high. This is because abortions are more likely to be performed in secret by quacks, using crude, unsafe methods.

**32. How many abortions are performed in developing countries per year?**

Documentation and accurate statistics are lacking in most developing countries. This is part of the problem of their parlous state of health infrastructure. Typically, the rates of abortion in developing countries are high. For example, an estimated 610,000 abortions are performed every year in Nigeria and almost 70% of these are unsafe or criminal abortions. The situation is similar in most developing countries, with criminal abortions taking the lion share.

**33. What are the common reasons for procuring criminal abortions in developing countries?**

Older women give reasons like having had enough children or being too old for pregnancy. Obviously, these reasons are not good enough, considering the danger in criminal abortion. This emphasizes the need for family planning education. Most girls procure abortions in developing countries because they are simply not ready to get pregnant. This may be because the girls are:

- Schooling
- Very young
- Not sure of ownership
- Ignorant that they are pregnant
- Afraid of reproach

**34. What are the common methods used for unsafe abortions in developing countries?**

The most popular method is dilatation and curettage (D&C) using all manner of sharp objects and metals, including spokes of bicycle wheels. Others include administration of injections, oral drugs, dangerous herbal concoctions and the insertion of harmful native herbal preparations into the vagina.

**35. What are the effects of herbal preparations?**

Abortionists use different unsafe methods in their desperate efforts to make money out of equally desperate young girls and women. Their crude methods commonly result in serious complications and the deaths of many young girls and women. Notable complications include serious genital tract infections which may progress to generalized infection or septicemia, bruises, burns, scar tissue formation, and deformity of the vagina, cervix and womb. Long term consequences include pelvic inflammatory disease, pelvic abscess, tubal blockage and infertility. These avoidable complications are as a result of the un-met needs for family planning and the absence of less restrictive laws on abortions where ever they occur.

### 36. What is the relative chance of death due to abortion in the USA and UK?

Deaths due to abortion are typically low in developed countries, due to the high level of care and non-restrictive laws. In the UK and the USA, similar situations obtain. This is in contrast with what happens in most developing countries, where the mortality rates due to abortion are usually high.

## DEAR DOCTOR:

### 37. If I must have an abortion, when is the safest time?

No time is completely safe to procure an abortion in pregnancy. However, if there is a medical indication for an abortion to be carried out, it should be done as early as possible, before 8 to 9 weeks of pregnancy, when the products of gestation can be sucked out easily from the womb. When pregnancies are older, complications are more likely, so it is advisable that you practice family planning immediately after the procedure, in order to avoid a repeat unwanted pregnancy.

### 38. If a doctor performs my abortion, does it make it safe?

When a doctor performs an abortion, he takes responsibility for ensuring that the abortion is properly done. The method of abortion, suitability and safety are important. Abortions performed by doctors should be safer than those performed by quacks, but no procedure is completely safe. The doctor must ensure that the instruments are sterilized properly and the procedure correctly done.

### 39. So what are the immediate complications of unsafe abortion?

The complications that may result from unsafe abortions are numerous depending on the methods used. I can mention two important immediate complications. The first is severe bleeding or hemorrhage. This usually happens while the abortion process is on-going and girls may bleed to death unless help comes quickly. The second is perforation of the womb and damage to abdominal organs. I can tell you that I have seen a girl's large intestines dangling from her vagina. The hapless 15-year old girl, suffered this as a result of a large perforation of the womb due to a criminal abortion performed by a quack downtown.

**40. Doctor I know that many young girls have died from complications resulting from unsafe abortions. What other immediate problems should I know about?**

Unfortunately, you are right. Injuries to the vulva, vagina and cervix often occur too. Here perforation or injury to the urinary bladder or rectum will result in uncontrollable leakages of urine or stool respectively. Incidences of serious infections or septicemia also usually happen a few days after procuring an unsafe abortion, leading to shock. This aspect is a major killer in developing countries.

**41. So there must be long term complications of unsafe abortions? What are they?**

The single most important long term complication is infertility, caused by tubal blockage. Others include: Scarring and narrowing of the vagina, scanty menstruation, cervical incompetence, complete stoppage of menstruation and severe pain during sexual intercourse.

**42. Doctor, please I have recurrent abortions, why is this happening to me?**

There are various reasons why you may have recurrent abortions or pregnancy wastage. The most common reasons are:

- Genetic problems - Genetic disorders may be inherited by the fetus from the mother, father or both parents. Very severe genetic problems are usually not compatible with life. In this case, abortions usually happen early in pregnancy, sometimes so early, that bleeding starts before the date of the next menstruation, so the woman may not realize that she was pregnant. Other genetic problems may allow pregnancy to survive for some weeks or months before ending in abortion. A few genetic problems allow the baby to survive but such babies suffer from various consequences of these problems, which include physical deformities, mental and behavioral abnormalities
- Infections - there are some infections that happen very early in pregnancy with far reaching effects on the development and well-being of the baby. The most severe consequence of this effect is abortion. If the infections are not adequately treated, they may result in pregnancy wastage. Such infections are more common in developing countries

- Chronic hormonal imbalance and metabolic disorders
- Cervical incompetence - The cervix is the neck of the womb. In a normal pregnancy, the cervix should be strong enough to ensure that it remains closed until the end of pregnancy when labor begins. In some women, the cervix is inherently weak and usually gives way at some point, due to pressure from the contents of the womb. This condition is called cervical incompetence. It usually manifests within the first 4 months of pregnancy and is a major cause of recurrent abortion.

### 43. So what should I do?

The first step is to visit your doctor to find out the reason for the recurrent abortions. To be able to assist you, it is important for the doctor to be familiar with the nature and timing of your pregnancy losses. Your doctor will order a series of tests in order to determine the reason for your recurrent abortions and once the reason is known, he or she should be able to assist you in most cases.

The tests and investigations involve:
- Detailing your history and physical examination: This should include examining the neck of your womb
- Blood tests: Some blood tests are important. These include hormonal analysis and tests for the presence of lupus anticoagulant and anti-cardiolipin antibodies. Other blood tests are those that rule out diseases like severe diabetes, syphilis, toxoplasmosis, rubella etc. which are important causes of repeated pregnancy losses
- HSG and Ultrasound scan: HSG means Hystero-salpingogram. It is an X-Ray test done to examine the womb, fallopian tubes, and cervix. Ultrasound scan may also be done
- Gene analysis: This may be done on you and your husband. If you see the doctor during the time of abortion, samples from the tissues of the fetus may also be taken for genetic analysis

### 44. Can you please tell me what causes cervical incompetence?

The causes of cervical incompetence fall into 2 categories. Firstly, some women are born with this inherent condition, so it is congenital. For this class of people, it is suspected that the cervix lacks power due to the absence or deficiency of some muscles or connective tissues, especially collagen. The reason for this is not known. Exposure of some female babies to some drugs such as diethylstilbesterol while in the womb, has been associated with congenital abnormalities, including malformed fallopian tubes, cervix and cervical incompetence.

Secondly, some women develop this condition. This may be as a result of aggressive dilatation of the cervix with large cervical dilators (more than size 9). This is commonly done by quacks that perform criminal abortions. Sometimes, cervical incompetence may occur due to tears and injuries to the cervix or forceful use of instruments like the forceps during difficult childbirths.

### 45. What are the chances that this type of pregnancy loss will occur to me again?

With one spontaneous abortion, the chance of another spontaneous abortion is about 25%. This risk increases with the second and third abortions. Women like you who have had more than 3 successive spontaneous abortions are said to be suffering from habitual abortion. There are modalities of treatment for cervical incompetence. Sometimes, following proper investigation and correct diagnosis, the neck of the womb may be tied early in pregnancy. I suggest that you see a gynecologist to evaluate your situation. This is necessary in order to make a proper diagnosis that will help you as early as possible in your next pregnancy.

### 46. Are there conditions when doctors must compulsorily perform abortions?

Yes. There are some situations where pregnancy can endanger the health of a woman and in such instances, allowing pregnancy to continue may lead to disaster and death. In most cases, this is due to pre-existing health conditions in such women. Conditions where pregnancy should be terminated or stopped through abortion include:

- Primary pulmonary hypertension
- Marfan's syndrome with involvement of the Aorta (the largest blood vessel in the body)
- Coarctation of the Aorta
- Severe narrowing of the mitral valves of the heart
- Previous history of heart attack or heart attack during pregnancy
- Other serious heart problems like the Tetralogy of Fallot or the narrowing of the Aorta

In most of the conditions above, the chance that the mother will die during pregnancy or childbirth may be as high as 15% or more. There are also instances in pregnancy, when the baby is so much deformed or seriously affected by other diseases, such that it makes no sense to allow pregnancy to be carried to term. Nowadays, all efforts should be made by the doctor using the various imaging techniques, like ultrasound and other investigations, to confirm diagnosis before abortion is embarked upon.

**47. If I exercise during pregnancy, can it lead to an abortion?**

Ordinary low intensity exercises should not cause abortion, however, high intensity, unaccustomed exercise may be dangerous. If there have been previous ominous events earlier on in pregnancy, like bleeding, lower abdominal pain or drainage of liquor, it is wise to avoid exercise until the doctor gives you the clearance to do so. In such instances, walking gently around the compound and resting in between should be harmless. If you are not sure whether a particular type of exercise will harm your pregnancy, it is better to avoid it. The risk may not be worth taking.

**48. Doctor, I aborted a 9 weeks old pregnancy 5 days ago because I was not prepared to have a baby yet. Now I feel a great sense of guilt and remorse. What should I do?**

It is not unusual to feel a sense of guilt after an induced abortion. This is natural. If you had had pre-abortion counseling, the doctor would have discussed issues surrounding abortion with you. These issues include:
- Explanation of the procedure of abortion and the complications that may arise
- Advice on alternatives to abortion, including allowing the pregnancy to go on to term
- Psychological issues like:
  - Guilt
  - Regret
  - Anxiety
  - How and where to get the required post abortion support and family planning
  - Post abortion follow-up

During the post abortion follow-up, the doctor will examine you to ensure that the womb is empty, no ongoing abnormal bleeding or related illnesses. Then also you have a chance of discussing your feelings. Sometimes, women need emotional support and interval counseling to help them overcome post abortion psychological issues. It is appropriate therefore that you consult your doctor and discuss your feelings with him. Your doctor should be able to counsel you or refer you to centers where further counseling and support are available.

**49. Should doctors perform abortions against their wish, if it will save a woman's life?**

For personal, moral or religious reasons, a doctor may not be willing to perform an abortion and it would be good practice to refer the woman to another doctor or center where an abortion can be procured. In most countries, it is quite possible to consult a directory and locate such centers and initiate an immediate referral.

# CHAPTER 6

# Family Planning

*"No woman can call herself free who dares not own and control her body. No woman can call herself free until she can choose consciously whether she will or will not be a mother."*
– MARGARET SANGER

### 1. What does family planning mean?

In practical terms, family planning means becoming pregnant only when you want to or when you are prepared for it. This is pregnancy by choice as opposed to pregnancy by chance. In other words, you have planned it from the beginning. In medical parlance, family planning refers to the various methods of preventing unwanted pregnancy.

### 2. What is the appropriate size of a family?

It depends on several factors. These include the health and age of the woman, as well as the socio-economic status of her family. On the average, a family size of 6 or less is good i.e. mother, father and four children. In the developed countries, family sizes are generally smaller than those in developing countries but it appears that the higher the social status of a couple, the smaller the family size.

### 3. Why do some couples have large families?

There are so many reasons. Many couples have large families because they believe that children are blessings from God and should therefore not be limited. Some couples equate children to wealth, so the more they have, the wealthier they feel. Others have many children, because although they believe that some may die, they expect a reasonable number to survive. Some couples end up with large families because of gender imbalances. More often, after several female births, the preference is for a male child, however, gender discrimination is the worst reason for a woman to risk a pregnancy that may cost her life. Other reasons include:

- Poor education
- Ignorance
- Rural life - rural dwellers are more likely to have large families than well-educated urban women
- Polygamy – where there are many wives, there are also likely to be large families
- Religious influences - Muslims are more likely to have larger families than Christians

### 4.    Is there any association between a large family and poverty?

Yes. Most couples with large family sizes are likely to be poorer and of low socio-economic status. With poverty, many children have poor or no education and may encounter more challenges in life.

### 5.    What effect does a large family have on the health of women?

From the information made available by the Guttmacher institute (www.guttmacher.org), an average family in the USA has 2 children. When a woman gets pregnant frequently, the physiological stress depletes her health because pregnancy and labor are very strenuous. This is apart from the associated poverty, difficult life and poor education of the children.

### 6.    What is the recommended interval between pregnancies?

It is advised that women leave a clear interval of 18 months to 2 years or more between successive pregnancies. This is to allow the body sufficient time to rest, recover from the stress of the previous pregnancy and return to the non-pregnant state as much as possible. The women will also have sufficient time to give quality care to their children and family members.

### 7.    What is the safe period?

Safe period refers to the time in a woman's menstrual cycle when she is least likely to get pregnant if she engages in unprotected sexual intercourse. However, practicing the concept of safe period is not a recommended family planning method. It is not safe or reliable.

### 8.    What is the fertile period?

This means the period of time in your menstrual cycle when you are more likely to be ovulating and therefore have an increased possibility of getting pregnant.

## 9. What are the various methods of family planning available?

There are many methods of achieving family planning. The important thing is that the method chosen must be suitable for the particular woman. So, the methods vary according to the circumstances of the individual woman or man and the best judgment of the doctor. Family planning methods can be grouped into natural methods and other methods that require the use of interventional materials like drugs, condoms, etc. The natural methods are more acceptable to certain religions. This is a chief advantage. These methods include:

- Natural Methods: These are family planning methods practiced without the use of any drugs or devices. They are the withdrawal method (Coitus interuptus) and abstinence
  - Withdrawal Method or Coitus Interuptus: In this method, the man withdraws from the vagina quickly before ejaculation. This means that sexual intercourse is interrupted. This is the oldest method but it is difficult to achieve. It is not recommended because it is not reliable at all
  - Abstinence: This means staying away from sexual intercourse until you are ready to become pregnant (total abstinence) or abstaining from sexual intercourse on the days near your time of ovulation (Rhythm method). Total abstinence is understandably effective but difficult. It is also not reliable because you may not be able to comply
- Other Methods:
  - Pills: The 2 main types are the Combined Oral Contraceptives (COC) and Progesterone Only Pills (POP). They are cheap, widely available and reliable. There are varieties of each type
  - Barrier Methods: e.g. male condoms and female condoms; they are worn before sexual intercourse. They are popular and widely used. There are other advantages that can be derived apart from preventing unwanted pregnancy
  - Intra Uterine Contraceptive Devices (IUCDs): These include all the devices placed in the womb for the purpose of preventing pregnancy e.g. Cu-T, Mirena etc.
  - Injectables or Contraceptive Injections: They are hormones, given as injections at intervals e.g. Depo provera is given every 2-3 months
  - Spermicides: These are chemicals that kill spermatozoa
  - Sterilization: This is the method of preventing pregnancy by obstructing the lumen of the fallopian tubes in women or cutting and tying off the vas deferens in men.

## 10. In what major ways do contraceptive methods prevent pregnancy?

The prerequisites for pregnancy are that ovulation must take place first and the sperm must travel up the fallopian tube to fertilize the female egg, forming a zygote or an embryo. The embryo must travel down the tube to implant in the womb. In principle therefore, most family planning methods work to prevent these key events from happening. Family planning methods work in 5 main ways:

- Prevention of Ovulation: Without ovulation, there is no female egg available to be fertilized by the spermatozoa. Therefore, pregnancy cannot occur
- Prevention of Fertilization: The egg and the spermatozoa do not make contact, so fertilization does not take place
- Prevention of Implantation: Some contraceptives cause thickening of the cervix and inner lining of the womb (endometrium) so that implantation of the embryo becomes difficult. Also, spermatozoa find it difficult to swim in such a hostile environment
- Spermicides: These are chemicals that kill spermatozoa directly
- Sterilization: This involves tying the fallopian tubes in females or the vas deferens in males; that is, blocking the fallopian tubes or the vas to ensure that there is no conveyance pipe for either sperm or embryo

## 11. What is the pill?

The 'Pill' is a hormonal tablet taken to prevent pregnancy. There are 2 main types. The first is the combined oral contraceptive pill (COC) which contains estrogen and progesterone. The second type is the progesterone only Pill (POP).

## 12. How does the combined oral contraceptive (COC) work?

Combined oral contraceptives work in 3 main ways:

- COCs suppress ovulation in 90--95% of women by preventing the occurrence of the LH surge which is necessary for ovulation to happen. In other words, they prevent ovulation and therefore there is no egg available for fertilization
- COCs change the pattern of endometrial development and make it difficult for the embryo to implant.
- COCs change the cervical mucus so that it is difficult for sperm to swim through

    It is important to note that the effect of COCs last for about 24hrs. It is therefore necessary to take them at precisely the same time. In the worst case scenario, the variation in timing should not be more than two hours.

### 13. What are the other benefits of combined oral contraceptives?
The extra benefits are:
- Reduction in the monthly menstrual blood loss; this is beneficial to those who have heavy menstruation
- Conservation of your eggs since there is no ovulation while you are on the pill
- Improvement or reduction of thyroid diseases, arthritis and osteoporosis

### 14. In what other ways does the COC help me, apart from preventing pregnancy?
Most family planning pills come in sachets which contain 28 tablets. The tablets commonly have two colors, 21 of which have one color while the other 7 have a different color. The first set of 21 tablets with the same color is the actual family planning pills. They are supposed to be started on day 1 of menstruation and should be finished by day 21. Between days 22 and 28 the last 7 tablets are swallowed. These are iron tablets (usually brown in color) which help to make blood during the last 7 days of the cycle, thereby preventing anemia which may result from menstrual blood loss. The other benefits are that the COC helps to reduce the amount of blood loss which is of additional benefit to women who have heavy menstrual flow. Lastly, pills help to normalize irregular menstruation, so they occur at fairly regular intervals.

### 15. What are the contraindications to COC?
Family planning methods are usually chosen by family planning providers and doctors, after due consideration of the objectives of the family planning, duration, mode of action, and side effects of the various methods available. These usually include careful history taking, examination and investigation, after which the doctor should be able to determine which method is most suitable. This will avoid or reduce the side effects and complications.

Those that should not use combined oral contraceptives include women with:
- Severe migraine
- Severe hypertension
- Uncontrolled diabetes
- Blood clotting disorder or thrombosis
- Serious heart ailments
- Chronic liver diseases
- Estrogen - dependent tumors
- Sickle cell disease and sickle cell anemia

- Inflammatory bowel disease
- Severe depression
- Diabetes

## 16. How does COC prevent anemia?

Apart from being an effective family planning method, COC prevents anemia in 2 ways:

- By reducing the amount of blood loss during menses, COC prevents iron deficiency anemia. This is important in women who have heavy menstrual flow
- Most COC packages contain 7 brown tablets which are taken during the last 7 days of the cycle. These tablets are iron tablets that help to make more blood

## 17. Do pills protect against diseases?

Yes. Pills protect against the following diseases:

- Benign conditions of the breast such as lumps
- Pelvic inflammatory disease
- Ovarian cysts
- Cancers of the womb and ovary
- Arthritis or chronic joint pains

## 18. What are the common problems that I may experience while on COC?

The COCs are suitable for most women and many do not have serious complaints while using them. However, you may feel nauseated or even vomit while on COC. You may also experience weight gain, increased discomfort and fullness in the breasts, especially in the first few months. The pills are associated with reduced menstrual blood flow. Therefore, women with scanty flow may experience further reduction in their menstrual losses. You should also be aware of some other complaints, even though they are not common. These include headache, mood change, depression, leg cramps and loss of interest or reduced desire for sexual intercourse. Women with scanty menstrual blood loss are not advised to use the pills.

## 19. What is the relationship between life span, smoking and the pill?

Smokers who are on the pills (COC) are more likely to die earlier than non-smokers e.g. at age 40 years. Smoking while on the pills is associated with mortality rate of over 31 per 100,000, while non-smokers on the pills have a much lower mortality rate of about 11 per 100,000.

**20. Will the COC affect the use of other drugs?**

Yes. There are some drugs that should not be used while on COCs. These include:
- Antibiotics
  - Cephalosporins
  - Ampicillin
  - Tetracycline
  - Rifampicin
- Griseofulvin
- Carbamazepine

**21. Does COC disturb sleep?**

In a few women, COC may affect sleep patterns negatively. This is not a common complaint, but it is necessary for women to have adequate sleep, so complaint of inability to sleep may be worrisome. It should be made known to the doctor.

**22. Does COC cause any other side effects?**

One of the unwanted side effects of the pill is weight gain. Many women on the pill experience this problem. The weight gain is due in part to the fact that the pills increase water retention in the body. If you are unduly worried, you should see your doctor for advice. Your doctor may recommend other suitable methods of family planning.

**23. Does COC cause hypertension?**

In some women, COC may disturb the renin-angiotensin-aldosterone system which is important in regulating blood pressure. Consequently, in up to 50% of women, the use of COC may result in high blood pressure. This may be a reason to stop the use of COC. Happily, the high blood pressure is usually reversed once the COC is stopped.

**24. What about thrombo-embolism?**

Thrombo-embolism is a form of blood clotting disorder. COC may increase the amount of proteins in the blood, including coagulation proteins. This results in higher risks of blood clotting, thrombus formation and thrombo-embolism.

**25. Who can utilize COC?**

Combined oral contraceptive pills are suitable for most women provided there are no conditions that disallow them. So most women are welcome!

## 26. Who should not use COC?

There are conditions that may preclude a few women from using COC. Those who should not use COC include:
- Smokers who are 35 years and above
- Women who previously suffered from heart attack or stroke
- Women with blood clotting or bleeding disorders
- Women with history of deep venous thrombosis
- Women with liver diseases
- Women suffering from severe migraine

Also, it is advisable that women who have the following conditions should avoid COC as much as possible to avoid complications. These conditions include:
- Breast cancer
- Obesity or overweight
- Sedentary lifestyles and occupations
- Systemic illnesses like
  - High blood cholesterol
  - High blood pressure
  - Disease of the heart valves

Most pills have instruction leaflets that should be read carefully before making a decision. Your doctor will also be happy to guide you.

## 27. How does POP work?

Progesterone Only Pills (POPs) mainly work in 2 ways:
- To make the cervical mucus difficult for the sperm to swim through
- To prevent implantation by creating a hostile endometrium

POPs also prevent ovulation, but in addition, they act on the lining of the womb cavity to prevent implantation or embedment of the embryo. POPs thicken the mucus secretion from the cervix and make it scanty so that it becomes difficult for spermatozoa to swim through. POPs are generally taken once daily for 21 days while iron tablets complete the remaining 7 days of the cycle.

## 28. What are the advantages of POP?

The benefits of POP include:
- Reduction of heavy menstrual blood loss but they can cause stoppage of menstruation in about 15% of women

- Reduction of menstrual pain and cramps
- Possibility of protection against cancer of the womb
- Reduction of endometrial thickness: When the endometrium is too thick, POP helps to reduce endometrial thickness thereby facilitating embryo implantation. This condition is called endometrial hyperplasia, which is associated with heavy menstrual loss and infertility

### 29. What are the main drawbacks of POPs?

They could cause irregular spotting or breakthrough bleeding in some women, resulting in great embarrassment. POPs can also cause amenorrhea or stoppage of menses, especially in older women.

### 30. Who can tolerate POPs?

POPs do not contain estrogen, therefore women in whom estrogen are contraindicated can use POP. These include those at risk of heart and other blood disorders due to the actions of estrogen. So POPs are suitable for:
- Women who have hypertension
- Women who smoke
- Women who have pre-existing risk of thrombo-embolism
- Women with migraine headache

### 31. Which one is more effective, COCs or POPs?

Both are good. The choice depends on which is most appropriate for the affected woman. Generally, COCs are more effective than POPs. The probability of failure of family planning is less with the COC. The failure rates of COC and POP are 0.1 and 2 per 100 women respectively.

### 32. What could cause unexpected bleeding while women are on COCs and POPs?

Bleeding or spotting outside menstruation is called break through bleeding. This happens in many women on the pill especially during the first 3 months of usage. The reasons for these include:
- Missed pills
- Diarrhea
- Vomiting
- Infections of the lower genital tract
- Other gastrointestinal tract diseases which reduce the absorption of the pills

### 33. What are the reasons for the failure of these pills?

Failure may occur for many reasons. For the pill to be effective, it must be absorbed from the gut and enter the blood stream. Absorption may be poor if the woman has diarrhea or vomiting. Poor digestion may also hamper absorption. Some drugs, such as antibiotics and anti-epileptics make the pills less efficient. Forgetfulness is another reason. Some women may forget to take their pills and may skip them for 1, 2 or 3 days. During such days they are not protected from pregnancy. In order to help women to remember to take their pills, they are usually advised to tie the timing of taking the pills to an important daily event, such as dinner or last activity before bed time.

### 34. Are pills and Hormone Replacement Therapy (HRT) the same thing?

No, they are not. You are probably confused because they both contain hormones. The differences are that:

Pills are formulated for family planning purposes. They are used for the sole aim of preventing unwanted pregnancy in women in the child bearing age group, that is, 18-44 years. Almost all of those who use family planning are women who still menstruate. In HRT, the tablets are used in women who are older and have stopped menstruation. These women have passed the age of pregnancy, so there is no need for family planning. The aim of HRT is to replace the deficient hormones, especially estrogen, in order to reduce the adverse effects of the hormone deficiency state. So, the aim of contraception is prevention of unwanted pregnancy, while the aim in HRT is to prevent the effect of estrogen deficiency.

### 35. What are the injectables?

These are hormonal injections given into the muscles in order to prevent pregnancy. They are usually injected deep in the muscle. From this site, the drug is released steadily into the body system in little quantities. The most common is medroxy progesterone acetate popularly known as depo-provera. Depo injections are usually given within the first 5 days of menstruation. Their actions last for 2 – 3 months after which a repeat injection is given.

### 36. What are the advantages of injectables?

The advantages are:
- Ease of administration; once in 2 – 3 months
- No particular motivation is required for the woman to continue once the injection is given
- It is effective

### 37. What are the disadvantages?

The major problems are:
- Irregular menstruation or breakthrough vaginal bleeding which may be worrisome and embarrassing

- Amenorrhea: This may cause severe anxiety and confusion as to whether or not the woman is pregnant. The woman may be miserable during the period of waiting for her menses to return
- Headache
- Bloating
- Weight gain
- Delayed fertility: There may be a delayed return to fertility of an average of 9 months when the injections are stopped

## 38. Are injectables suitable for all women?

In choosing contraceptive methods, women should take into consideration whether they want family planning for a short or long period or even permanently. Those who want temporary family planning will discontinue when they need to get pregnant again, while those who have completed their families are more suited to longer term family planning methods like injectables or permanent methods such as sterilization.

## 39. What are implants?

Implants are structures impregnated with hormones that are usually buried under the skin for the purpose of family planning. The hormones are released into the body in minute quantities for a specified period of time.

## 40. How do they work?

The implants are hormones and work by suppressing ovulation.

## 41. What are the main advantages of implants?

There are several but they include the following:
- They are effective
- Women do not need special motivation to continue with the method once implants are in place
- Women are in control of their bodies as far as fertility is concerned
- Return to fertility is prompt, because the hormones in implants like levonorgestrel (LNG) disappear from the body within 48 hours
- Without the fear of pregnancy, confidence is boosted and this may promote sexual pleasure

## 42. What are the disadvantages?

The disadvantages are few and include:
- Pain during and after insertion
- Swelling at the site of implantation
- Probability of infection
- Problems attributable to the hormones are irregular menstruation and break through bleeding

- They do not protect against sexually transmitted infections
- In some cases, fertility may not return quickly after discontinuation

### 43. What about male condoms?

Male condoms are widely popular and available in most parts of the world. There have also been tremendous improvements in the quality of condoms such that greater satisfaction and ease of use is now possible. The male condom is a barrier method. When ejaculation takes place, semen is released inside the condom instead of the vagina. Therefore, the sperm does not meet the egg and fertilization is not possible. In this way, pregnancy does not occur.

### 44. What are the things to note when using condoms?

In order to guarantee maximum efficacy, the following tips are beneficial:
- It must be worn correctly: To cover the full length of the erect penis
- It must be worn when there is erection before thrusting into the vagina
- It must be carefully examined for damage or tears before fixing
- In case it bursts or gets torn, the sexual act should be discontinued immediately

Beware! Some men play tricks by withdrawing the condom gradually, so that they end up releasing sperm into the vagina which the woman may not notice immediately.

### 45. What are the main advantages of condoms?

The condom has several advantages apart from preventing unwanted pregnancy. These are:
- It can be used by all categories of men
- It is cheap and widely available
- It is simple to wear
- It protects against sexually transmitted infections including HIV
- It is almost devoid of side effects
- It is not a drug, so it does not affect body systems
- It is effective when used correctly

### 46. Are there any side effects?

Of all the family planning methods apart from withdrawal method, the condom most probably has the least side effects. Some of the side effects or complications are:
- Condoms may cause irritation and itching of the penis in some people, who may actually be reacting to the rubber material used in making them
- Condoms may get torn or burst inside the vagina during sexual intercourse and discharge semen into the vagina

- Some men truly complain that it is cumbersome for them and psychologically, it puts their minds off sexual intercourse. This reduces their sexual pleasure

## 47. Who can use male condoms?

The vast majority of men can use condoms. Condoms are suitable for all except perhaps those that are not willing to use it. Some who don't like to use condoms give various reasons including:
- Condoms are cumbersome
- They disrupt the rhythm of sexual activity
- They make sexual intercourse un-natural
- They reduce sexual enjoyment and pleasure

## 48. What about female condoms?

Female condoms are worn over the neck of the womb or cervix. They work by covering the space through which semen enters the cervix, so that fertilization cannot take place since sperm does not meet the female egg. Female condoms come in different sizes, according to the size of the cervix and a woman must find the one that fits her cervix perfectly. They are far less popular than male condoms.

## 49. Are there any advantages?

The main advantage is that the woman is in control of planning her family, so the man cannot play any pranks. Also, when correctly fitted, it prevents sexually transmitted infections including HIV. It is also an effective method if used correctly.

## 50. Who can use female condoms?

Almost all women are suitable candidates. The issue is that most women do not want to go through the rigors of learning how to fix it correctly, since it may involve trying out different sizes, in order to find a suitable one. For other women, the availability of other equally effective methods that are less cumbersome makes female condoms less attractive.

## 51. What is the main disadvantage of female condoms?

Female condoms must be correctly worn on the cervix. This may be difficult. The woman must first find the correct size and then be trained on how to wear it. Some women find this strange and may be discouraged. The act of fitting the condom may also be messy and not convenient, especially if she needs to fix it when the sexual partner is already intimately aroused.

## 52. What is the diaphragm?

The diaphragm is a barrier method that needs instruction on the correct use. It is usually inserted before coitus and left in the vagina for at least 6 hours after coitus. It should be removed not later than 16 hours after coitus to reduce the risk of infection. Diaphragms are usually used in combination with spermicides to improve its efficacy.

## 53. What are the advantages of the diaphragm?

It is cheap and makes the woman to be in control of her own family planning, unlike the male condom with which the man can play tricks. Also, it may protect from sexually transmitted infections.

## 54. What are the disadvantages of diaphragm?

The main disadvantages are:
- The woman must be trained in the correct way to fit it in
- It should be left in place for some time and must not be forgotten inside beyond 16 hours, otherwise it may result in increased vaginal discharge or higher risk of infection
- Insertion may be viewed as a cumbersome ritual leading to discouragement

## 55. What are Intrauterine Contraceptive Devices (IUCDs)?

Intrauterine Contraceptive Devices (IUCDs) are popularly called Coils. They are objects inserted into the womb cavity to prevent pregnancy. There are 4 main types:
- The Inert type: Those made of inert substances or materials like plastic or rubber and inserted into the womb for variable lengths of time. Inert coils are no longer used
- Hormone impregnated devices: These normally contain progestogens for continuous release into the womb cavity
- Metal bearing devices: They act by preventing implantation of the embryo in the inner wall of the womb; some have other substances like copper added to them to make them more effective. Others contain hormones, e.g. progesterone
- Mirena IUD: highly effective with low failure rate

## 56. How does an IUCD work?

Doctors are not too certain about how IUCDs work to prevent pregnancy. However, they may work by:
- Preventing implantation of the embryo
- Causing early abortion of the implanted embryo

### 57. For how long can an IUCD like Copper-T be left in the womb cavity?

The duration depends on the type of IUCD. Copper-T can be left for a variable length of time, provided that there are no reasons to prematurely discontinue its usage e.g. severe vagina bleeding or pelvic pain. However, it is recommended that it should be left for not longer than 7 years in the womb. If there is need to continue after 7 years, the Copper-T should be changed to a new one.

### 58. What are the advantages of IUCDs?

The advantages are many and far outweigh the problems. The major benefits are:
- They begin preventive action immediately after insertion
- They are cheap and widely available
- They do not require any motivation for the woman to continue to use it once inserted
- They are effective
- Women can resume fertility and become pregnant once they are removed, which means that there is no delay in getting pregnant

### 59. What are the complications of IUCDs?

Women are usually told and appropriately counseled on the few complications before being offered. The problems include:
- Infection – Many women on IUCDs experience increased vaginal discharge and womb infections
- Heavy menstruation - With IUCDs, there is increased likelihood of heavy and more prolonged menstruation and irregular vaginal bleeding
- Painful menstruation – IUCDs are associated with lower abdominal pain, cramp or worsened pain during menstruation
- Bleeding - Bleeding after insertion and intermittent lower abdominal pain may occur in some women
- Missing IUCDs - The coil may be lost or unreachable after insertion or may migrate further inside from its former position. Sometimes, it may migrate through the wall of the womb to lie in the pelvis or lower abdominal cavity. This is an understandable cause of anxiety in women, since missing IUCDs sometimes need to be removed through surgical operations

Despite these complications, the IUCD is a popular method of family planning, especially in women who may wish to become pregnant soon after discontinuing family planning. Fertility is usually resumed once the coil is removed.

## 60. Which women can use an IUCD for family planning?

This method is suitable for:
- Women who have never been pregnant before with low risk of sexually transmitted infections (those with single sexual partners)
- Women with mutually single sexually partners
- Women who desire family planning for more than 2 years
- Smokers older than 35 years of age
- Women who are breastfeeding
- Women who have high risk of blood clotting disorders
- Women who are afraid of using drugs, especially hormonal drugs
- Women with poor compliance with other family planning methods
- Older women who decline sterilization

## 61. What are spermicides?

Spermicides are chemicals which are usually inserted into the vagina in order to immobilize and destroy sperm cells. They are usually inserted well ahead of sexual intercourse. The best known spermicide is probably nornoxynol-9, which comes as a vaginal pessary. Other spermicides come as vaginal foam, tablets, gels, cream, etc. Spermicides are commonly combined with a barrier method like the diaphragm for improved efficacy.

## 62. What are the disadvantages of spermicides?

The disadvantages are:
- Spermicides are not highly effective
- Spermicides may cause irritation in both sexual partners
- Women may experience burning vaginal sensation due to Spermicides
- Spermicides may increase the quantity of vaginal discharge
- Spermicides do not prevent sexually transmitted infections including HIV

## 63. What is the rhythm method?

The rhythm method entails having sexual intercourse when the woman is most likely not to become pregnant during her menstrual cycle. This means avoiding sexual intercourse around the time of ovulation.

## 64. What are the advantages of the rhythm method?

This method, though not effective, is widely practiced and attractive to the adherents of some religions. The main advantage is that it is the closest any family planning can get to natural coitus. It is not influenced by anything external or artificial.

## 64. What are the disadvantages?

The rhythm method can only be practiced if the woman has an accurate estimation of her ovulation time. This is only suitable for a few women because their cycles must be regular and predictable. Consequently, the failure rate is high because of the inability of many women to abstain totally during the ovulation period or inability to predict the ovulation period correctly.

## 65. Is the withdrawal method a family planning method?

Yes, but it is not a reliable family planning method. The failure rate is high. It requires severe discipline, especially on the part of male sexual partners, who may not be able to successfully withdraw. It is not recommended.

## 66. What is sterilization?

The fallopian tube is the pipe that naturally conveys semen to the female egg. Fertilization takes place at the tail end of the fallopian tube. It also conveys the embryo back to implant in the womb. In sterilization, the tube is obstructed or cut at a suitable point along its length. This obstructs the natural movement of semen and ensures that sperm cells cannot contact the female egg. Therefore, fertilization and hence pregnancy, cannot take place. To achieve interruption, apart from cutting or dividing the tubes on both sides, the fallopian tube can be tied or obstructed by using special clips or rings. Female sterilization is a very effective method of family planning. It should also be permanent and considered by women who are sure they do not desire pregnancy anymore. It is meant to be irreversible.

## 67. Which conditions make sterilization necessary?

These conditions include:
- Women for whom pregnancy constitutes serious danger which may result in death, for examples, those with serious heart diseases or hypertension
- Women who have completed their families and are sure that they do not want more children
- In developing countries, women who have had 4 Cesarean sections or more are usually advised to stop child bearing because of the high risk of womb rupture
- It is usual to recommend that women who have delivered many children should put a permanent stop to childbearing to prevent complications during future pregnancy, labor and after child birth, especially if 35 years or older

## 68. Is sterilization a suitable family planning method for every woman?

Sterilization is not suitable for all women. Those who should not consider sterilization as a family planning method include the following:
- Single women
- Women who have not completed their families
- Women who desire to stop childbearing for a while or are not sure whether they may change their minds concerning pregnancy in future
- Women in unstable or insecure relationships
- Women who have never been pregnant before
- Women who have no living child
- Women who have depression or other mental problems
- It is also not advisable to agree to sterilization during periods of grief such as loss of a husband or beloved partner as this may not be an appropriate time to take such an important decision

## 69. What are the disadvantages of sterilization?

There are several possible disadvantages:
- Some women may require anesthesia, which could involve consequent complications
- It is an operation which might cause:
  - Infection
  - Bleeding
  - Injury to other organs during the sterilization procedure
- Some women may change their minds and request that the procedure be reversed. This may be difficult or not effective.

## 70. What are the complications of sterilization?

- It involves an operation which is either a laparoscopy or a laparatomy. The mortality rate is 4 – 15 per 100,000 mainly due to problems associated with anesthesia
- It is basically irreversible but when successfully reversed, more than 15% of women experience ectopic pregnancies

## 71. Which women should consider sterilization?

They include:
- Women with chronic severe medical conditions
- Women with large numbers of children
- Women who are at risk of womb rupture if they become pregnant again
- Women who chose sterilization for social reasons

### 72. How popular is family planning in developing countries?

Actual figures are not available in many developing countries, but the percentage of women who practice family planning is low. For example, in Nigeria, certainly less than 10 % of women utilize one method of family planning or the other, excluding abstinence. This utilization is very low considering the number of deaths and serious complications arising from illegal abortions due to unwanted or unplanned pregnancies. This is the opposite of what happens in the developed countries where family planning is more or less the norm.

### 73. Do the traditional methods like family planning rings work?

In many local communities all over the world, there are traditional ways of preventing unwanted pregnancy such as rings, charms etc. This is common in the developing countries. However, they do not seem to work and are not recommended. There is no scientific basis for their perceived efficacy in the women who use them.

### 74. Some women insert native herbs and chemicals into the vagina as a method of family planning, are these effective?

This is a dangerous practice. They are not family planning methods and the consequences are usually very serious. They may cause extensive burns, ulceration and scars in the vagina, womb and even the urinary bladder, resulting in serious pelvic pain, dripping of urine and infertility. Please, do not attempt this.

### 75. What is post coital douching?

Some women jump out of bed soon after ejaculation in order to wash out the sperm quickly before it enters the womb. This act of washing out the vagina is called post coital douching. Douching may be done using water, chemicals like spermicides, vaginal pessaries and other preparations apart from water. This is called chemical douching. However, post coital douching is not a recommended method of family planning.

### 76. Why is douching not effective?

After ejaculation, spermatozoa move rapidly from the vagina into the womb and the tubes within seconds. Also, the womb contracts to suck them in. So, millions would have gone in before you wash them out. Therefore, washing does not prevent pregnancy and may cause infections and increased vaginal discharge.

### 77. Is breastfeeding a method of family planning?

No. It is not a recommended method. However, when a woman is breastfeeding exclusively, the process of suckling prevents ovulation and more often, ovulation is suppressed and menstruation does not occur. This is called lactation amenorrhea. Therefore, the possibility of pregnancy during exclusive breastfeeding is much reduced. The absence of ovulation and menstruation can last for about 6 months. Please, note that this is not true for all women and it may fail to protect you at any time. For this reason, once a woman becomes dry after childbirth and wishes to resume sexual intercourse, she should discuss her family planning needs with her doctor. Always remember that it is quite possible for you to become pregnant while breastfeeding.

## DEAR DOCTOR:

### 78. Why is it important for me to plan my family?

It is obviously better for a woman to become pregnant when she is medically, psychologically, socially, and financially prepared. When pregnancy is planned, the outcome is more likely to be better for the mother, her baby and family. A planned family is more capable of coping with the social and economic demands of life. Consequently, the whole family enjoys a better quality of life.

### 79. What are the consequences of lack of family planning?

Failure to plan your family will result in unwanted pregnancy and families that are too large. In many communities, most young women resort to procuring abortions. In the process, many women lose their lives or suffer severe complications, sometimes leading to serious health issues, including infertility and death.

### 80. How great is the burden of family planning in the USA?

According to the Guttmacher institute in the USA (www.guttmacher.org), there are about 61m women in the reproductive age group (15-44 years). Of these, about 43m or 70% are at risk of unintended pregnancy. The risk of unintended pregnancy is highest in teenagers between 15-19 years and lowest in women 40-44 years.

## 81. What are the commonly used family planning methods in the USA?

From the statistics made available by the Guttmacher institute, in 2014, the percentages of women and men on the more common family planning methods in the USA are as follows:

| FAMILY PLANNING METHOD | PERCENTAGE |
|---|---|
| The Pill | 25.6% |
| Female sterilization | 21.8% |
| Male condom | 14.3% |
| IUD | 11.8% |
| Male sterilization | 6.5% |
| Withdrawal method | 8.1% |
| Injectables | 3.9% |
| Vaginal ring | 2.4% |
| Ovulation time | 2.2% |
| Patch | 0.2% |
| Implant | 2.6% |

## 82. At what age do you advise that I start family planning?

In principle, any girl or woman who is sexually active and does not desire pregnancy should use some form of family planning regardless of her age.

## 83. So should girls adopt family planning on attaining puberty?

Technically speaking, it is the best way to prevent unwanted pregnancy in young girls. At this time, these girls are inexperienced and in transition to adulthood. In some communities, lack of family planning is one of the reasons why criminal abortion is common among young girls, especially high school students. However, family planning issues should be handled with care because of inexperience and adolescent behavior.

## 84. What about sex education at puberty?

Sex education at the time of puberty and adolescence is a sensitive matter. Some parents shy away from discussing it because of the fear that it may cause immorality or promiscuity. This is in line with the fact that adolescent girls are fond of trying out what they have heard, seen online or on TV, without thinking of the consequences. On the other hand, it may be dangerous and counterproductive if their parents don't teach or inform them at all. Girls may have no other option than to seek information elsewhere, especially from the internet. This is obviously dangerous. Perhaps in order to strike a balance, a fair policy is to answer their questions as decently as possible. If they ask, they really want to know and you should not keep them in the dark. If they do not ask questions, they may already have something to hide so parents should watch their girls closely and participate keenly in their activities so they can give appropriate guidance at the right time.

### 85. My boyfriend says there is a safe period. Is it true?

Safe period refers to the time in a woman's menstrual cycle when she is least likely to get pregnant if she engages in unprotected sexual intercourse. However, practicing the concept of safe period is not a recommended family planning method. Tell your boyfriend that it is neither safe nor reliable.

### 86. When is my fertile period?

You are most fertile during the period of time in your menstrual cycle, when you are more likely to be ovulating. This means you have an increased possibility of getting pregnant.

### 87. How do I know my fertile period?

There is no time in your menstrual cycle when you are 100% certain of the exact day of your ovulation. Therefore, your fertile period spans a few days before and after your calculated date of ovulation. It is only fairly possible to calculate your fertile period when your menstrual cycle length is regular, that is, every 28, 30 or 32 days etc. To calculate this, follow the steps below:

Step 1: Subtract 14 days from your cycle length.

Step 2: Subtract and add 2 days from your answer to Step 1 above.

For example, for a 30-day cycle, subtract 14 days. This leaves 16 days, 16 − 2 is 14 while 16 + 2 is 18. Therefore, the fertile period for a regular 30-day cycle, will lie between the 14th and 18th day of the cycle. At this period, you are not safe. Please, note that this is a rough estimate and you should not use it as a family planning method. Rather it is used for the purpose of timing sexual intercourse in order to achieve pregnancy.

More Examples:

| Length Of Cycle | Subtract 14 Days | Subtract 2 Days | Add 2 Days | Unsafe Period |
|---|---|---|---|---|
| 22 | 8 | 6 | 10 | 6th—10th days |
| 24 | 10 | 8 | 12 | 8th—12th days |
| 26 | 12 | 10 | 14 | 10th—16th days |
| 28 | 14 | 12 | 16 | 12th—16th days |
| 32 | 18 | 16 | 20 | 16th—20th days |
| 36 | 22 | 20 | 24 | 20th—24th days |

**88. If I missed my family planning pills for 1 – 2 days, what do I do?**

You should take the pills you missed as soon as you remember and continue with the rest of the tablets in the sachet as usual. However, if your menses does not come when expected, please consult your doctor. You may need to do a pregnancy test to find out if you are pregnant. Extra precautions should be taken for the next 7 days, especially where there is also vomiting. Vomiting will reduce absorption of the rugs add render may render them less effective in preventing pregnancy.

**89. If am on family planning like pills or injections and become pregnant, should I terminate the pregnancy?**

You do not need to terminate the pregnancy. Most family planning methods will not affect your unborn baby. However, if you are using the pills or injections, you need to stop it as soon as you discover that you are pregnant and see your doctor immediately.

**90. The doctor said I could not use the coil because it may worsen my heavy menstruation, so instead I was given pills. Is this okay?**

Coils or IUCDs are not suitable for some women. It is contraindicated in women like you who bleed heavily during menses, because it is most likely to increase the severity of the bleeding. On the other hand, the pill normally reduces menstrual flow by up to 50%, so it is beneficial in your own case. Therefore, your doctor is right. Coils are not advisable for those who have conditions like:
- Pelvic infection or pelvic inflammatory disease
- Irregular menstruation
- Masses in the womb such as fibroids

- Existing chronic pelvic pain
- Existing menstrual pain
- Heavy vaginal discharge

**91. What if I get pregnant while the coil is in my womb?**

This happens in some women when family planning fails to prevent pregnancy but you do not need to procure abortion because of this. This is because in most cases, the baby and the coil will peacefully coexist in the womb. Most times, the coil will come out or be expelled during delivery but you need to inform your doctor about your situation as soon as possible.

**92. Doctor, since I started using the pill, I have noticed copious vaginal discharge. What do I do?**

It is usual for some women to experience this complaint when on the pill. Of all the methods of family planning available, the pill and IUCDs may increase offensive and worrisome vaginal discharge. This increased discharge is one of the undesirable side effects of the pill. It is advisable that you discuss this issue with your doctor. There are many other family planning methods that are equally effective and do not increase vaginal discharge.

**93. My sexual partner assured me that he withdrew just before ejaculation and did not release semen inside me. However, I am doubtful. Doctor, can I still get pregnant?**

It is quite possible. The period of orgasm starts before the final ejaculation. During orgasm, there are multiple, short squirts of semen preceding the final big splash. These little squirts contain sperm cells and it is possible that a few sperm cells could find their way down the fallopian tubes. If the sexual act has happened during your time of ovulation, pregnancy is quite possible. It is dangerous to rely on the withdrawal method as a means of family planning. After such an experience, you should contact your doctor for advice on emergency contraception.

**94. If I had sterilization and changed my mind to have one more child, could the sterilization be reversed?**

Yes. It is possible to reverse it, but your chance of getting pregnant may be quite difficult. Reversal also depends on the method used to achieve the initial sterilization. Sterilization is meant to be permanent. This type of problem signifies poor decision making on your part or inadequate counseling by your family planning provider.

**95. Does family planning reduce enjoyment of sexual intercourse?**

No. family planning does not reduce libido or the degree of enjoyment during sexual intercourse. Rather, it removes the fear of unwanted pregnancy and protects against diseases. It increases confidence and brings about increased relaxation and satisfaction during sexual intercourse.

### 96. How do I know which method of family planning is most suitable for me?

There are many methods of family planning, but the particular method chosen has to be suitable for the individual woman. It should be the most effective and suitable method, with the least side effects. For this reason, it is not always good to procure family planning drugs over the counter. Your healthcare provider should guide you. So ask questions if you are in doubt. You should be able to find a method suitable for you.

### 97. Doctor, please can you provide an insight into how effective these family planning methods are?

One way to do this is to look at the True use failure rates (TUFR) of the various family planning methods. The TUFR is denoted as a percentage of 100 women in whom a particular method will fail and result in pregnancy. This is on the assumption that the women have used the family planning method correctly. The table below published by the Guttmacher institute (www.guttmacher.org) in the USA shows the TUFR of some family planning methods.

| FAMILY PLANNING METHOD | FAILURE RATE |
|---|---|
| Combined pills | 7% |
| Progestin only (minipill) | 7% |
| LNG (levonogesterone) | 0.1-0.4% |
| IUCD (Cu-T) | 0.8% |
| Implant | 0.01% |
| Depo – provera injection ("Shot") | 4% |
| Patch | 7% |
| Condom (with lubricants) | 13% (male) & 21% (female) |
| Cervical cap & spermicides | 17% |
| Spermicides | 21% |
| Coital interception | 30% |
| Safety period | 2-23% |

| Female sterilization | 0.5% |
|---|---|
| Male sterilization | 0.15% |

### 98. What is the most reliable family planning method?

Of course, with total abstinence from sexual intercourse, if it is at all possible, the chance of pregnancy is zero. However, it requires great self-discipline by you and your partner. It is not a popular or practicable method for obvious reasons. Among the other family planning methods, one of the most effective is combined oral contraceptives (COC). It is also acceptable to most women.

### 99. If I refuse to use any of these family planning methods, what are the chances that I may become a victim of unwanted pregnancy?

If you do not use any contraceptive method, the risk of unwanted pregnancy is 60 – 70%. That's a big price to pay!

### 100. If I have sudden unplanned sexual intercourse, is there any form of family planning that can be done quickly?

Yes, some family planning methods are designed to take care of such emergency situations. They are called emergency contraceptives. There are 2 main types:

- Pills: These may be high doses of combined oral contraceptives (COC) or progesterone only pills. They must be taken within the first 72 hours following unprotected sexual exposure. They should be repeated 12 hours after the initial dose. The progesterone only pill (POP) is more effective than the combined oral contraceptive pills (COC). POP can reduce the risk of pregnancy by about 85%.

- Copper intrauterine contraceptive device is the second method. When inserted not later than 5 days after such sexual intercourse, it is also effective

In all cases of emergency contraception, it is advisable to do a pregnancy test at about 21 days from the date of sexual exposure. It is also good to report the incident to the doctor for further advice.

### 101. How soon can I get pregnant after discontinuing family planning?

It depends on the type of family planning that you used. With family planning methods like pills, IUCDs and barrier methods, return to fertility is immediate. With other methods such as the injectables, there may be some delay. With sterilization, the fallopian tubes are tied. This is meant to be a permanent family planning method, so don't do it unless you are sure you no longer desire pregnancy.

**102. If I intend to get pregnant in the near future but desire short term family planning, which method will be most suitable for me?**

There are a few family planning methods that may be suitable. These include the monthly oral contraceptive pills and barrier methods. Male condoms for your partner are also appropriate as they are effective and protect you against sexually transmitted infections. An IUCD like a Copper-T, though effective as a temporary method, is not recommended for young and single women. Whatever your age may be, please visit a family planning clinic or your doctor for further guidance.

**103. If am on family planning like pills or injections and become pregnant, should I terminate the pregnancy?**

You do not need to terminate the pregnancy. Most family planning methods will not affect the unborn baby. However, if you are using pills or injections, you need to discontinue as soon as you discover that you are pregnant and see your doctor immediately.

**104. My menstruation is irregular, so do I still need to use family planning?**

Yes. Irregular menstruation does not prevent pregnancy. You may become pregnant unexpectedly if you do not use family planning. The combined oral contraceptive is particularly suitable for you, because in addition to preventing unwanted pregnancy, it will also make your menses become regular.

**105. Should I have a Dilatation and Curettage (D&C) done if I miss my period?**

No. A D&C is not a family planning method. It is dangerous if it is not recommended or performed by the doctor. Unfortunately, this practice is very common in developing countries. There are many other reasons why you may miss your period. Some women believe that their menstruation should come at the same date every month. This is not necessarily true. In teenagers, for instance, it is normal for menstruation to be irregular, even psychological or emotional upsets may lead to delayed menses. The first step is to wait for 1-2 weeks and see if the menses will come. If it does not, and you are sexually active, you should run a blood pregnancy test to see if you are pregnant. If you go hurriedly to procure D&C when you are not actually pregnant, the inner lining of your womb may be damaged, which could result in your inability to menstruate again. It is better to prevent pregnancy through family planning than to abort it.

**106. Is abortion a method of family planning?**

No. The goal of family planning is to prevent pregnancy from occurring and not to terminate it. It is therefore wrong to set a goal of preventing unwanted pregnancy, through criminal abortion. Each time unwanted pregnancy occurs, it is a reminder of an un-met need for family planning. Abortion and the dangerous consequences are the prices you pay when you fail to use family planning.

## 107. Why is menstruation sometimes delayed, after discontinuing family planning?

This is more common with long term contraceptive injections like Depo provera. This is due to the fact that even when the injections are stopped, some amount of drugs still remains in the body and the effect disappears slowly over time.

# CHAPTER 7
# Uterine Fibroids

*"We cannot confront the massive challenges, of poverty, hunger, disease and environmental destruction, unless we address issues of population and reproductive health."*
– THORAYA OBIAD

### 1. What are uterine fibroids?
Fibroids are abnormal growths or tumors which usually occur in multiples, within the womb. They are hard and appear like onions when cut.

### 2. What causes uterine fibroids?
The exact cause of uterine fibroid is unknown. Some doctors believe that fibroids develop as a result of abnormal changes in some of the muscle cells of the middle layer of the womb. In medical parlance, this type of change is called mutation.

### 3. What are fibroids made of?
Fibroids are made of muscle cells of the womb. Despite the fact that they may make women bleed heavily, they have poor blood supply.

### 4. From which part of the womb do they grow?
The womb has three 3 layers. These are the inner and middle layers and the outer covering. The inner layer, to which pregnancies attach, is also called the inner lining of the womb. It is soft, well supplied with blood, and contains many glands. This is also the layer that is shed during menstruation in the non-pregnant womb. The muscle layer consists of muscles of the womb, and blood vessels and has the ability to contract and relax. Excessive relaxation of the muscles may cause bleeding during and after childbirth. It is from this muscle layer that fibroids develop.

## 5. How common are fibroids?

Fibroids are the most common tumors in women in the African environment. It is present in up to 60% of women above 25 years of age. In general, fibroids are seen in about 50% of women during operations on the womb, including those women who do not ordinarily appear to have fibroids before surgery.

## 6. At what age do women develop fibroids?

Fibroids are not common in females below the age of 18 years. It tends to show up from about the age of 24 years and beyond, when women are at their prime. In many women, there is usually a positive history of fibroids in the mother and other female siblings.

## 7. Can fibroids also be found outside the womb?

Yes. Fibroids can be found on other structures apart from the womb. For example, fibroids can be found in the broad ligaments, which is a structure adjoining the womb.

## 8. How are fibroids classified?

Fibroids are usually classified according to their locations in the womb. That is, whether they are located outside the womb, in the wall or in the cavity. Using this method, there are 3 main types:
- Intramural: When located within the muscular wall of the womb
- Subserous: When located predominantly bulging on the outside
- Submucous: When located predominantly in the womb cavity

Other less common types include:
- Pedunculated: When attached to the outside wall by a stalk
- Intracavitory fibroid polyp: These are located inside the womb cavity and connected by a stalk
- Cervical: When found in the cervix or neck of the womb.

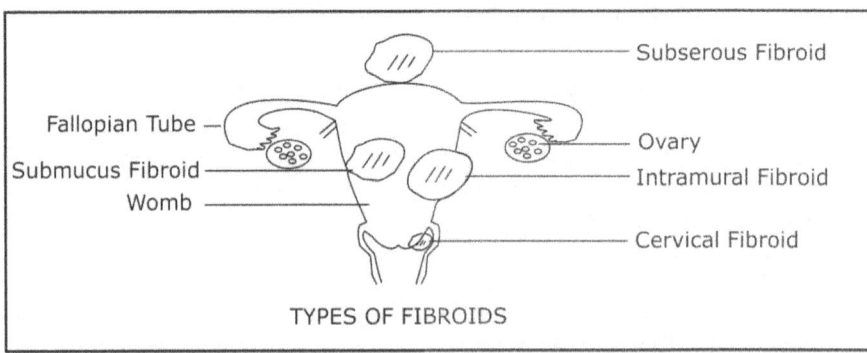

TYPES OF FIBROIDS

## 9. What are the risk factors for the development of fibroids?

The following factors increase a woman's risk of developing fibroids:

- Race - Fibroid is more common in the Black race. Black women are nine times more likely to develop fibroids than Caucasians. Also, the fibroids in Black women are more numerous and bigger than those found in Caucasians
- Family and relations - In some families, fibroids are common among females. This means that if a mother has fibroids, her daughters also have an increased risk of developing fibroids. This is contrary to the situation in Caucasian families
- Estrogen hormone - The growth of fibroids seems to be partly dependent on the availability and abundance of the estrogen hormone. Estrogen acts like some kind of fertilizer that enhances the rapid growth of fibroids; thus the more abundant the estrogen, the faster the rate of growth of fibroids. For this reason, the development of fibroids usually happens in younger women who are still bearing children; say between 24 - 44 years of age. At this period, there is abundant estrogen
- Obesity - Women who are overweight tend to be at a higher risk of developing fibroids, because obese women usually have higher estrogen hormone levels which may increase the risk of developing fibroids
- Infertility - Many women who are infertile also have fibroids. This is common in the African environment. Commonly, the fibroids are big and many. The function of the womb is to carry pregnancy. Since fibroids are common in infertile women, it thus appears that a womb that is not pregnant with a baby is most probably going to be "pregnant" with fibroids.

Other women who may have a higher risk of developing fibroids include:

- Those who have diabetes
- Those who have hypertension
- Those who attain menopause late
- Those on prolonged use of estrogen drugs
- Those with existing diseases of the lining of the womb

## 10. Can I develop fibroids even after menopause?

After menopause, there is estrogen deficiency and the growth of fibroids slows down. It may actually shrink in size. It is not common for fibroids to appear for the first time in women who have attained menopause.

## 11. What are the effects of fibroids?

The effects depend on the location, number and sizes. They include:

- Big tummy – In the African environment, some women have huge, multiple fibroids. These makes their tummies appear big, as if they are pregnant. This appearance runs contrary to their actual situation because many of them are infertile
- Heavy menstrual flow - Fibroids are associated with heavy bleeding, usually with pain, during menstruation. This may be prolonged and the woman may bleed for several days or weeks. It is sometimes irregular and comes on and off. The episodes are usually associated with the appearance of blood clots. This may lead to chronic anemia or shortage of blood. The woman may not be able to venture out of her home or go to her office in order to avoid unexpected bleeding episodes. Her life may be miserable and she may be too weak to carry out her daily chores
- Irregular vaginal bleeding - The main complaint in a few women may be only irregular vaginal bleeding
- Lower abdominal pain - Many women complain of lower abdominal pain associated with fibroids. The pain varies in intensity from mild discomfort to severe lower abdominal pain, which may be associated with other complaints. It may be described as cramps or dull in nature. It is usually felt in front but may sometimes be felt at the lower back. It may also move around the waist and down the lower limbs
- Pressure symptoms giving rise to:
    - Swollen legs - Big fibroids usually compress the blood pipes of the legs and waist region. Because of this blockage, blood returning from both legs cannot flow freely. It becomes more or less stagnant. Water from the blood then finds its way into the tissues of the feet and legs which become swollen. The swelling is more during the day when the woman is standing and less in the morning when she gets up from bed
    - Dilated skin blood vessels - Visible blood vessels in the legs and feet may begin to appear due to blockage and distention of the blood pipes. The distended pipes appear tortuous and ugly. They are called varicose veins. This may be cosmetically embarrassing to some women
    - Frequent urination - Large fibroids may compress the urinary bladder in the pelvis and reduce its volume. With the reduction in volume, the bladder fills up in a shorter time and the woman feels the urge to urinate more frequently
    - Retention of urine - The urinary blabber and womb are both located in the pelvic cavity. Sometimes, the bladder may not be able to empty its urine if it is blocked or incarcerated at the bladder neck by fibroids. Therefore, the bladder gets distended with accumulated urine which cannot be emptied. This is a very painful condition and usually warrants urgent visits to the doctor. Sometimes, the fibroids may partially compress the bladder. All

these reduce the total capacity of the bladder and it fills up with urine within a very short time. In this situation, the woman feels the urge to urinate more frequently. This may be worrisome and embarrassing. This is called urgency
- Kidney related challenges - Fibroids may sit on the ureters and compress them. The ureters are pipes that bring urine made in the kidneys to the urinary bladder. When they are compressed, urine accumulates in the ureters and with time, flows backwards into the kidneys, where it collects to form cystic masses called hydronephrosis. This can result in pain at the lower back or loin. Hydronephrosis may cause kidney damage unless the condition is noticed early and corrected
- Constipation - Sometimes, fibroids do compress the large intestines so that stool cannot pass down to the anus. Because of this stagnation, more water is absorbed from the stool which becomes hardened. The woman becomes constipated and may need medical attention
- Infertility - Many women who have symptomatic fibroids also suffer from infertility, although there is no proven cause and effect relationship between fibroid and infertility. In principle, if the fibroids seem capable of preventing the woman from getting pregnant, then they should be removed through surgery
- Weakness - Severe weakness and dizziness may be experienced due to anemia because of chronic vaginal bleeding from fibroids and poor appetite, as the woman battles with her pain. This may lead to progressive weight loss and general ill health

## 12. Do all fibroids cause problems?

No. About 50% of women with fibroids do not have any complaints. Many of these women therefore do not need treatment

## 13. When is it necessary to treat fibroids?

Treatment becomes necessary when the fibroids are causing problems. Some are so large that women become embarrassed, because people think they are pregnant. Sometimes when they cause severe and prolonged bleeding during menstruation or in between menses, it may result in anemia (shortage of blood) or dizzy spells. Women should also be treated when fibroids cause pressure symptoms, discomfort and severe pain. When they are suspected to be the cause of infertility, they should be removed.

## 14. What are the main ways of treating fibroids?

There are 3 main methods of treating fibroids. These are: surgery, drug treatment, radiological intervention and other methods. The best method is chosen by the doctor depending on certain considerations, which include the type of symptoms, the age of the woman and whether the womb has to be preserved or not. The womb is preserved usually if the woman still desires to become pregnant.

- Surgery: Open abdominal surgery is commonly performed to remove fibroids. This operation is called myomectomy. Surgery may also be done through laparoscopy. Sometimes, it is possible to remove chips of fibroids through the use of an instrument called a hysteroscope. This procedure is suitable for small fibroids. If a woman has completed her family, the womb should be removed through an operation called hysterectomy. This solves the problem once and for all
- Drugs: Drugs are also used to treat pain and reduce bleeding due to fibroids. The type of drugs used depends on the problem. The injections may be taken monthly or at longer intervals according to the doctor's prescription. Some drugs are also used to shrink fibroids
- Interventional methods: These include the various radiological methods of stopping or reducing the growth of fibroids. This is done by reducing the blood supply to the fibroid in order to starve it. Some of these methods include:
  - Uterine artery embolization: Blocking the blood supply to the fibroid to stifle the growth
  - Uterine artery ligation: This is a new and effective method of ligating the uterine artery. It was pioneered by this author as a member of a research team at the Lagos State University Teaching Hospital in Lagos, Nigeria. This simple, cost effective procedure was done by tying up the uterine artery at the level of the internal opening (internal os) of the cervix through the vagina. It achieved a remarkable 50-86% reduction in the sizes of majority of fibroids within 1 year. This method is beneficial in low technology locations, especially in developing countries

## 15. What is the most common treatment of fibroids?

The most common treatment is an operation which is performed on the womb to remove the fibroids. During this operation, called myomectomy, the surgeon removes as many lobes of fibroids as possible, especially the big ones. It is usually not possible to remove all the lobes when operating so it is common for fibroids to re-occur, either as a result of the untouched lobes or from new lobes. Unfortunately, fibroids will re-occur in about 25% of cases after fibroid operation, which is a major drawback to myomectomy.

## 16. What are the problems with myomectomy?

The main danger is that of uncontrolled bleeding during surgery. This may require transfusion of many units of blood and if it does not stop, the entire womb may have to be removed in such an emergency. This becomes an issue because the woman only wakes up to be told that she no longer has a womb. The other issue is that of the reoccurrence of fibroids. This happens in 25% of women after myomectomy. Myomectomy is also associated with adhesion formation in the pelvic and womb cavity.

### 17. Are there other procedures that are less painful than open surgeries?

Yes. If you are afraid of operations, your doctor may suggest less painful procedures like hysteroscopic resection or laparoscopic (pinhole surgery) removal of the fibroids. Laparascopic surgeries are less painful and the wound heals faster, but large fibroids are not suitable for laparoscopy. One remarkable disadvantage of laparoscopy is that it offers a limited operating field and makes the total surgical removal of fibroids more difficult. The issue of scar tissue or adhesion formation after such a procedure is also a big concern, as this may result in blockage of the fallopian tubes, causing infertility. With laparoscopic removal and many adhesions, future operations in the abdominal cavity become more dangerous and risky.

### 18. What is laparoscopic myolysis?

This is one of the procedures used to remove or reduce fibroids during laparaoscopy. The fibroid lobes are chopped and grinded with an instrument called a Morcillator. The fragments are then taken out in bits through the barrel of the hysteroscope. Other emerging treatments for fibroids include radio frequency ablation.

### 19. Are there injections than can be used to treat fibroids?

Yes, some drugs are used in the management of fibroids. They are given as injections taken at intervals. They work by shrinking or reducing the size of fibroids. However, the fibroids do not disappear completely. These drugs are useful only in a few instances. For example, they may be given for a period of time, to a woman who has large fibroids, before performing the fibroid operation. This will shrink the fibroids and reduce bleeding during surgery. Also, the injections may be used as an alternative to surgery in a woman who is near menopause. This is because once menopause sets in, the fibroid stops growing due to lack of estrogen - the 'fertilizer' that helps fibroids grow. The major disadvantage of these injections is that when they are stopped, the fibroids often grow back. Secondly, menstruation may stop altogether due to the effects of the injections. To some women, especially Africans, this side effect may be a big issue. This is because culturally, some women value menstruation and will do everything possible to continue menstruating, or ensure that their menses is re-established within a reasonable time. Drug treatment for fibroids is consequently a temporary measure and not as popular as myomectomy.

**20. What is the best treatment?**

The best treatment is to remove the womb, especially if the woman has had all her children. The fibroids alone can be removed if the womb needs to be preserved; however, in many cases, the fibroids may re-occur. Other methods using radiology and laparoscopy are gaining prominence.

**21. Are there any other drugs part from the injections already mentioned?**

Drugs like Mifepristone, (Ru486) can be used to shrink fibroids but the use is not as popular as Gonadotropin releasing hormone analogs (GnRH). Again, there is evidence that fibroids may shrink more permanently with systemic administration of substances like Alpha interferon. This is good news, but it is yet to be deployed widely for this purpose.

**22. What are the problems that fibroids may cause during pregnancy?**

In many cases, fibroids do coexist peacefully with pregnancy. However, fibroids in some cases may be associated with problems during pregnancy. The common problems include:

- Bleeding - fibroids may be associated with heavy bleeding during pregnancy. The bleeding episodes may be prolonged and erratic in nature. Bleeding in pregnancy is one important reason that should compel you to see your doctor immediately. Delay may lead to loss of too much blood. This may cause anemia and jeopardize the health of your baby
- Placenta problems – the presence of fibroids may cause placenta previa and placenta abruptio. The term placenta previa means that the placenta is in the lower part of the womb. In this position, it may cause bleeding or block the birth canal so that the baby cannot be delivered naturally without operation. With placental abruptio, there is bleeding from the placenta; thus oxygen supply and nutrition are cut off from the baby. In severe abruptio, the baby usually dies quickly inside the womb
- Abortion and premature labor - fibroids are associated with increased risks of abortion and premature labor. These ultimately lead to the delivery of premature babies. Premature babies face many challenges of survival outside the womb. Many of these babies die after delivery depending on the severity of the prematurity, the associated challenges and level of medical care
- Operation - fibroids increase the risk of operation during pregnancy. Because of issues like bleeding, mal-presentation, placenta problems etc. the probability that the doctor will perform operations to deliver the baby is higher. Surgical operations expose the woman and her unborn baby to further dangers

- Mal presentation - when fibroids are big and located right inside the womb, they may disturb the baby from swimming freely inside the womb. If they are located near the neck of the womb, they may not allow the baby's head to come down towards the birth canal. This type of bad positioning is called mal-presentation. If this situation persists till the time of labor, it may block the baby from being safely delivered through the birth canal. This is called obstructed labor

## 23. In terms of rate of growth, how do fibroids behave in pregnancy?

Most fibroids experience a 'growth spurt' during pregnancy due to pregnancy hormonal influences, so most pregnant women experience an increase in the sizes of existing fibroids.

## 24. Do fibroids degenerate during pregnancy?

In some instances, fibroids may cause severe pain as a result of degenerative changes inside them. There is a type of degeneration that is important to pregnancy called red degeneration. In about 5-10% of cases, red degeneration causes severe pain which usually results in hospital admission during pregnancy. Other types of degeneration are hyaline, cystic, mucoid degenerations and calcification. However, they are not peculiar to pregnancy even though they may happen.

## 25. Do fibroids cause infertility?

Yes, they may. If the fibroid is large and located in the uterine cavity, it may disturb implantation of the embryo or compete for space with pregnancy. This may lead to pregnancy wastage. Also, it has been observed that fibroids are associated with pelvic inflammatory disease (PID). Tubal blockage resulting from PID is the most common cause of infertility in developing countries. Furthermore, fibroids may sit and compress the fallopian tubes due to their locations. All these reasons are debatable. There are many women with large multiple fibroids who have successfully carried pregnancy to term. Very large multiple fibroids are seen more often in African women.

## 26. Why do fibroids sometimes cause pain?

There are 3 reasons why a woman with fibroid may have pain. These are:
- Degeneration: This happens when the blood supply of the fibroid is cut-off or becomes insufficient, maybe because of its large size
- Torsion of a pedunculated fibroid. This means that the stalk attaching the fibroid to the womb is twisted. This cuts off the blood supply and results in an excruciating pain
- Sarcomatous change or transformation into cancer

### 27. So, fibroids can become cancer?

It is difficult to suspect that fibroid is transforming into cancer because it is a rare occurrence but they can transform into a type of cancer called sarcoma. This is a very rare occurrence that happens in about 0.3 - 0.7% of cases of fibroids. In other words, the chance that fibroids will transform into cancer is less than 1 case out of every 1000 cases. However, when a previously small, harmless fibroid suddenly begins to grow rapidly and cause severe pain with increasing intensity, you should visit the doctor. It may turn out to be cancerous!

### 28. Can fibroids be cured?

The only way to cure uterine fibroid is to remove the womb completely.

### 29. What are the self-help measures that may help me?

Fibroids can pose many problems, but in about 50% of cases, there may be no complaints. The most common complaints are bleeding, lower abdominal enlargement and pain. Women complain of pain more commonly during menses. Measures that may be beneficial include:

- Appropriate medication: In all cases where a woman is bleeding severely, it is necessary to visit the doctor for treatment or reassurance, unless you already have your doctor's prescription to stop or reduce such bleeding. So, if you are experiencing heavy bleeding, take your drugs and see your doctor without delay. Family planning drugs tend to reduce menstrual blood loss
- Pain killers: Simple analgesics or pain killers may be tried. If you are used to antispasmodic drugs, you can also try this. If the pain does not abate with simple pain killers, you should see your doctor
- Heat therapy: This may also be useful. This is usually done by placing a hot water bottle on the lower tummy for some minutes at a time. Care must be taken to avoid skin burn or accidental opening of the lid of the water bottle. This measure may be complimented by a hot beverage of your choice. Heat improves blood supply to the womb and relieves discomfort in some women
- Regular exercise: This is generally beneficial to good health and has been suggested to reduce discomfort and pain. Surely, exercise increases the ability to cope with stress. So, for maximal effect, try and exercise regularly even outside menses
- Primrose: There are claims that the use of primrose alleviates the symptoms of fibroids generally. You may wish to try this out

# DEAR DOCTOR:

**30. How do I know if I have fibroids?**

Complaints which may suggest that you have fibroids include prolonged or heavy menstrual bleeding, irregular vaginal bleeding, low abdominal pain, especially during menstruation, enlarging tummy and the feeling of a hard swelling or mass in the lower abdomen. These are the common complaints and may show up early, more often in association with inability to conceive. However, in 50% of fibroid cases, there may be no complaint at all.

**31. What tests should I do if I suspect that I have fibroids?**

The first step is to see a doctor about your complaints. Apart from examining your tummy, the doctor will order some tests. The most popular test for fibroids is the ultrasound scan. This is a painless test without any side effect. It diagnoses tumors or masses of the womb with good accuracy. Ultrasound scans are affordable and available currently in many diagnostic centers or clinics. On rare occasions, when the doctor is not sure of the problem, you may be asked to undergo a Computed tomography scan (CT), or a Magnetic Resonance Imaging (MRI) test. These are expensive and may not be readily available or affordable. Apart from these, fibroids may be appreciated or identified when performing Hysterosalpingography (HSG), Laparoscopy and hysteroscopy tests.

**32. What determines the type of treatment that I may have to undergo for my fibroids?**

There are some issues that may guide your doctor in choosing the type of treatment that is suitable for you. These include:
- Your major complaint - Excessive bleeding, severe pain, painful menses, large or bloated abdomen due to the bulging fibroid mass etc.
- Location of the fibroids and their sizes
- Your age
- Menses or nearness to menopause
- Fertility issues - whether you have completed your family or not

If a woman has completed her family, the perfect treatment is to remove the womb.

**33. My doctor said that I have sub-serous fibroids. Will this prevent me from getting pregnant?**

No. Sub-serous fibroids are located outside the muscular wall of the uterus. They grow outside the wall and are on the external surface of the womb.

Sometimes, they may even be connected to the surface of the womb by a stalk or pedicle. They do not cause infertility or affect pregnancy.

### 34. What about sub-mucus fibroids?

Sub-mucus fibroids are located inside the womb cavity. They may bleed irregularly for prolonged durations and cause confusion and difficulty in your ability to estimate your ovulation time. Bleeding also makes it difficult for the embryo to attach to the womb properly. Also, embryos cannot be implanted or attached directly on a fibroid because fibroids are hard masses (like onions), unlike the normal womb lining that is soft and well supplied with blood. Therefore, sub-mucus fibroid can cause delay in achieving conception.

### 35. I am 32 years of age. I have fibroids, but I do not suffer any problem due to the fibroids except that I cannot conceive. Should I go ahead and have an operation to remove them?

Yes. It is appropriate, even though you do not have any complaints. Generally, doctors do not remove fibroids if they do not cause problems. The association between fibroids and infertility has not been proved completely. However, if there is no other reason for your infertility, after thorough investigations, surgical removal of the fibroids may be beneficial. Where the cause of infertility is unknown, pregnancy can be achieved in about 40% of cases after surgical removal of fibroids. So, it is advisable that you remove the fibroids.

### 36. I am convinced that my big tummy is because of pregnancy and not fibroid, but all my pregnancy tests have proved negative. I am confused, what is the way out?

In all cases, fibroids can be detected through tests. The presence of fibroids makes the womb bigger or bulky. It is therefore possible to detect most fibroids by undergoing tests like ultrasound scans. This is the most common test performed to detect fibroids and it is highly accurate in most cases. Other tests like MRI or CT scan are much more expensive. They are usually done when ultrasound tests are not conclusive or when there is doubt. Fibroids are real and not spiritual. It is always good to pray and commit one's health to God, but it also necessary to take the right treatment once the doctor has made the diagnosis. Prayer does not disturb treatment. It is certain that the correct diagnosis is fibroids, not pregnancy.

### 37. The doctor said I am at risk of developing problems during labor because I have fibroids, so he has recommended surgery. What should I do?

Fibroids can cause problems during labor and after delivery. Fibroids that are located at the neck of the womb or cervix can make it more difficult for the baby to pass through the birth canal. Safe delivery may then be difficult. This may cause obstructed labor. Secondly, there is the possibility of excessive bleeding during and after delivery. This is because the fibroids may reduce the ability of the womb to contract firmly and prevent bleeding. For these reasons, your doctor is right, especially if your baby is also mal presenting, as a result of the fibroid.

### 38. Is it possible for me to prevent fibroids?

Doctors still don't know what causes fibroids. It is only when doctors know the cause that preventive measures are possible. As of now, there is no way to prevent fibroids from occurring. It is not a preventable disease. There are suggestions that regular exercises are beneficial in preventing fibroid. However, this has not been proven.

### 39. Does eating red meat cause fibroids?

There are suggestions that regular consumption of red meat increases the risk of fibroids, although there is no sure proof that this is true. However, it is a known fact that the consumption of red meat increases the risk of other diseases including hypertension, heart diseases, and stroke. The contribution of red meat to the risk of diseases is confusing as of now. Anyway, it is advisable to reduce the consumption of red meat to a moderate amount, if it cannot be avoided totally.

### 40. Is massaging by hand a treatment method for fibroids?

In some parts of the world, there are native health practitioners who engage in the practice of physical massaging of the tummy as a treatment for fibroids. Such native practitioners are found in African communities like the southern part of Nigeria. There is no evidence that massage treatment works. As such, it is not recommended.

### 41. Do fibroids cause pain during sexual intercourse?

Yes. It is not unusual for fibroids to cause pain during sexual intercourse. This may occur when fibroids are located in the lower part or the neck of the womb. The intensity of the pain may be increased if the pelvis is also congested due to constipation, retention of urine or pelvic infection. However, you need to visit your doctor for proper identification of the cause of your pain as there are other conditions that may be responsible for this type of complaint.

# CHAPTER 8
# Polycystic Ovarian Syndrome (PCOS)

*"Being a girl today can be tough. That's why 'Chicken Soup for the Girl's Soul' is so amazing. Each story shows you that other girls are going through the same thing as you are and that you are not alone"*
– CATHERINE LEE

### 1. What is Polycystic Ovarian Syndrome (PCOS)?

PCOS means Polycystic Ovarian Syndrome. PCOS is a condition seen in women mostly in the child bearing age group. As the name implies, most doctors regard this condition as a syndrome rather than a disease. Syndromes are usually diagnosed when a person shows a unique combination of clinical features that may suggest a problem, condition or disease. The recognized clinical features or complaints in women with PCOS are:

- Infertility
- Lack of ovulation
- Menstruation upset
- Obesity
- Excessive hair growth in the body
- Many small, immature follicles in the ovaries

### 2. What is the cause of PCOS?

Doctors are not exactly sure of the cause of PCOS. However, some problems are known to be common to women with PCOS. These findings include:

- Elevated luteinizing hormone (LH) level and a relatively lower Follicle Stimulating Hormone (FSH) level in the blood
- Excessive amounts of androgen hormones, these cause:

- Poor growth of eggs, poor egg quality and ovulation disturbances
- Excessive hair growth in the body called hirsutism
- Chronic Acne or pimples
- Excess weight gain
• Women with PCOS have insulin insensitivity, resulting in high levels of insulin, which encourage the production of excessive male hormones (hyper-androgenism)

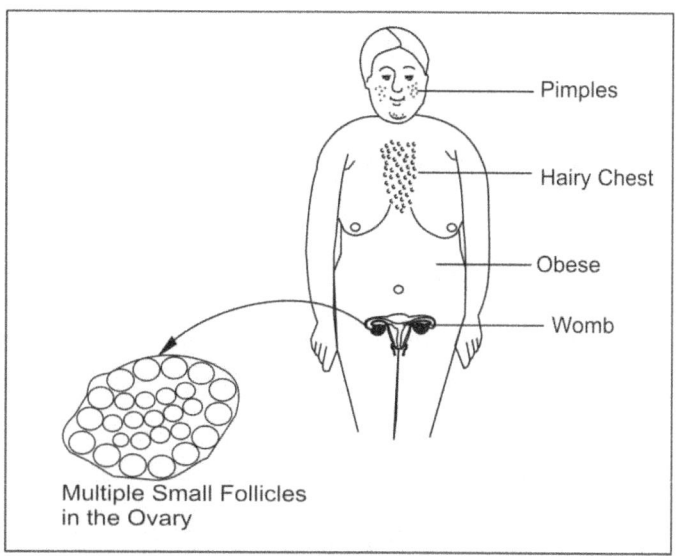

## 3. How common is PCOS in the USA?

PCOS is a common condition that affects 10 – 20% of women between the ages of 18 and 45 years globally. In the USA, about 5 million or more women have PCOS. PCOS is the most common hormonal imbalance associated with infertility globally. According to the Center for disease control and prevention (CDC), PCOS is the most common cause of female infertility in the USA.

## 4. Can PCOS also affect young girls?

Yes. PCOS has been diagnosed in girls as young as 10 years.

## 5. Which complaints are commonly associated with PCOS?

Most women who have PCOS should have 2 or more of the complaints listed below. However, a remarkable percentage does not complain of any problems and they are not sick. PCOS may be discovered during examinations such as an ultrasound scan of the ovaries or blood hormone evaluations. The complaints include:
- Infertility

- Irregular menstruations or no menstruation at all
- Inability to ovulate
- Obesity or overweight
- Excessive hair growth on the body:
  - Face
  - Abdomen
  - Chest
  - Limbs
- Excessive dandruff
- Male pattern of baldness
- Stubborn acne or pimples
- Oily skin
- Skin flaps in the neck and armpit
- Thick dark brownish skin around the neck, on the breast, arm or thigh

## 6. What findings may suggest that I have PCOS?
- Ultrasound scan will reveal enlarged ovaries with:
- Many small cysts or immature follicles. The enlarged ovaries may cause lower abdominal pain or discomfort. The scan may also reveal that the lining of the womb or endometrium is thick.
- Blood work:
  - Elevated leutenising hormone (LH) far and above the level of follicle stimulating hormone (FSH). Usually the LH: FSH ratio will be more than 2:1
  - Elevated androgenic hormones e.g. testosterone, DHEA, androstenedione
  - Elevated insulin due to insulin resistance; this is associated with dark patches of thick skin that looks velvety. The skin patch is called acanthosis nigricans in medical parlance
  - Elevated blood sugar
  - Evidence of no ovulation

## 7. Why does PCOS upset menstruation?
Many women with PCOS have elevated amounts of male hormones or androgens. Male hormones are the hormones that are normally found in higher quantities in males than females. Examples are testosterone, DHEAS etc. The elevated male hormones are not good for the eggs in the ovaries, because they prevent the eggs from attaining proper growth and maturity, like the eggs in normal women. Eventually, small, immature eggs increase substantially in both ovaries and are typically arranged in a circular manner at the outside margin of the ovaries. These eggs are in a male dominated hormonal environment and of poor quality. The name PCO is therefore so derived; it means 'many cysts' in the ovaries.

### 8. What about hirsutism?

The second effect of elevated male hormones (androgens) is the growth of excessive hairs on the body. Androgens cause excessive hair growth in places like the tummy, chest and limbs. Women with PCOS also have male pattern baldness and their hair growth pattern also resembles that found in males.

### 9. Why do women with PCOS fail to ovulate?

In women with PCOS, despite the presence of many follicles, the ovaries lack the required hormones for the follicles to mature. For a normal ovulation, the eggs must be fully mature. Consequently, women with PCOS may rarely ovulate or may not ovulate at all. The hormone called progesterone is also deficient in PCOS women, causing the menstrual cycle to cease or become irregular. When a woman does not menstruate for prolonged periods of time, eventually, the inner lining of the womb becomes thicker than normal. So, women with PCOS do not ovulate, may not menstruate at all and if they do, they are usually irregular.

### 10. When is a woman said to have a Polycystic Ovary (PCO)?

In PCO, there are 8 or more follicular cysts which are arranged like a ring at the outer part of the ovary. The follicles are usually less than 10mm in diameter when viewed with an ultrasound scan. A PCO is not used as a good criterion in diagnosing PCOS because some women who are perfectly normal also have PCO.

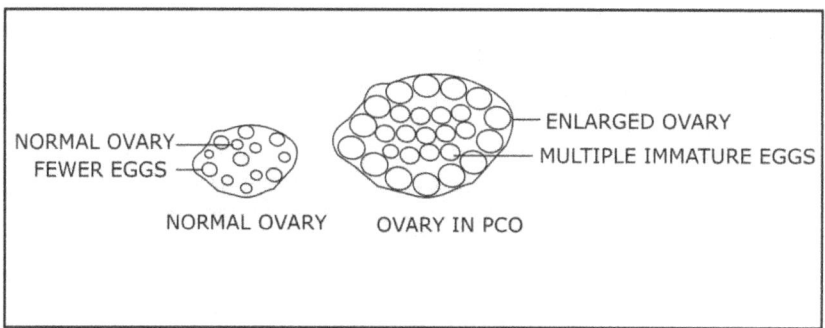

### 11. What are the 2 most important criteria for the diagnosis of PCOS?

The 2 most important requirements are:
- Excessive androgen levels
- Chronic lack of ovulation

## 12. What are the health risks associated with PCOS?

There are some other health problems that women with PCOS may have. PCOS increases the risks of:
- Heart attacks and Stroke
- Increased amount of bad cholesterol
- Hypertension
- Type II diabetes
- Diabetes in pregnancy
- Brief stoppage of breathing during sleep (sleep apnea)
- Endometrial hyperplasia which may lead to womb cancer
- Mental illness – anxiety and depression

## 13. How can I prevent these complications?

It may take some time for doctors to suspect or diagnose PCOS. Most women will present when problems such as infertility are already being experienced. However, the earlier the diagnosis is made and management started, the better the chance of preventing complications or reducing the severity of the condition. Some of the steps that may reduce health risks include:
- Regular exercise and dieting to prevent and reduce obesity, as well as amounts and effects of bad cholesterol
- Early treatment will produce better results with infertility
- Reduced risk of hypertension
  - Reduced risk of heart attack
  - Reduction in the severity of hirsutism
  - Reduced the risk of diabetes

## 14. What is the importance of PCOS in infertility?

In the developed countries like the USA, PCOS is about the most common cause of infertility in women. Globally, PCOS is the most common hormonal imbalance in women. In the developing parts of the world like sub-Saharan Africa, the most common cause of infertility in women is blockage of the fallopian tubes caused by sexually transmitted infections. However, PCOS is also the most important hormonal problem.

## 15. What are the goals of treatment of PCOS?

There are 3 main goals that doctors hope to achieve when managing PCOS. They are:
- To restore ovulation and normal menstruation; this may resolve infertility
- To reduce the severity of excessive hair (hirsutism) and acne
- To prevent the development of endometrial cancer in the womb

## 16. What is the remedy for ovulation problems?

Lack of ovulation is managed by drugs which stimulate the ovaries and promote maturity of the eggs to achieve ovulation. The common drugs in use are:

- Clomiphene: This is the most commonly used ovarian stimulant. It achieves ovulation in the majority of women with PCOS. They are given as tablets and should be prescribed by your doctor
- Follicles Stimulating Hormone (FSH): This is less commonly used; it is useful when clomiphene fails to achieve ovulation. They are given as injections
- Metformin tablets: This is another alternative that is used where clomiphene alone fails to achieve ovulation. Metformin is effective when combined with clomiphene. Metformin is a drug originally used to lower blood sugar in diabetes. Its usefulness in PCOS is probably because many PCOS women have high blood sugar (hyperglycemia). Metformin lowers male hormones in the body and since it also reduces body weight, it is useful in controlling obesity
- IVF: Ovarian stimulation drugs can result in multiple pregnancy with the attendant complications during pregnancy, childbirth and thereafter. Currently, more women undergo IVF as treatment for their infertility. IVF also offers a chance to reduce the incidence of multiple pregnancies by reducing the number of embryos transferred. Even though multiple pregnancy is regarded as risky and undesirable in the advanced world, many women in developing countries, especially in Africa, regard multiple pregnancy as desirable multiple blessings from God.
- Weight loss: Where women are overweight, adequate and controlled weight loss may restore ovulation in some women. Even a loss of 10-15lbs may be helpful. Weight loss usually involves a carefully planned weight loss program involving exercise and dieting, over a period of time. Such programs are usually combined with drug treatment
- Ovarian drilling: This is performed through laparoscopy. This procedure is performed using a diathermy which uses small currents to destroy little portions of the ovary at various points. Doctors believe that ovarian drilling helps to reduce male hormones and facilitate ovulation. This type of procedure is less commonly done on women now because of the availability of more effective treatments that improve ovulation

## 17. What are the remedies for irregular menstruation?

This is commonly treated with family planning pills. This works for most women. It makes the menses come at predictable intervals, most commonly every 28 – 30 days with a normal or reduced flow. If the woman wishes to get pregnant, the family planning pills can be used for a short period of 2 – 3 months and then, fertility treatment can be started by the doctor. This is a common situation because many women with PCOS have infertility challenges and desire pregnancy.

### 18. How is obesity managed?

Obesity is managed via introduction of weight reduction programs. This usually involves:
- Low calorie diets: 1000 – 1500 cal/day
- Diet planning: To reduce calorie intake and increase consumption of vegetables, fruits, whole grains and supplements. Saturated fatty food and processed foods which usually contain salt should be avoided
- Exercise: To burn excess calories and improve overall fitness
- Metformin (Glucophage): Glucophage helps in weight reduction in some women with PCOS. Metformin can be used even if the woman does not have hyper-androgenism or obesity
- Weight control alone may sometimes be all that is required in some cases of PCOS. However, in most cases, weight control is combined with other drug treatments for improved efficacy. These lifestyle modifications should be life-long in order to derive full benefits

### 19. How is the excessive hair growth in PCOS managed?

Hirsutism or excessive hair growth is caused by excessive androgens. Some women are worried by the unusual appearance of excessive hair in many parts of their bodies. However, complaints of excessive hair growth are less than complaints about infertility. There are many ways to deal with excessive hair on the body. These include:
- Drugs: Anti-androgens like finasteride, spironolactone and cyproterone are useful. Anti-androgens reduce hair growth, but they are not approved for this purpose in the USA. However, women who are planning pregnancy or who are already pregnant should be careful about taking anti-androgen drugs because male babies may be feminized in the womb. All women taking anti-androgens should be closely supervised by their doctors
- Creams, such as vaniga can be applied on the face to reduce embarrassing facial hair
- Laser removal of hair is also practiced
- Electrolysis can also be used to remove hair
- Mechanical methods like shaving are appealing to some women

# DEAR DOCTOR:

**20. How do I know if I have PCOS?**

Many women with PCOS are not sick, so they do not have any complaint. The condition is diagnosed more commonly when such women consult their doctors because of infertility or irregular menstruation.

**21. I was diagnosed with PCOS but with my doctor's assistance, I was able to have two children. Now that I have attained menopause, am I risk free?**

Not totally so. It is good that you were able to achieve pregnancies and have children of your own. At menopause, some of the health risks still persist and may in fact get worse. Women with PCOS have higher risks of heart attacks, strokes etc, even after menopause.

**22. My sister was previously diagnosed with PCOS. Does it run in families?**

Yes. PCOS may be found to be more common among women in the same family or close relatives. The explanation for this is not exactly clear. The current thinking is that PCOS may be partially genetic.

**23. Can PCOS affect my pregnancy?**

Yes. Apart from causing infertility, PCOS may affect pregnancy in many ways. The effects on pregnancy include:

- Multiple Pregnancy: Multiple pregnancy is common in PCOS because the ovaries are usually artificially stimulated to produce multiple eggs for multiple ovulation. Some consequences of multiple pregnancy are increased risks of:
  - Miscarriage and abortions
  - Hypertension and eclampsia
  - Gestational diabetes
  - Premature delivery
  - Difficult labor and delivery which may lead to surgical operations
  - Complications in newborn babies

Some of these effects may also be partly due to the drugs used in the treatment of PCOS such as metformin.

PCOS may be the culprit: Aside from the complications that may arise due to multiple pregnancy or drugs, babies of women with PCOS ordinarily have

increased independent risks of complications in pregnancy, childbirth and after birth. These risks include:
- Abortion and miscarriage
- Premature delivery
- Congenital abnormalities
- Neonatal complications
- Neonatal death

**24. Where can I get help if I have PCOS?**

A good idea will be to discuss your challenges with your doctor as much as possible. Sometimes, sharing your concerns with close and responsible persons that you trust can lessen your emotional stress. There are also many support groups in many communities. You should be able to locate one near you with the help of your doctor or clinic.

CHAPTER 9

# Endometriosis and Adenomyosis

*"Hopefully in the next couple of generations.....they're going to have the right treatments and this will no longer be an issue"*

– MOLLY QERIM

### 1. What is endometriosis?

Endometriosis is a medical word that denotes the presence of endometrial tissues outside the womb. The normal location of endometrial tissues is the lining of the womb cavity. In endometriosis, endometrial tissues are found in many other parts of the body, outside the womb cavity.

### 2. How does endometriosis get outside the womb cavity?

Nobody knows. Doctors and scientists are still not sure how endometrial tissues get deposited in the various parts of the body. Few suggestions have been put forward to try and explain this. Some of the suggestions are:

- Embryonic origin - Very early, when a baby is formed in the womb, some cells have the same origin and ability to form other types of cells of the various parts of the human body at any time, if the cells experience the right stimulation. Doctors who believe in this suggestion argue that with the right stimulus, cells that share the same origin with endometrial cells of the womb will undergo the same changes like their counterparts inside the womb, no matter where they are located in the body. It therefore means that if a woman has endometriosis in the ovaries, eyes, brain, etc., when she bleeds during her normal menstruation, there will also be bleeding in the ovaries, eyes, brain etc
- Backward flow - When a woman menstruates, the menstrual blood which contains shed endometrial tissues with glands and other cells, flow out through the vagina. However, if for any reason, the menstrual blood is blocked from coming out, the menses accumulate and then

flow in the opposite direction and eventually through the canal of the fallopian tubes. Once outside the fallopian tubes, the blood can then be deposited on the ovaries, urinary bladder, rectum and other surrounding structures. This suggestion makes sense but it cannot explain the deposits in distant places like the brain

- Transplantation - Some scientists believe that endometrial tissues can be carried from one place to another when a surgeon operates on parts that contain endometrial tissues. This makes sense when we consider endometriosis in old scars of surgery
- Immune system - Some doctors believe that the failure of the immune system of women with endometriosis to destroy endometrial cells located outside the womb is responsible for endometriosis
- Hormones - One of the normal functions of estrogen hormone in the first half of the menstrual cycle in women is to stimulate the growth of the cells of the inner lining of the womb. Because of this function, some doctors believe that endometriosis may be due to estrogen action

There are a few other suggestions but none of these have been able to explain the occurrence of endometriosis at all the sites. So the debate goes on.

### 3. How many layers does the womb have?

The womb has 3 layers. These are the outer, middle, and inner layers. The outer layer is the thin, cellophane–like covering of the womb, while the middle layer is the muscular layer. The inner layer is called the endometrium. The endometrium is made up mostly of glands and other tissues.

### 4. What is the importance of the endometrial layer?

The endometrial layer is where pregnancy attaches to the womb and grows. The main function of the womb is to house the baby during pregnancy. When a woman is not pregnant, she menstruates. Menstruation represents the inability of a woman to achieve pregnancy in a particular menstrual cycle. Of the 3 layers of the womb, only the endometrial layer has the ability to grow back when it is shed. During menstruation, the endometrial layer is shed and comes out as menstrual blood loss or menses. The glands and other tissues immediately start to grow back to form a new endometrial layer. This ability to re-grow is important and efficient to the extent that even if endometrial tissues are located outside the womb, they can grow and also undergo changes that normal endometrial lining inside the womb go through, during a menstrual cycle.

### 5. Where are the common sites of endometriosis?

The most common site for endometriosis is the surface of the ovaries.

Other sites are the:
- Uterosacral ligament, which is a structure that attaches the uterus to the sacral bones at the back of the pelvis
- Fallopian tubes and broad ligaments
- Urinary bladder
- Intestine, especially the sigmoid colon and rectum
- Surface of the uterus, cervix, vagina, and vulva.
- Umbilicus
- Old scars of operation

Less commonly, endometriosis may be deposited in distant organs like the brain, lungs, kidneys etc.

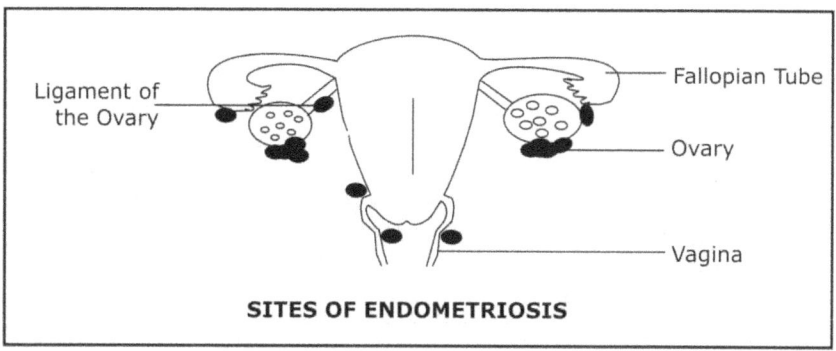

**SITES OF ENDOMETRIOSIS**

### 6. How common is endometriosis?

It is common. Some doctors believe that endometriosis occurs in up to 7% of women, but the actual frequency is not known. Endometriosis is more common in women with infertility. The belief of most doctors in the past was that endometriosis was almost a disease of Caucasian women or the Western world. However, more cases have been seen increasingly in Black women too. Thanks to the availability of equipment and expertise, currently, laparoscopy for infertility is performed more frequently in the developing world. It is estimated that more than 5 million women suffer from endometriosis in the USA alone.

### 7. What age group is more likely to have endometriosis?

Endometriosis is more common in young women in the age bracket of 30-45 years. So, as long as a woman is still menstruating, endometriosis and its various problems remain a possibility.

## 8. What are the risk factors for endometriosis?

There are some identified factors that increase the risk of endometriosis in a woman. These include:

- Race – Caucasian women are at a higher risk of endometriosis than Black women and African Americans
- Infertility - Endometriosis is more common in women with infertility
- Familial - The condition may run in some families. If your mother, sister or close relative had endometriosis, then you may be at a higher risk
- Menstrual patterns - Women who have prolonged duration of menses or short menstrual cycles of less than 28 days are at higher risks of endometriosis

## 9. How does endometriosis cause infertility?

Endometriosis results in bleeding, inflammation and scar formation. Endometriosis reduces fertility potential in the following ways:

- Cyst formation: Each time endometriosis deposits on the surface of the ovary, bleeding occurs and because not all the blood can get out, cysts are formed. With repeated bleeding into the ovary, the blood clots and cakes to various extents. These form characteristic chocolate cysts in the ovaries. They are called chocolate cysts because their contents appear like brown chocolate. The consequence is the gradual destruction of the ovarian tissues including the eggs, so that the fertility potential of the woman is reduced
- Inflammatory response: Endometriosis is associated with formation of extensive scar tissues. Scar tissue can totally cover the surface of the ovary. Therefore, even when eggs are released during ovulation, it is not accessible to the male sperm and fertilization does not take place. Scar tissue also has the destructive effect of gumming organs and other tissues together. When the fallopian tubes are gummed together, it results in tubal blockage
- Poor alignment of the womb: Scar tissue formation may cause the womb to be poorly aligned and its orientation distorted
- Reduced frequency of sexual intercourse: This may be as a result of severe pain experienced by the woman during sexual intercourse. Inadequate sexual exposure is one of the factors that delay pregnancy

## 10. What are the main complaints in women who have endometriosis?

There are many women in the community who have endometriosis without any complaint whatsoever. The condition may be diagnosed accidentally during routine examinations or investigations by doctors. Many cases like this are diagnosed during the procedure of Laparoscopy. The complaints of women suffering from endometriosis largely depend on the part of the body where the deposits are located. The major complaints are:

- Pain - this is the most common complaint. The pain usually occurs during menses. It usually starts just before menstruation, gets to a peak during menses and then reduces gradually. The severity of the pain varies from one woman to another. Pain during menstruation is called dysmenorrhea. The pain may be so great and horrible to the extent that life becomes miserable for the woman during menses. Such women are most anxious as the menses approach. Endometriosis also causes pain during sexual intercourse, if the deposits are around the vagina or rectum. This becomes worrisome if the woman has to abstain from sexual intercourse, in order to avoid pain. Pain may be experienced at other sites including lower back, tummy and when passing urine
- Menstrual problems - Endometriosis can cause spotting or irregular bleeding in between your menses at times you don't expect. You may also experience prolonged and heavy menses. Some women may experience bleeding from sites of endometriosis like the umbilicus or old scars of operations. Bleeding from the belly button may happen suddenly and be embarrassing
- Infertility - Endometriosis is associated with increased risk of infertility. It destroys the ovaries where the eggs are produced and can block the fallopian tubes. In the Western world, about 15% of all women with infertility challenges have endometriosis
- Other complaints - include passage of blood in the urine or stool, diarrhea etc., depending on the location and extent of the endometriotic deposits.

## 11. How common is infertility in women with endometriosis?

Endometriosis is more common in women in the reproductive age group and where it has been diagnosed in such women, as many as 30% also have difficulty in achieving pregnancy.

## 12. What about the pain during sexual intercourse?

Pain during sexual intercourse is called dyspareunia. Sexual discomfort is experienced by quite a number of women with endometriosis. This type of pain is usually felt deep in the vagina and the lower back. Dyspareunia is usually due to endometriosis in the vagina or the rectum. Associated back pain maybe felt when the uterosacral ligament is involved. This ligament joins the back of the womb to the sacral bone of the lower vertebral column. Unless this complaint is properly and quickly treated, it may lead to avoidance of sexual intercourse, which may degenerate into marital disharmony. The doctor must be consulted immediately for remedy.

### 13. What is the association between pain during sexual intercourse and infertility?

Some women have severe pain during sexual intercourse. This is called deep dyspareunia. This pain is due to deposits of endometriotic tissues at the back wall of the vagina and the rectum. Up to 70% of women who experience severe deep dyspareunea also have infertility challenges.

### 14. Is there a relationship between food and endometriosis?

There is no evidence as of now that the consumption of any particular food causes endometriosis. Also, there is no evidence to suggest that if you avoid a particular food, your risk of endometriosis will be lower.

### 15. Can endometriosis be transmitted?

No, Endometriosis is not an infection. It cannot be contracted or transmitted from one person to another.

### 16. What are the modalities of treatment for endometriosis?

Treatment of endometriosis can be through an operation or medically through the use of drugs. These two methods can be combined depending on the type of complaints and the findings of the doctor during investigations. Medical treatment is more popular especially in less severe cases of endometriosis.

### 17. What is the main objective of treatment of endometriosis?

Most women suffering from endometriosis complain of severe pain either during menstruation or during sexual intercourse. A remarkable percentage of such women have difficulty in getting pregnant. Therefore, the two main objectives of treatment are to reduce the pain to the barest minimum and achieve pregnancy faster.

### 18. What is the best treatment for endometriosis?

The type of treatment largely depends on your complaints and whether you desire pregnancy or not. The most important thing is to reduce or stop menstruation so that the endometrial cells responsible for endometriosis are not stimulated. The main options are:

- Drugs - there are many drugs that may be beneficial depending on the type of complaint
    - Hormonal drugs - here pregnancy is not desired, family planning pills are helpful. They are used in a continuous manner such that the woman menstruates less frequently. The endometrium is therefore rested since it is not shed as monthly or cyclical menstruation. Family planning pills are also useful in reducing the amount of blood loss and making the menses occur in a more regular

manner. Gonadotropin releasing hormone agonists (GnRH) are also widely used to treat endometriosis. They work by reducing the amount of estrogen in the body
- Danazol - This is one of the most popular drugs
- Depo-provera
- Aromatase inhibitors
- Analgesics - to reduce pain

- Open Surgery - operations can be performed to remove endometriotic tissues and ovarian cysts in selected cases. During surgery, scar tissues and adhesions are also removed
- Infertility treatment - the gynecologist will assess the condition and make the best treatment plan for achieving pregnancy. Depending on the extent of the disease, the doctor may wait to see if the patient can achieve pregnancy naturally; otherwise, the doctor may stimulate the ovaries and perform assisted conception. This may include intrauterine insemination or in vitro fertilization (IVF). Endometriosis is associated with a lower rate of pregnancy so patience is required while the doctor tries to helps you achieve pregnancy. Ultimately, the doctor will decide which treatment is most suitable for the patient

## 19. Which is the most popular treatment?

The most popular medical treatment of endometriosis is done through the use of gonadotrophin releasing hormone (GnRH) analogs. There are many forms of these hormones. Examples are Buserelin, Goserelin (Zoladex) and Naforelin (Synarel). These drugs are effective but expensive.

Some doctors have achieved good results with the use of oral contraceptives pills taken in a continuous manner. Another important drug used in the treatment of endometriosis is danazol.

## 20. How does GnRh work?

GnRh analogs work by suppressing the hormones of the pituitary gland. Consequently, most women will not ovulate or menstruate. This means that endometrial tissues are not shed for as long as the effect lasts.

## 21. What are the side effects of GnRh analogs?

GnRh analogs have many side effects. The manifestations may vary from one individual to another and the specific type of analog used. Some of the important side effects are:
- Low estrogenic state – which manifests as:
  - Hot flashes
  - Reduced bone mass (osteoporosis)
  - Loss of libido
  - Vaginal dryness

- Androgenic effects – which may manifest as increased:
  - Weight gain
  - Acne or pimples
- Muscle Pain
- Hirsutism or excessive abnormal hair growth
- Male voices - the voice may become more masculine (hoarse and deeper)

## 22. What is danazol?

Danazol is also widely used in the treatment of endometriosis. It is a steroid hormone related to the hormone called testosterone. Danazol is effective in reducing the symptoms caused by endometriosis and the tablets are used daily for a prolonged time, sometimes for over one year.

## 23. What are the side effects of danazol?

Danazol has several side effects including:
- Amenorrhoea
- Acne and pimples
- Weight gain
- Muscle cramps
- Loss of libido
- Hot flashes
- Voice changes
- Hirsutism
- Reduction in breast sizes

## 24. What types of surgery are performed for endometriosis?

Surgery may be performed to investigate pain, determine the extent of endometriosis or the cause of infertility. The types of surgery include:
- Laparoscopy
  - To determine the extent of disease and destroy the deposits as much as possible
  - To reconstruct and realign pelvic organs
- Laparoscopy and Laser destruction of endometriosis
- Surgical severance of nerves in order to reduce pain.

## 25. What is adenomyosis

In the normal womb, the 3 layers have distinct boundaries. This means that the outer, middle and inner layers can be clearly identified. The middle layer is the muscular layer while the inner layer or endometrium consists of glands, blood vessels and lining cells. In some women, the tissues of the endometrium are also found in the middle layer. This means that instead of muscles alone, the middle layer contains pockets of endometrial glands. This condition is called adenomyosis.

## 26. Where in the wall of the womb is adenomyosis more common?

Adenomyosis enlarges the womb and it is most commonly seen in the posterior wall.

## 27. When are women most likely to experience adenomyosis?

Adenomyosis is more common in middle age, usually between 30-50 years.

## 28. With respect to location, what is the difference between adenomyosis and endometriosis?

In endometriosis, the endometrial tissues are deposited outside the womb in organs like the ovaries, surfaces of the urinary bladder, pelvic walls etc. On the other hand, in adenomyosis, endometrial tissues are deposited *inside* the muscular layer of the womb. Adenomyosis is also called endometriosis interna just to emphasis that the deposits are still inside the womb.

## 29. What are the usual complaints that come with adenomyosis?

Many women who suffer from adenomyosis do not have complaints. A higher percentage of these women have had children, but it is usual for some to experience delays in getting pregnant. If there are complaints, the two most likely problems are:

- Pain – The woman may experience pain or lower discomfort during menstruation. The pain typically gets worse during menstruation. The woman may describe it as" cramps" and may be able to localize it to the womb. Occasionally, pain may also occur during:
    - Sexual intercourse
    - Stooling
    - Urination
- Menstruation problems – It is usual for women suffering from adenomyosis to experience heavy menstruation. They may bleed heavily for a prolonged period of time. Sometimes, bleeding may occur in an irregular manner

In addition, women may experience the following:
- There may be stomach upset and diarrhea, but this is less often
- Anemia may be present due to prolonged and heavy menstrual flow
- Some women experience numbness in the fingers and toes

### 30. What is the best way to diagnose adenomyosis?

In 80% of cases, ultrasound scans can sufficiently diagnose adenomyosis. Magnetic resonance imaging (MRI) tests are more accurate but they are far more expensive.

### 31. What are the conditions commonly associated with adenomyosis?

Adenomyosis is closely related to endometriosis. Fifty percent of women with adenomyosis also have endometriosis. Similarly, about 50% of women with adenomyosis have fibroids. While many women with adenomyosis have no issues bearing children and may in fact have had multiple births, in some women, adenomyosis may be associated with infertility. In such women, the rate of miscarriage may be up to 50%.

# DEAR DOCTOR:

### 32. How do I know if I have endometriosis?

There are some features that could make you suspect endometriosis. If any of your close relatives has been diagnosed with endometriosis, then your risk may be higher. Other features include:

- Pain - Complaints of pain during menses, sexual intercourse and lower back pain
- Menstruation - Excessive bleeding during menses and irregular menses
- Infertility - the inability to achieve pregnancy
- Investigations - The doctor may order an ultrasound scan for you, which may detect ovarian cysts and other masses and collections in the pelvis. Sometimes, other forms of imaging like MRI may be done. The most definite test is laparoscopy which is a "look-see" procedure. This will enable the doctor to examine the womb, ovaries, fallopian tubes, urinary bladder and other organs for endometriosis

Despite your suspicions, it is your doctor that makes the final diagnosis. Therefore, it is advisable to see your doctor as soon as you can, so that treatment can start as early as possible.

**33. I experience severe pain during my menses. The doctors have confirmed I have mild endometriosis. If my endometriosis is mild, why then is the pain so severe?**

Your doctor is right. Endometriosis is associated with lower abdominal pain, back pain and pain during sexual intercourse. However, the severity of pain does not always correspond with the extent of endometriosis because some women with extensive endometriosis may have mild pain. In contrast, women with less extensive endometriosis may complain of serious pain. It is not clear why this is so.

**34. Why do I experience pain during sexual intercourse?**

Pain during sexual intercourse is called dyspareunia. Sexual discomfort is experienced by quite a number of women with endometriosis. This type of pain is usually felt deep in the vagina and the lower back. Dyspareunia is usually due to endometriosis in the vagina or the rectum. Associated back pain maybe felt when the uterosacral ligament is involved. This ligament joins the back of the womb to the sacral bone of the lower vertebral column. Unless this complaint is properly and quickly treated, it may lead to avoidance of sexual intercourse, which may degenerate to marital disharmony. The doctor must be consulted immediately for remedy.

**35. Can I get pregnant if I have endometriosis?**

It is possible. This depends on many factors, especially the severity of the disease. However, most women with endometriosis experience delay and difficulty in achieving pregnancy. It is advisable to plan your pregnancy as early as possible, since the disease and its complications may get worse, making pregnancy much more difficult.

**36. Is there any relationship between endometriosis and social status?**

Yes. Endometriosis is common in women of high socio-economic status. Most often, these are affluent single women in their thirties who are yet to bear children. Such women are usually highly educated and tend to place their careers over and above child bearing.

**37. How do I know if I have adenomyosis?**

It is difficult to know because in as many as 30% of women, adenomyosis is diagnosed accidentally, perhaps when the doctor is investigating other diseases or during operations. Many cases of adenomyosis are identified during routine ultrasound scans of the womb.

## 38. What is the ultrasound scan likely to reveal in adenomyosis?

The features that may suggest adenomyosis on ultrasound scans are:
- Small cystic masses in the muscular layer of the womb - these are endometrial glands
- Small, irregular, shiny structures in the muscular layer of the womb- The endometrial plate may also be irregular or crooked. The normal endometrial plate is usually seen as a straight line in the middle of the womb during an ultrasound scan
- Sections of the womb may be seen to be bulging without any clearly identifiable mass

## 39. How can I benefit from treatment of adenomyosis?

If you do not suffer from pain or menstrual upset, you may not need to be treated. It is also possible for doctors to selectively remove identified spots of adenomyosis during laparoscopy. The best treatment for problematic adenomyosis is removal of the womb (hysterectomy). Severe pain during menses may warrant the use of analgesics. The treatment of menstrual upset should be planned and executed by the gynecologist. Some drugs including gonadotropin releasing hormone analogs and family planning pills are beneficial in some cases. However, since many cases are diagnosed accidentally, if you have unexplained pain during menses, menstrual upsets or prolonged delay in achieving conception, you should see a gynecologist for proper assessment and treatment.

# CHAPTER 10
# Infertility

*"From the outside looking in, you can never understand it. From the inside looking out, you can never explain it"*
— SARAH KAY HOFFMAN

### 1. What is infertility?
Infertility is the failure of a couple to achieve pregnancy despite adequate, unprotected sexual intercourse. Usually, the couple should have lived together for at least 12 months.

### 2. What do doctors mean by adequate sexual intercourse?
This means 2-3 occurrences of unprotected sexual intercourse by the couple per week. This should be appropriately timed so that it is more frequent around the time of ovulation. It is therefore important for the woman to be able to identify her time of ovulation. Regarding adequacy of sexual intercourse, it is important that couples live together in harmony.

### 3. Is infertility a disease?
Most people who have infertility challenges are not physically ill. Apparently, they appear to enjoy good health. It is therefore appropriate to regard infertility as a condition rather than a disease. It is more dignifying for doctors to address infertile couples as clients rather than calling them patients. This may also be more pleasant and reassuring to the couples.

### 4. How many types of infertility are there?
Infertility is classified into primary and secondary. Primary infertility means that the woman has never achieved pregnancy in her marriage or relationship. That is, she has never been pregnant before. Secondary infertility refers to a situation where a woman who has been pregnant before finds it difficult to achieve pregnancy again.

## 5. How common is infertility?

Infertility is more common than it appears to be. This is because in many cases, people are not admitted to hospital or confined to bed just because they are infertile. So, unless they decide to visit a hospital or complain to healthcare providers, there is no certain way to identify them. Currently, The Center for Disease Control and Prevention in the USA (2018), estimated that about 6.1 million or 10% of women between the ages 15 – 44 years have difficulty in achieving pregnancy or retaining pregnancy in the USA. Africa and other developing countries of the world bear far greater burdens of infertility. Unfortunately, statistics on infertility is lacking in most developing countries, due to poor health infrastructure and lack of accurate documentation.

## 6. At what time should a couple get worried or seek treatment for infertility?

Normally, 80% of couples achieve pregnancy within the first 12 months of living together. Therefore, a couple should seek help from a doctor if they fail to achieve pregnancy after 12 months of adequate, unprotected sexual intercourse.

## 7. Must couples wait for 12 months before consulting the doctor?

Not always. There are some situations where couples do not need to wait that long. Some women have pre-existing conditions that may prevent pregnancy and might have been diagnosed before marriage. These conditions include:
- Previously diagnosed tubal blockage
- Women who do not ovulate regularly
- Polycystic ovarian syndrome (PCOS)
- Inappropriate lactation
- Other hormonal imbalance problems
- Menstruation problems
- Multiple uterine fibroids
- Endometriosis and adenomyosis
- Advanced age at marriage - already 30 years or above
- Past history of frequent miscarriages or unintended abortions in previous relationships.

Some men also have conditions that were diagnosed before marriage. These may require urgent attention and include:
- Low sperm count, low motility, or abnormal sperm forms
- No sperm at all
- Erectile dysfunction

The list above is not exhaustive but in all such circumstances, the doctor should be consulted as early as possible. Starting infertility treatment early may facilitate pregnancy, so once you are married you should forge a common front to resolve infertility issues. Unfortunately, some women would rather hide these problems from their husbands due to the uncertainty about what the man's reaction may be.

## 8. At what age is a woman maximally fertile?

In women, the chance of achieving pregnancy is greatest in the late teens and early 20s that is, between 18 and 24 years of age. Fertility declines with age and after 35 years this chance is remarkably reduced.

## 9. Who is to blame for infertility, is it the woman or the man?

Unfortunately, in certain communities, women are usually blamed by men for being the causes of infertility. This is not fair, because women are responsible in just 30% of cases. Men are equally, responsible in 30% of cases. The man and woman are jointly responsible in another 30%. These sum up to 90% of all cases of infertility. The cause of infertility is unknown in the remaining 10%. Since men are as guilty as women, public health education for couples regarding the causes of infertility is very important and men should be encouraged to cooperate and support their wives in order to achieve good results.

## 10. Why do some men blame women for their inability to get pregnant?

This blame has no basis, but this attitude is more common in Africa and other developing countries. It is a way of intimidating women in marriage and should be discouraged. Many men claim that they had had children previously by other women or got impregnated some women in the past, before they got married. This is selfish and may not be valid. Only a DNA paternity test can conclusively tell which man truly owns a pregnancy.

## 11. Is it true that some cases of infertility cannot be treated?

Yes, it is true. After thorough investigations, a small percentage of infertile couples will still have their problems unresolved. Such infertility cases are referred to as being idiopathic or of unknown cause. This is the situation in about 10% of cases of infertility. For this category, assisted reproductive technology (ART) or test tube baby technology (IVF) may be appropriate. For unresolved cases child adoption may be considered. Unfortunately, many couples go from one hospital to another looking for solutions until financial resources are exhausted and advanced age has crept in. In developing countries, IVF acceptance is growing but adoption is still largely unpopular. This situation requires proper public education in order to increase awareness and acceptance of IVF and other available options.

## 12. Does sexual behavior have a part to play in infertility?

Women who have multiple sexual partners run a higher risk of contracting sexually transmitted diseases. These may lead to pelvic inflammatory disease (PID) and tubal blockage, which is the most common cause of infertility in developing countries.

## 13. What causes tubal blockage?

Tubal blockage is the most common cause of infertility in females in most developing countries. More than 45% of cases of infertility are due to tubal blockage. This is due to the high prevalence of sexually transmitted infections (STI) caused by the following:

- Gonorrhea
- Syphilis
- Chlamydia infections
- Trichomonas infection
- Staphylococcus infection
- Others - Although it is rare, tubal blockage can sometimes be congenital or inherited. Occasionally, while still in the womb, female babies may be exposed to drugs such as diethylstilbestrol and as such, could risk damage and mal-formation of their reproductive organs.

## 14. What are the complaints that may suggest tubal problems?

Although tubal blockage may not be linked to specific complaints, they are one of the long term consequences of genital tract infections. Most women with tubal blockage have had recurrent episodes of sexually transmitted infections resulting in PID, with the attendant copious, foul smelling vaginal discharge and waist pain. Such patients typically have multiple sexual partners or past histories of criminal abortions and their condition is discovered in hospital, when they complain about their inability to become pregnant.

## 15. What are the treatment options for blocked tubes?

When one tube is blocked, in theory, the chance of pregnancy is reduced by 50%. When the two tubes are blocked, the chance that a woman will achieve pregnancy naturally is zero, because it is impossible for the sperm to come in contact with the female egg. So, fertilization cannot take place. In the past, the remedy was to unblock the canal by forcefully blowing water or gas through the tubes. Some doctors also perform operations in order to open up the lumen of the tubes. Sometimes, the blocked aspect may be cut and the good ends joined together. One of the cut ends may also be re-implanted into the womb. All these measures are old-fashioned and performed less often now, because they yield poor results. Assisted reproductive techniques (ART) or more commonly In Vitro Fertilization (IVF) is now available in many parts of the world. In vitro fertilization (IVF) is currently the best treatment when both tubes are blocked.

### 16. What is Hysterosalpingogram?

Hysterosalpingogram or HSG is an X-ray test done to check the patency of the tubes and the state of the womb cavity. Tubal blockage is the most common cause of infertility in developing countries and HSG is an important test in the investigative process.

### 17. What alternative is there to HSG?

Laparoscopy and dye tests are not only good alternatives to HSG but are also superior to HSG in diagnosing tubal blockage. In this procedure, a small cut is made under the navel through which an instrument called a laparoscope is passed. This instrument pipes light into the tummy and facilitates a direct view of organs like the tubes, ovaries and womb. During the procedure, which is usually performed under anesthesia, a dye such as methylene blue is passed though the cervix and tubes. In a normal patent tube, the dye flows through the tubes, spilling over at the far end near the ovaries, thus enabling a direct view of the dye. A doctor can then confirm tubal patency and rule out tubal blockage. Pelvic adhesions, hydrosalpinx, ovarian cysts, abscesses, and endometriosis can also be corrected simultaneously and the conditions of other pelvic structures equally assessed.

### 18. Which complaints are likely indications of ovulation problems?

Perhaps it is right to say that the most common complaint in women who have anovulation (medical term for the inability to ovulate), is infertility. Many women with anovulatory cycles only get to know of the problem when they go to hospital to investigate their infertility. However, there are a few complaints that may suggest that a woman is probably not ovulating. These include:
- Irregular menstruation
- Excessive and inappropriate breast milk secretion outside pregnancy and breastfeeding
- Absence of signs of imminent ovulation like wetness, stretchable cervical mucus, rise in basal body temperature and mid cycle ovulation pain. These signs are presumptive and some women do not experience them.

### 19. Are there any simple tests or signs that may indicate whether or not ovulation has taken place?

There are some simple tests that may suggest ovulation. These include:
- Cervical mucus

- Basal body temperature: This should be done early in the morning on waking up. The temperature should rise by about 1oc over the readings of the days preceding ovulation, if ovulation has occurred. In environments where infections and febrile illnesses such as malaria and typhoid fever are common and the literacy level is low, the value of basal body temperature as an ovulation monitoring method is reduced
- Use of urine dip stick: Luteinizing hormone (LH) testing can also be done on your early morning urine at about the mid cycle to detect the LH surge. This shows up as a typical color change in the strip which suggests ovulation. Such strips are widely available in most pharmacies
- One-sided low abdominal pain at mid cycle. This pain may be due to ovulation from the ovary on the same side
- These are all indirect tests of ovulation. The surest evidence that ovulation took place is when pregnancy is achieved

## 20. What is the appearance of cervical mucus discharge during ovulation?

At the time of ovulation, the discharge is much increased, more watery and quite elastic. It can be stretched between the fingers and women feel generally wet. With experience, many women who ovulate regularly can recognize this type of mucus. However, non-recognition does not always mean that ovulation has not taken place.

## 21. Why do some women fail to ovulate?

There are certain prerequisites that must be met for ovulation to take place and they involve three important structures. These are the:
- Hypothalamus
- Pituitary gland
- Ovaries

In order to understand their relevance, let us consider their roles.

The hypothalamus is the command center for the pituitary gland. It sends commands to inhibit or enhance the release of the hormones of the pituitary gland. Its functions can be adversely affected by diseases, physical stress, emotional upsets, and drugs. The pituitary gland produces hormones that stimulate the eggs in the ovaries. Many of these eggs develop every month, one, or occasionally more, matures and is released during ovulation at every cycle. So, the main function of the ovaries is to produce eggs. When things go wrong with the hypothalamus, pituitary, or the ovaries, their functions may be adversely affected. Depending on the severity of the problem, the chances of ovulation may be reduced. Sometimes, ovulation may not occur at all because of a variety of problems, including:
- Hypothalamus problems:

- Infections - encephalitis and meningitis
- Tumors or space occupying masses including cancers
- Physical stress - highly demanding sports, energy sapping work schedules
- Emotional stress or upsets - grief due to the loss of a husband, social and financial insecurity, un-met official and personal goals
- Pituitary problems:
  - Infections
  - Tumors – microadenoma, which causes excessive prolactin hormone secretion
  - Pituitary failure – which may follow severe blood loss
- Ovarian problems:
  - Hormonal imbalances - polycystic ovarian syndrome (PCOS) and hyperprolactinaemia
  - Infections
  - Ovarian failure
  - Pre-mature menopause
  - Resistance ovary - when eggs are insensitive to follicle stimulating hormone
  - Tumors or deposits in the ovary - ovarian cysts, endometriosis, tuberculosis, destruction of the ovary by talcum powder and cancer
- Other reasons are:
  - Endocrine disorders - thyroid disorders especially hypothyroidism
  - Drugs
  - Contraceptives
  - Injectables
  - Anti-cancer drugs
- Severe or chronic illnesses:
  - Cancer
  - Tuberculosis
  - Severe sickle cell anemia
  - Uncontrolled diabetes
  - Chronic blood loss
- Severe weight loss, less than 25% of the ideal body weight, starvation, anorexia nervosa
- Severe weight gain or obesity is also associated with anovulatory cycles
- AIDS

It is obvious therefore, that if a woman cannot achieve pregnancy because she does not ovulate, she must see the doctor for proper evaluation and treatment. Unfortunately, many women resort to self-help by procuring all sorts of un-prescribed drugs especially clomiphene citrate.

**22. Doctor, is it true that fallopian tubes may not be efficient even though they are not blocked?**

Although the most common problem linking fallopian tubes to infertility is tubal blockage, there are some infections that destroy the lining of the tubes without blocking the canals. Consequently, cells lining the tubes can no longer help in sperm and embryo movement and nourishment. This is the situation in genital tuberculosis. Women should therefore bear in mind that tubes must be patent as well as functional. This is an important consideration for doctors when evaluating the HSG X- ray films of the fallopian tubes of infertile women.

**23. Are there any drugs that can help restore ovulation?**

Yes, but most of the drugs work by stimulating the ovary or reducing hormonal imbalance, e.g. clomiphene, parlodel and other ovulation enhancing injections. However, you should realize that these drugs should be used only if they are prescribed for you by the doctor. You should also know that the inability to ovulate is just one of the causes of infertility. There are many other reasons for infertility. You are therefore advised to see your doctor for proper evaluation of your condition and appropriate treatment. The following list comprises the common drugs that women with infertility challenges are likely to be given depending on the cause of infertility.

- Clomiphene citrate tablets – It works by stimulating the ovaries
- Follicle stimulating hormone (FSH) injection. This stimulates the follicles in the ovary, ripening them in readiness for ovulation at about mid cycle. They must be prescribed by the doctor
- Gonadotropins -The Human urine of women who have attained menopause contain high concentrations of FSH and LH. These hormones are extracted from the urine and given as injections to stimulate the ovaries in the treatment of infertility. Gonadotropins can also be synthesized in the laboratory and given as injections
- Gonadotropin releasing hormone (GnRH) - is naturally produced by the hypothalamus in the brain. GnRH is also synthesized in the laboratory. It acts to release FSH and LH from the pituitary gland. FSH stimulates the ovary
- Bromocriptine – Excessive amounts of the prolactin hormone in the blood prevents ovulation and is called hyperprolactinemia. Bromocriptine (Parlodel) reduces the level of prolactin in the blood and enhances ovulation
- Metformin - Some women have a condition called polycystic ovarian syndrome (PCOS). One of the features of this syndrome is insulin resistance, which results in high insulin concentration in the blood.

This condition is called hyperinsulinemia and the use of metformin enhances ovulation in women with PCOS

## 24. How effective is clomiphene in resolving ovulation problems?

In about 70% of women, ovulation is achieved with the use of clomiphene tablets only. Of these, pregnancy occurs in 40% of women. When clomiphene fails to resolve ovulation problems, other drugs can be used as already listed. The most popular alternative is Follicle stimulating hormone (FSH) injections.

## 25. For how long can I continue to take clomiphene?

Clomiphene is a good drug that is widely used for ovarian stimulation. However, it is suspected that when the ovaries are stimulated in multiple cycles for a long time, the result is chronic ovulation of multiple eggs, leaving the ovary heavily depleted. Secondly, the risk of cancer of the ovaries may be increased. Consequently, it is recommended that clomiphene should not be used for more than 6 months or 6 consecutive cycles. Unfortunately, this very important drug has been subjected to great abuse by some women in their quest to achieve pregnancy. They buy various brands of clomiphene citrate over the counter without doctor's prescriptions and worse still, such women use the drug wrongly and for a prolonged time.

## 26. What are the side effects of clomiphene?

Women on clomiphene may experience some side effects. The side effects experienced vary from one woman to another. The important common side effects include:

- Hot flashes: About 10% of women will experience sudden occurrence of hotness and sweating while on clomiphene
- Distension or bloating of the tummy with a general feeling of weight gain
- Breast pain: About 2% of women on clomiphene complain of breast tenderness, pain, or discomfort
- Mood swing: The mood changes between dullness to excitement and irritability. At such times, the woman may complain that she feels just sick without being able to give any tangible reason
- Dizziness
- Headache: This may be experienced by some women. Severe headaches which are associated with vision problems or migraine are dangerous. Once this type of complaint happens, the doctor must be told immediately. This type of headache usually warrants that the drug be discontinued
- Hair loss: Some women experience loss of hair while on clomiphene. This is known as alopecia in medical parlance
- Multiple pregnancy: In up to 5% of women, use of clomiphene will result in multiple pregnancy. These are either twins or sometimes

more, which in some developing countries, are regarded as multiple blessings. Medically speaking, multiple pregnancy is associated with higher risks of complications to the mother and babies. The best situation is to be pregnant with one baby at a time.

## 27. How serious or dangerous can these side effects be?

Clomiphene should not be used unless it is prescribed and supervised by a doctor. Despite its benefits, incessant or prolonged use is dangerous because apart from leaving the ovaries exhausted, it may have other harmful long term consequences.

The severity of the complaints vary from mild, moderate, to severe depending on each woman. Any complaint must be made to the doctor or health care provider as soon as possible. However, a complaint of blurring of vision called scotoma, requires immediate stoppage of the drugs because it may lead to serious health consequences including blindness. The doctor must be informed immediately.

## 28. How does clomid cause cancer?

The reason is not clear, but there is a growing concern among doctors and scientists that prolonged use of clomiphene may result in a higher risk of ovarian cancer due to incessant ovulation. Devastated ovaries may also lead to other major health consequences.

## 29. What is hyperprolactinemia?

This is a medical word that means excessive amounts of prolactin in the blood. High prolactin levels suppresses ovulation, causing infertility.

## 30. What are the causes of hyperprolactinaemia?

There are many reasons why a woman may suffer from hyperprolactinemia. The majority of cases occur for unknown reasons and are said to be idiopathic or of unknown cause. The most Important reasons are:
- Tumors:
  - Bronchogenic cancer
  - Cranio-pharyngioma
  - Pituitary stalk tumor
- Infections:
  - Meningitis
  - Encephalitis
- Stress: Emotional and physical
- Drugs:
  - Sedatives and tranquilizers, e.g. chlorpromazine and diazepam
  - Anti-anxiety of amytriptiline

- Anti-hypertensives: e.g. methylidopa, resepin
- Cardiac drugs
- Cimetidine
- Metoclopropamide
- Diseases:
  - PCOS
  - Endometriosis

## 31. How does one test for hyperprolactinemia?

After interviewing a woman and performing a physical examination of the breast, doctors usually require hormonal estimations or hormonal profiles. The most important is the estimation of blood prolactin values; values above the normal range confirm hyperprolactinemia.

Most women with hyperprolactinemia usually visit the doctor with one or more of these complaints:

- Inappropriate milk secretion from the breast
- Irregular menstruation
- Inability to conceive

## 32. What are the treatment modalities for hyperprolactinemia?

The most common drug used to reduce blood prolactin level is bormocriptine (parlodel). This drug reduces prolactin secretion from the pituitary gland. When the prolactin level is reduced to normal, the woman may resume ovulation spontaneously and the menses should become regular once more.

Sometimes, the level of prolactin may be extremely high. In this situation, doctors usually want to ensure that such a high level is not due to a tumor of the pituitary gland in the brain which produces prolactin. It is common to request a computed tomography (CT) or X-ray of the skull to ascertain if this is true. In many cases, such tumors result in a remarkable enlargement of the pituitary gland. In this situation, an operation is performed to remove the tumor or trim down the size of the pituitary gland. This is a delicate operation performed by specialist surgeons.

## 33. Is it possible for a woman to menstruate without ovulation?

Yes, it is quite possible to menstruate even when ovulation has not taken place. This type of menstruation is regarded as anovulatory menstruation and is more common in obese women, young adolescents in the immediate years following puberty, and those with hormonal upsets. Women who have regular menstruations are more likely to experience normal ovulation, so irregular menstruation may be a pointer to the fact that a woman is not constantly ovulating.

## 34. What are the side effects of Parlodel?

Women on Parlodel (bromocriptine) do complain of various side effects. Some are common while others are less common and individualized. The more common side effects include:

- Headaches
- Dizziness or drowsiness
- Tiredness
- Dryness of the mouth
- Stuffy nose
- Loss of appetite
- Nausea and vomiting
- Stomach problems:
  - Stomach pain
  - Constipation
  - Diarrhea
- Inability to sleep
- Tingling sensations
- Numbness and cold fingers
- Mood change, anxiety, and unhappiness
- Blood pressure: may cause hypertension or hypotension depending on the individual

## 35. With respect to infertility, what are the major differences between developed and developing countries?

In most developed countries, the environments are clean and the prevalence of sexually transmitted infections are much lower, so problems like tubal blockage are much less common. Secondly, women live longer in developed countries. This means that more women will experience difficulty in ovulation because ovulation generally becomes more difficult and irregular in older women. The third reason is that whereas most African women get married early, and tend to have simple life styles, in the developed world, women tend to get married later in life because of career issues and they have more complex and stressful lifestyles. Physical and emotional stress prevents ovulation.

## 36. Is there any age at which pregnancy is not possible?

The recommended optimal time for pregnancy is from about the age of 22 up to 34 years but in a practical sense, any girl who has started menstruation, and any woman that is still menstruating and ovulating can become pregnant. Consequently, pregnancy is possible in healthy women, between the ages of 11 and 52, if ovulation can still take place. However, when a young girl starts to menstruate, for the first few cycles, she may not produce eggs, so the chance of pregnancy is less at this time. Such cycles are said to be anovulatory. For this same reason, older women do not get pregnant easily around the time of menopause but it is advisable to practice family planning, in order to prevent unwanted pregnancies.

### 37. What are the causes of infertility in women?
The causes are many, but they can be summarized as follows:
- Ovulation problems
  - Failure of egg production and release
  - Failure of egg and sperm to meet each other
- Failure of embryo transport
- Failure of embryo to attach to the womb and grow (implantation failure)
- Inadequate sexual intercourse or wrong timing of sexual intercourse

Under each of these sub-headings there are various causes. In the African environment, the commonest cause of infertility is tubal blockage caused mainly by sexually transmitted infections. In most parts of the developed world like the USA and other western countries, the most common cause of infertility is ovulation problems.

### 38. What are the high-risk factors that increase infertility in women?
There are several, including:
- Stress - physical stress from hectic work schedules, grief and other emotional upsets
- Substance abuse:
  - Tobacco
  - Alcohol
  - Heroin, cocaine, etc.
- Obesity
- Excessive weight watching or being underweight which may affect models and fashion conscious ladies. Anorexia nervosa, a medical condition in which young girls and women have deliberate aversions to food, is more common in the developed world. This is, to the extent that some are so afraid of adding weight that they repeatedly force themselves to vomit deliberately. They also engage in acts like putting their fingers into the back of their throats to cause irritation and vomiting. The goal is to remain slim or avoid getting fat at all cost
- Sexually transmitted infections - which are more common in women with multiple sexual partners, can result in pelvic inflammatory disease (PID) and tubal blockage, when poorly treated or neglected

### 39. Which chronic illnesses may increase the risk of infertility?
Some long standing illnesses can increase the risk of infertility or worsen the existing condition, if treatment is delayed.

These include:
- Chronic PID
- Uncontrolled diabetes
- Genital tuberculosis
- AIDS
- Thyroid gland disorders like Hypothyroidism and Hyperthyroidism

## 40. Does yeast infection cause infertility?

Yeast infections of the genital tract are common in women and may result in a troublesome, itchy sensation and offensive odor. However, it does not usually cause tubal blockage or infertility.

## 40. How do fibroids cause infertility?

Fibroids can cause infertility in 2 main ways:
- Due to their size and locations: If the fibroids are big and located near the junction between the tubes and the womb, they may sit on the tubes and compress them, causing tubal blockage. When fibroids are located right inside the womb cavity, proper implantation of the embryo becomes difficult
- Fibroids may also cause severe bleeding: This may result in early pregnancy losses. Unfortunately, many women wait until fibroids have grown to very big sizes before seeking medical help or even accepting treatment

## 41. Does staphylococcus cause infertility?

Staphylococcus is a germ which is harmful to the genital tract. However, the role of staphylococcus as a cause of infertility has been over-publicized in some communities, especially in sub-Saharan Africa. Despite causing genital tract infection, staphylococcus is not a prominent causative germ of severe PID that commonly leads to tubal blockage. Germs like Chlamydia and gonorrhea are more notorious for causing PID and tubal blockage.

## 42. How does polycystic ovarian syndrome (PCOS) affect infertility?

Polycystic ovarian syndrome (PCOS) is the most common form of hormonal imbalance in women. In the developed countries like the USA, the disturbance of ovulation due to diseases such as PCOS is the most common cause of infertility in women. When women have PCOS, they have plenty of immature, poor quality follicles in a male dominated hormonal environment, which creates an abnormal situation for the proper development of female eggs. In the developing parts of the world like sub-Saharan Africa, the most common cause of infertility in women is the blockage of the fallopian tubes, while PCOS is the most important hormonal problem.

### 43. Does weight affect fertility?

Obesity is a significant public health issue which is more rampant in the affluent and developed countries. Severe obesity has negative impacts on several organs and systems in the body. Obese women have a higher risk of experiencing ovulation problems ranging from irregular ovulation to complete stoppage of ovulation for long periods of time. Many women also suffer from other associated disorders that link weight to menstruation complaints.

### 44. What lifestyles or occupations can lead to infertility?

There are many lifestyles that may negatively affect fertility in women. These include:
- Obesity
- Smoking
- Alcoholism
- Deliberate excessive weight loss
- Stress
- Use of talc powder around the waist area
- Undue delays in getting married
- High socio-economic status
- Multiple sexual partners
- Limiting body weight like run-way models
- Drugs: Many drugs, especially those used in the treatment of cancer, destroy eggs
- Infections: Some male occupations increase the risk of sexually transmitted infections. These include long distance truck drivers who frequently have casual, unprotected sexual intercourse. Such men may then pass these infections to their spouses.

### 45. How does lifestyle and occupation affect infertility?

One of the occupational or lifestyle issues is the negative effect of stress on infertility. The hypothalamus is the command center that signals the pituitary gland in the brain, to release follicle stimulating hormone (FSH) and leutinizing hormone (LH). Both are needed to stimulate the ovaries to produce eggs for the purpose of ovulation. Since the hypothalamus is highly sensitive to physical and emotional stress, tension in any form can cause dysfunction of the hypothalamus which may result in the disruption of ovulation.

### 46. How do infections and cancers of the pituitary cause infertility?

Infections disrupt the production and release of stimulating hormones from the pituitary gland. The non-release or inadequate release of the follicle stimulating hormone and the leutinizing hormone, may result in inadequate stimulation of the ovaries. This means that, for as long as the infection remains untreated, the woman will experience anovulatory cycles.

Sometimes, she may fail to menstruate altogether. Cancers invade and destroy ovarian tissues so that the quantity of eggs and secretary capacity of the ovaries are reduced. Some cancers are also known to secrete hormones like prolactin which leads to hyperprolactinemia and subsequent suppression of ovulation.

### 47. Does having crawling sensations all over the body cause infertility?

No. This is not a recognized cause of infertility. It is more or less a psychological issue in infertile women. Similarly, some women feel that hotness in the lower abdomen may be the cause of their infertility. These reasons may underline the intensity of their emotional or psychological desires to achieve pregnancy. In all cases of doubts, the doctor should be consulted for evaluation and treatment.

### 48. Does watery sperm cause infertility?

No, this is also not an identified cause of infertility. In fact, a normal semen sample should liquefy or become watery within 1 hour of ejaculation. If this does not happen, it is possible that the semen quality is poor. Imagine that it is easier for a fish to swim inside water than mud. Thick semen is like mud. It reduces the ability of sperm cells to swim, yet the sperm cells need to swim fast enough and straight, to meet the eggs for the purpose of fertilization.

### 49. If the sperm flows out of the vagina soon after intercourse, can this cause infertility?

No, it does not. However, semen regurgitation from the vagina is a common complaint by many infertile women in developing countries. Ejaculation is a forceful and spontaneous act. Once semen is deposited in the vagina, the sperm cells swim so fast, that within seconds, millions of sperm cells are already well on their way in the cervical canal and onward into the womb and fallopian tubes. In 30 minutes, sperm can be found in the fallopian tubes. The amount flowing out is of no clinical significance. It is perfectly normal and women who do not have infertility issues will most probably confirm that they experience semen regurgitation too. Those who are worried about this may stay lying down for a while after sexual intercourse but remember not to waste precious time trying to figure out how to solve this problem because it does not contribute in any way to infertility.

### 50. When the womb bends backward, does it cause infertility?

No, it does not. This condition is called retroversion of the uterus or womb. Retroverted wombs may cause low back pain and waist pain or discomfort especially during menstruation, but not infertility.

### 51. Does excessive weight cause infertility?

Yes, there is a relationship between obesity and infertility. In excessively fat women, poor ovulation and irregular, infrequent menstruation are common. For these reasons, infertility is more common in obese women.

### 52. Can severe weight loss reduce my chance of pregnancy?

Yes, severe weight loss, perhaps due to illness, excessive exercise, starvation or deliberate vomiting called anorexia nervosa, may result in the inability to ovulate or menstruate. This happens when the body weight drastically falls below the ideal body weight. In order to ovulate, women need at least 17% of body weight as body fat while about 20% of body weight as fat is needed in order to menstruate normally. So, women suffering from severe weight loss and excessively slender women may experience difficulty in ovulation and menstruation.

### 53. Does breast milk outside pregnancy or breast feeding cause infertility?

Yes, about 30% of women who have such inappropriate breast milk secretion do not ovulate regularly and have problems with menstruation. This means that not all women who suffer infertility do so because of excessive milk secretion. Unfortunately, many women and quacks over-emphasize this condition, and waste precious time trying to dry up the milk in the breasts, when in actual fact, it may not be the cause of infertility. Women who experience this problem should see their doctors for proper investigation and treatment.

### 54. Does diabetes cause infertility?

Diabetes is an important systemic illness and a significant public health issue globally. If diabetes is well controlled, it should not affect fertility. The issue with diabetes in most developing countries is that many diabetic women report late to hospital. In such cases, complications would have set in, making pregnancy difficult and more risky.

### 55. Does hypertension cause infertility?

There is no direct relationship between controlled hypertension and infertility. Severe hypertension may upstage the body systems and have a damaging effect on other body functions. So, well-controlled hypertension should ordinarily not affect fertility.

### 56. What about thyroid gland enlargement?

When the thyroid gland is functioning below normal, the condition is called hypothyroidism. In severe hypothyroidism, ovulation and menstruation may stop, leading to infertility. When the gland is functioning above normal, the condition is called hyperthyroidism. In this condition, menstruation may become irregular, scanty or stop completely. If the woman becomes pregnant, there is an increased risk of abortion and the growth of the baby in the womb may be impeded. This may also result in intra uterine fetal death.

### 57. What is endometriosis?
The inner lining of the womb is called endometrium. The endometrium is typically shed regularly during menstruation. Endometriosis is a condition where the endometrial tissues are present outside the womb cavity. In the past, doctors in Africa and other developing countries used to think that endometriosis was more common in Caucasians than Black women. However, more laparoscopies are being performed to address infertility in many developing countries, so more women are now diagnosed with endometriosis.

### 58. What are the common sites for endometriosis?
The ovary is the most common site where endometriosis forms cysts filled with brownish fluid, which appears like chocolate. Other pelvic structures like the utero-sacral ligaments of the womb, pelvic peritoneum, urinary bladder, umbilicus and bowels may be involved. Externally, endometriosis can be found at the navel and old operation scars in the abdomen.

### 59. Does endometriosis cause infertility?
The reason for the appearance of endometrial tissues outside the womb is unknown, so the answer to this question is not clear. However, endometriosis is associated with serious scar formation in the pelvis and other sites. Scar tissues could lead to distortion of female reproductive structures which may result in reduced fertility. Of course, endometriosis destroys the ovaries and reduces ovarian reserve, which will in turn, reduce ovulation and affect fertility.

### 60. What is PCOS?
PCOS is an acronym for polycystic ovarian syndrome. This is a condition seen in women mostly in the child bearing age group. Women with PCOS more often present to the doctor because of their inabilities to achieve conception. The clinical features or complaints in majority of women with PCOS are:
- Infertility
- Anovulation
- Amenorrhea and Menstruation upset
- Obesity or overweight
- Excessive hair growth
- Many small immature follicles or cyst in the ovaries

### 61. What are the complaints in women with endometriosis?

The condition is associated with infertility and therefore infertility may be the main reason that brings a woman to the doctor. Other complaints include heavy menstruation and moderate to severe waist pain during menses. Some women may experience pain during sexual intercourse. The pain is usually described as 'deep' in the pelvis or waist. At the time of menses, there is bleeding at the sites where the endometriotic tissues are deposited. So, some women may bleed from the umbilicus and abdominal operation scars etc. The bleeding normally stops when menstruation is over. Many women with endometriosis may not have any complaint and the condition may be discovered accidentally during laparoscopy or surgery.

### 62. Who are those more likely to suffer from endometriosis?

Those who commonly suffer from endometriosis include:
- Caucasian girls and women between 25 to 40 years of age. It is less common in Blacks
- Infertile women; those who have never been pregnant before and women of low parity
- Women of high socioeconomic status, professionals, and the wealthy

### 63. What is oligospermia?

Oligospermia means low sperm count. This is a medical term used to describe a situation where the sperm concentration in the ejaculate is less than 15 million per ml. When the concentration is less than 5 million per ml, the man is said to have severe oligospermia. In such circumstances, the couple may find it difficult to achieve pregnancy naturally, unless the condition is treated.

### 64. What are the causes of low sperm count?

There are many reasons why a man may have low sperm count. In some cases, the reason may not be apparent after extensive investigations. In such cases, the low sperm count is said to idiopathic. Some genetic diseases are associated with low sperm count:
- Idiopathic
- Genetic
- Familial
- Infection
- Hormonal problems
- Systemic diseases
- Stress
- Lifestyle: smoking, alcoholism etc.
- Environmental issues
- Drug abuse

### 65. What is the solution to low sperm count?

The remedy for low sperm count depends on the identified reason, although in a remarkable percentage of men with low sperm count, the cause may not be apparent. Current technology can however be helpful and there are various treatments:

- Infections: Many cases of low sperm count are due to genital tract infections, especially the sexually transmitted infections. For such infections, proper diagnosis and early treatment with appropriate antibiotics usually restore or improve sperm count
- Drugs: there are some drugs that stimulate the production of sperm cells. In appropriate cases, such drugs may be prescribed by the doctor after thorough investigations
- Life style modifications: In cases where low sperm count is due to environmental conditions like hot temperatures such as bakers and fish mongers, a change or modification in work routines like staying away from heat, may improve sperm count. In the same manner, stoppage of cigarette smoking and excessive alcohol consumption may also improve sperm count
- Surgical Operations: This may be necessary in some instances. The reduction of blood vessels around the testis may be necessary to improve sperm formation and sperm count
- Intra-cytoplasmic sperm injection (ICSI): This procedure is performed as an integral part of an IVF procedure. It is useful and can be deployed to achieve good fertilization in many people with moderate to severe low sperm counts. Similarly, intra-uterine insemination (IUI) can be done to achieve pregnancy in cases of mild and some cases of mild to moderate low sperm counts

Other treatment modalities generally derive from individual cases. For example, a man may experience low sperm count as a side effect of drugs prescribed for other reasons or as part of an ongoing illness. Such cases are amenable to the stoppage of the offending drugs or treatment of the illness.

### 66. What is Azoospermia?

This medical terminology is used to describe a situation where a man has no sperm in the ejaculate. This means that when seminal fluid analyses (SFA) are performed in the laboratory, no single spermatozoon will be found. This condition is worse than oligospermia. In this type of situation, donor sperm may assist women to get pregnant through intra uterine insemination (IUI) or IVF.

### 67. What is SFA?

SFA is an acronym for seminal fluid analysis. It is the most important test that enables men determine whether or not they are infertile. When doctors advise men to examine their semen in a laboratory, they are interested in 3 important parameters which were approved by the World Health Organization (WHO) in 2010.

These are:
- Sperm Count: This refers to how many sperm cells are contained in 1ml of the seminal fluid. Normal seminal fluid should contain at least 15 million sperm cells per ml. When the count is less than 15 million, it is referred to as low sperm count.
- Motility: This refers to the ability of the sperm cells to move. In a normal seminal fluid, 32% of sperm cells should be motile and exhibit fast and forward movements.
- Morphology: This refers to the percentage of normal forms that is contained in 1ml of seminal sample. In a normal seminal sample, at least 4% of the sperm cells should be normal in appearance.

Count, motility, and morphology are the 3 most important parameters of a semen sample. Other less important parameters include volume, total count, and the pH of the seminal fluid sample.

## 68. What are the World Health Organization (WHO) parameters?

Some parameters were agreed upon in 1999 but in the light of new scientific evidence, they are now obsolete.

The minimum values of the most important parameters of both the 1999 and 2010 seminal fluid analysis, as defined by the World Health Organization (WHO), are depicted in the table below:

| PARAMETER | (WHO, 1999) | (WHO, 2010) |
|---|---|---|
| Volume | 2ml | 1.5ml |
| Count or concentration | 20 million/ml | 15 million/ml |
| Motility | 50% | 32% |
| Morphology | 14% | 4% |

The WHO (1999) parameters were taken as the standard by all doctors before the WHO (2010) parameters were implemented. Some doctors still use the WHO (1999) parameters, especially in the developing countries. The WHO (2010) parameters are now being used because the parameters were arrived at by studying the sperm parameters of over 4000 fertile men, a far larger sample size than the 1999 studies. The WHO (2010) parameters are now regarded as standard in interpreting SFA results by doctors.

## 69. What is ICSI and how can it help men with fertility challenges?

ICSI is an abbreviation for intra cytoplasmic sperm injection. It is a procedure used in the treatment of men with severe low sperm count or motility, during IVF. In a typical or routine IVF procedure, about 75,000 high quality motile spermatozoa or more are needed for every single female egg or oocyte, from which only one will penetrate and fertilize the egg. This explains why millions of good quality spermatozoa are needed for normal fertility in men, who require a minimum concentration of 15 million per ml of seminal fluid. Since this may be impossible for men with low sperm count, during an ICSI procedure, a special inverted microscope with a micro manipulator is used to pick one high quality spermatozoon at a time. This is then injected into one female egg. In this way, the number of spermatozoa needed is equal to the number of eggs available. For example, if 10 eggs need to be fertilized, only 10 good quality spermatozoa are required and for 12 eggs, only 12 spermatozoa are needed. ICSI is now generally regarded as a universal IVF solution to low sperm count.

## 70. How many types of ART are there?

ART is an acronym for assisted reproductive technology. Assisted reproductive technology (ART) encompasses all the procedures performed to artificially facilitate fertilization of the female eggs by sperm cells or generate embryos in the laboratory. The types of ART currently available include in-vitro fertilization (IVF), gamete intra-fallopian transfer (GIFT) and Zygote intra-fallopian transfer (ZIFT). Intra-uterine insemination (IUI) is a procedure commonly performed by many doctors to treat infertility, but strictly speaking, IUI is not an assisted reproductive technique. It is a medically assisted conception procedure.

## 71. What other procedures are involved in ART?

There are a few additional procedures that are done in order to improve the success rate of IVF. A particular procedure is only chosen if the doctor is convinced that it will help. The common ones include:

- Intra-cytoplasmic sperm injection (ICSI): This is the solution to low sperm count
- Percutaneous epididymal sperm aspiration (PESA): During this procedure, sperm cells are aspirated from the epididymis through a small incision in the skin of the scrotum
- Testicular sperm extraction (TESE): Sperm cells can also be extracted from the tissues of the testis, especially when the sample from PESA fails to yield any sperm. PESA is normally performed before TESE
- Others include:
    - Hysteroscopy: To assess the womb cavity
    - Laparoscopy: to assess the pelvic and abdominal organs

## 72. Does tubal flushing or 'washing of the womb' help women become fertile?

No, it does not. Many women believe that washing or cleaning up the womb mostly through D&C will help them to achieve pregnancy. Actually, having a D&C done when there is no need may permanently damage the inner lining of the womb. Such women may stop menstruating because the layer being shed regularly during menstruation has mistakenly been scraped off during D&C. Do not insist on washing your womb if the doctor has not said so. Many women run into problems because they take counsel or advice from friends, relatives or quacks who are equally ill-informed.

## 73. What procedures are likely to be recommended before an IVF cycle is embarked upon?

Some women may need to undergo special investigations during the period before their IVF treatment cycles. These investigations may be needed to ascertain diagnosis or to correct problems in the womb, ovaries etc. Investigations such as sonohysterography (SONOHSG), laparoscopy, and hysteroscopy are the most important procedures commonly performed. During SONOHSG, a little quantity of sterile water or saline is instilled into the womb under direct view with the aid of an ultrasound scan. This test is used to assess the womb cavity for problems like fibroids, polyps, and adhesions. It also ascertains whether the cavity expands well or not. The Hysteroscope is an instrument which pipes light into the cavity after fluid has been instilled into the womb enabling accurate assessment. Some minor repairs like removing adhesions or small fibroids can be carried out at this time. During laparoscopy, a little incision is made under the belly button, to create a pinhole through which the laparoscope is passed into the abdominal cavity for direct visual access. Some minor surgical procedures may be carried out during laparoscopy, all of which improve the chance of success in IVF.

## 74. What is IVF?

IVF is an abbreviation that means In Vitro Fertilization. It is a highly technical procedure for the treatment of couples with infertility challenges. In this procedure, the woman and her husband first undergo investigations to determine the cause of infertility in order to choose the appropriate type of IVF. During IVF, the woman is given drugs which make her produce many eggs. Her womb also undergoes some preparations at the same time, to make it suitable for pregnancy. When the eggs in her ovaries are mature enough, they are removed or aspirated with a special needle. The eggs are then processed and mixed with the sperm of her partner in the laboratory and the mixture placed in an incubator. In 16 to 24 hours, a check is conducted to see if fertilization has taken place and embryos have developed. While the embryos develop further, they divide several times to form many human cells and a few of the good embryos (1 to 3) are then replaced in the womb. Two weeks after embryo transfer, a pregnancy test is carried out to determine whether or not pregnancy has occurred. If it turns out negative, then the procedure is deemed to have failed.

### 75. Is IVF an operation?

No, IVF is not an operation. Some of the procedures involve taking injections but the most painful aspect of IVF is the egg retrieval process, during which eggs are removed from the ovaries. For this procedure, patients are given a powerful pain killer injection to minimize pain. All the other procedures are not as painful and do not justify rejection of IVF. The advantages of IVF are far greater than the minimal pain.

### 76. What is the success rate of IVF?

Generally, the success rate of IVF is 15 to 35% depending on many important factors. These include the age of the woman, the quality and quantity of eggs, cause of infertility, the quality of the man's sperm and the quality and number of embryo replaced in the womb. The skills and experience of attending personnel, available equipment and overall quality of the program at the particular IVF center are also important factors. Success rates vary from one center to another and even in the same center, there may be significant differences between IFV batches.

Success rates are higher:
- In young women less than 35 years of age
- In couples with unexplained infertility
- When donor eggs are used
- With donor sperm generated embryos when the husband's sperm quality is very poor
- When blastocysts are transferred

Where there are repeated IVF failures, it seems that the greater the number of previously failed cycles, the lower the possibility of pregnancy in subsequent treatment cycles, unless the causes of such failures can be identified and corrected ahead of the repeat IVF treatment.

The chance that a woman will achieve natural pregnancy in any particular month is about 20%. Even if a couple takes their chances on a monthly basis for 12 consecutive months, the highest chance of achieving pregnancy naturally is 80%. It never gets to 100% percent. Since to some extent, reproduction in human beings is a wasteful process, the success rate of IVF is higher than the chance of achieving pregnancy naturally. The big difference and disadvantage is the high cost of IVF across the globe.

## 77. What are the major complications of IVF?

To a large extent, IVF is safe. The major complications are few. The most important is the ovarian hyper-stimulation syndrome (OHSS). OHSS occurs once in a while during IVF treatment cycles. In most cases, the OHSS is mild. If detected early, progression to severe OHSS may be avoided or prevented. Other complications that may occur during IVF include:

- Infections, especially while taking multiple injections and during egg retrieval from the ovaries
- Pain and abscess at injection sites
- Hemorrhage or bleeding during egg removal
- Side effects of the drugs used - dizziness, headache, nausea or vomiting
- Anemia or shortage of blood may occur as a side effect of the steroid drugs used
- Heartburn
- Amenorrhea - a small number of patients may experience a delay in menstruation or may fail to menstruate, if they have been down-regulated in a long protocol ovarian hyper-stimulation. Menstruation usually returns spontaneously as a rule but the period of waiting represents a time of great anxiety for many women
- Weight gain and bloating may be experienced by some women mainly as a result of the drugs used

Other side effects are minor and most probably individualized.

## 78. Can diseases be transferred through the IVF process?

It is important that embryos transferred during IVF are as healthy as possible so donors of sperm and eggs are made to undergo tests to exclude important diseases that could be transferred or inherited. These include genetic anomalies, hepatitis, syphilis, HIV infection, diabetes and tuberculosis. Blood groups (ABO and Rhesus), physical stature, appearance, complexion and educational attainments, are also taken into consideration. In some IVF centers, couples are allowed to bring their own donors or choose from a pool of donors but donors still need to be tested to ensure that they are safe and healthy.

## 79. I understand that OHSS is a dangerous complication in IVF. Can you please explain?

OHSS means ovarian hyper-stimulation syndrome. In the treatment of infertility, doctors normally give women drugs or injections to stimulate the ovaries in order to produce many eggs. This is routinely done during IVF, with the aim of producing just about the number of eggs needed, usually 7 to 12. Sometimes, a woman may produce too many eggs, far in excess of what is needed, most probably due to high dose of the ovarian stimulation drug or the woman's unique flare-up reaction, even to the usual dose. Normally, each stimulated or developing follicle produces a hormone called estrogen as it grows; the more the eggs, the more the estrogen produced. In OHSS, the woman has so many developing eggs, each producing estrogen. Hence both ovaries become abnormally enlarged and this causes lower abdominal pain or discomfort. There is excessively high estrogen in the blood. The exact cause of OHSS is still unclear but the features or complaints are well known. The important complaints include:

- Lower abdominal pain or discomfort
- Abdominal bloating or enlargement – the ovaries are enlarged and there is fluid collection in the tummy. This partially accounts for the bloating and pain
- Nausea (feeling of vomiting) and vomiting
- Dehydration: partially due to nausea, vomiting
- Fluid collection in many parts of the body
- Breathlessness - which may be as a result of fluid collection in the chest, strapping of the diaphragm by fluid in the tummy
- Electrolyte imbalance
- Weakness, fainting attacks and collapse may occur in severe cases
- Rarely, death may result if there is delay in recognizing or treating this syndrome

Unfortunately, the severity of OHSS is increased with worse consequences, if the woman becomes pregnant during the same IVF treatment cycle. Although there are not many major complications with IVF treatment, OHSS is one of the most significant.

## 80. What are GIFT and ZIFT?

In GIFT, gametes are deposited in the fallopian tube for fertilization to take place. After fertilization, the zygote produced continues further embryo development, as it is transported down the tube and eventually implanted in the womb.

In ZIFT, the fertilized egg or zygote is deposited in the fallopian tube. Further development of the embryo takes place down the tube on its way into the womb where it implants.

## 81. What is the role of IUI?

IUI is an acronym for intra-uterine insemination. In this procedure, the ovaries are stimulated with drugs such as clomiphene citrate. The aim is to produce about 2 to 3 eggs in both ovaries, which are monitored with ultrasound scans. Once the eggs are mature, an injection of human chorionic gonadotropin (hCG) is given, which causes ovulation within 2 days. Ovulation is usually confirmed by testing the woman's early morning urine with a dip stick test, to ascertain whether the LH surge, which normally happens at ovulation, has taken place. If ovulation is confirmed, then sperm cells from the husband or donor are further processed to get a better quality. The processed sperm is then deposited through a narrow tube into the womb cavity, from which it swims through the tubes to meet and fertilize the female egg.

IUI is performed in the following situations:
- Where the fallopian tubes are patent
- Where the husband has only minor problems with the sperm, e.g. low sperm count, fair morphology, and fair motility
- Cases of unexplained infertility

Where the husband's sperm is of very poor quality, a donor's sperm may be used or the couple is counseled for IVF with an intra-cytoplasmic sperm injection (ICSI).

## 82. What is meant by ovarian hyper stimulation?

Ovarian stimulation is one of the major steps in the treatment of infertility in women. The aim is to cause the ovaries to produce many mature eggs or follicles which can then be fertilized. In IVF, the aim is to produce an even greater number of eggs, 10 – 12 at a time. To achieve this, more effective or potent drugs are used at higher doses and for a longer duration than in IUI. This is called ovarian hyper stimulation. This is necessary in order to get a good number of high quality eggs that can be fertilized to produce an equally good number of high grade embryos. Unlike natural conception, where one embryo is desired, in IVF, 1 - 3 embryos may be replaced in the woman's womb with the probability that 1or 2 will implant. Lastly, ovarian stimulation is done in women who are infertile because they do not ovulate naturally for so many reasons. In many countries, the use of some ovarian stimulation drugs has been abused by many women, who resort to self-help and procure over the counter drugs. Apart from the danger inherent in using drugs that are not prescribed, such women invariably suffer self-inflicted adverse effects. The most widely abused drug in this category is clomiphene citrate, which is well known to most women. Clomiphene is recommended for use when indicated and for not more than 6 cycles. Chronic or extended use of clomiphene means prolonged stimulation of the ovaries, which not only seriously deplete the eggs but may also cause cancer of the ovary. Women are therefore advised to desist from such detrimental practices and seek their doctor's opinions rather than resorting to self-help.

# DEAR DOCTOR:

**83. Are children conceived through IVF as normal as children conceived naturally?**

There is no evidence at present to suggest that children conceived through IVF have more abnormalities than children born through natural conception. In vitro fertilization (IVF) children are normal and studies are currently going on in different parts of the world that focus on the medium to long term follow up of IVF children, to see if there could be associated abnormalities. At the present time, the general belief is that IVF is safe.

**84. Is there any age limit for women who wish to have IVF?**

Practically speaking, there is no age limit. Many women, in fact, have stopped menstruating or gone past the age of 50 years before accessing IVF. However, the woman must be medically fit to carry a pregnancy. Singleton pregnancy, as opposed to multiple pregnancy is better, even though from experience, women in this situation would want to have multiple pregnancies, in order to recover lost grounds. Pregnancy at old age is a high risk venture and must be managed as such, under specialist care. There are a few cases of women who have had successful IVF pregnancies in their 60th decade but it is not desirable to get pregnant beyond 45 years of age. In some countries, IVF is well regulated and the oldest age at which IVF is offered is often stated.

**85. If IVF fails, what else can be done since it seems to be the last option for me?**

One of the challenges of IVF treatment is what to do when it fails, especially when huge amounts of money have been spent. The psychological trauma and negative reactions are enormous, although these issues are usually explained to the couples during counseling sessions before and after each treatment cycle. Most couples would accept a repeat IVF treatment cycle after a period of rest. The cost is remarkably reduced, if frozen embryos are used for the repeat cycle. Many clinics also have policies that guarantee reasonable discounts on the cost of repeat IVF cycles. The question of what to do when there are repeated failures of IVF is problematic. Sometimes, the solution may be to use donor eggs, donor sperm or donor embryos if the couples are well disposed to these. Where failed treatments are due to problems in the womb or unknown reasons, using a younger surrogate may achieve success. When all else has failed, couples may be counseled for child adoption.

## 86. Is it advisable to try for multiple pregnancy during IVF treatment?

Singleton pregnancy is better than multiple pregnancy in terms of outcomes, for both baby and mother. Singleton pregnancy is associated with less risk during pregnancy and childbirth. With multiple pregnancy, almost all pregnancy-related risks are higher and worse. In the developed countries, the goal of pregnancy is to bear one baby at a time. Doctors regard multiple pregnancy as a complication or mistake because the higher the number of babies in the womb, the higher the risks. In some cultures, the socio-cultural orientation is such that many people regard multiple pregnancy as multiple blessings from God and in fact, pray for such. Some doctors transfer about 3 embryos during IVF just because all may not survive. However, sometimes 2 or more may survive, leading to multiple pregnancy. The rate of multiple pregnancy in IVF may be up to 20% or higher in some parts of the world. This is currently a great challenge to doctors. In the developed countries, there are strict regulations guiding the number of embryos that can be transferred at a time. The objective is to prevent multiple pregnancy in order to avoid the complications and cost.

## 87. Can I use IVF to select the sex of my baby?

The goal of IVF is to achieve conception and put smiles on the faces of couples with infertility problems; not minding whether the baby is a boy or a girl. In the civilized world, this is the norm. However, the sex of a baby may become important in cases of sex-linked or sex related diseases. This is because in some diseases, the sex of a baby may determine whether he or she will inherit the disease or not. In such instances, it is appropriate to determine the sex of the unborn baby very early in pregnancy so that the couples involved can be counseled and treatment instituted. Other important inherited or genetic diseases are also diagnosed at this time. Sometimes, this may require terminating the pregnancy. The process of prenatal diagnosis usually involves performing procedures like chorionic villus sampling (CVS) which entails the examination of samples of the placenta. Amniocentesis which entails the examination of fetal cells in the liquor early in pregnancy is another method. Some biochemical tests may also be done. These are usually done between the 9th and 14th weeks of pregnancy. Major complications of these procedures are infection, bleeding and abortion. In vitro fertilization offers the doctor the opportunity to diagnose these diseases and ascertain the sex of a baby much earlier, within the first 2-3 days after fertilization in the laboratory, through a genetic testing process called Pre-implantation genetic diagnosis (PGD). This enables the successful transfer and or replacement of embryos of the desired sex and those free of diseases. PGD can therefore be used to select embryos that are free of sickle cell disease, cystic fibrosis, female or male gender embryos. It also avoids the dilemma of having to terminate pregnancy because the replaced embryos have been pre-selected before pregnancy. This is a clear advantage over CVS and Amniocentesis. In some parts of the world, couples ask for IVF to be done just for the purpose of gender selection, for purely socio-cultural reasons, usually to select the male sex for reasons like lineage propagation and property inheritance purposes. This practice is common in parts of the world where a premium is placed on the male child and is clearly a serious form of gender discrimination that should be discouraged. In vitro fertilization should not be performed for the sole purpose of sex selection and with appropriate counseling, it is possible to persuade some couples to see children as invaluable gifts, irrespective of their gender.

### 88. Can IVF babies be delivered naturally or must delivery be through an operation?

IVF pregnancies are just as normal as natural pregnancies. Women who are pregnant through IVF can deliver normally without a Caesarean section. Operations are not compulsory unless there are medical grounds, however, many couples commonly request for Cesarean sections due to the circumstances surrounding their struggles to achieve pregnancy. These couples persuade the doctor to go the extra mile and do everything to ensure that the mother delivers safely. This emotion is understandable and the pregnancy can be described as a "precious pregnancy". Two other reasons which make Caesarean operations more common in IVF pregnancies are:

- Advanced age of mothers: In many cases, women who achieve pregnancy through IVF, are already above 35 years of age. For some of these women, normal labor is high risk and complications may develop rapidly. After thorough appraisal, the doctor may advise an operation
- Multiple pregnancy: The likelihood of multiple pregnancy is higher in IVF. This is because many doctors transfer more than one embryo. Multiple pregnancy has a higher risk of complications during pregnancy and delivery, including the death of both mother and baby. Although operations are more commonly performed in IVF pregnancies, caesarean sections are not compulsory unless the doctor thinks it is necessary.

### 89. If I go through IVF treatment, must I still undergo IVF for subsequent pregnancies?

Whether you will need to do IVF in subsequent pregnancies or not, depends mainly on the reason for your previous IVF. If you had your IVF because both fallopian tubes were blocked, then the only way to achieve pregnancy again will be through IVF. Seek your doctor's advice as soon as you are ready, for guidance.

There are some situations when repeat IVF may be a smarter and faster way to achieve pregnancy. Such situations include:

- Old age: many IVF patients are advanced in age and it may be unwise to waste more time trying to achieve pregnancy on their own. They

may need to decide as early as possible because success rates reduce greatly with advancing age
- Distant couples: In situations where couples live far away from each other and can rarely be together, the man's semen can be frozen and used for repeat IVF treatment cycles. This reduces logistic troubles, time and costs for the couple
- Left-over embryos: If there are frozen or left over embryos from the previous cycle, it is natural to use them for a repeat IVF cycle. This is much cheaper and wastes less time. In some cases, the reason for the first IVF may be corrected spontaneously, thereby normalizing ovulation problems due to hormonal imbalances. You may then be able to achieve pregnancy on your own

### 90. How can I improve my chances of success in IVF treatment?

Here are some of the tips that may help:
- Decide early: Once the doctor has confirmed that IVF is the appropriate treatment for you, do not waste precious time going from one hospital to another looking for alternatives, only to accept IVF when you are much older. All things being equal, success rates are higher in younger women
- Use of donor eggs or sperm: Your egg is as old as your age. Eggs of older women are more likely to be genetically abnormal and have less potential for pregnancy. Eggs from younger females are usually of higher quality with higher fertilization rates and they produce better embryos. So, you should accept a donor egg program if the doctor thinks it is a better option. Many women reject this important advice for sentimental reasons. In the same vein, don't refuse donor sperm, simply because you want your baby to resemble you
- Quality of program: The success of your program also depends on the quality of care. Ensure that you enroll in a high quality program at a center with a high success rate. Sometimes, this may mean paying a little more but it is better than wasting your hard earned funds. Get yourself the best because expertise, experienced personnel, equipment and treatment protocols are all important issues that affect the success of IVF programs. Ask questions and obtain as much information as you can before you commit yourself to the program. Also remember that big names may sometimes not be the best. Some smaller IVF centers may have better success rates and may be cheaper too.

### 91. I am 40 years old and have been scheduled for IVF. The doctor advises donor eggs because of the risk of having an abnormal baby. Is he correct?

Yes, your doctor is right because we regard any age above 35 years as advanced maternal age. The risk of abnormal births rises significantly, after women are 35 years old, due to increased genetic problems. Apart from abnormal babies, eggs from older women are more likely to produce low quality embryos, so attaining pregnancy is more difficult. It is therefore better to use eggs donated by younger women.

### 92. Can I have IVF treatment if I have fibroids?

Yes, you can. Although about 40% of fibroid cases are associated with infertility, after surgical removal about 40% still achieve pregnancy. The important considerations are the locations of the fibroids and their sizes. There are three places where fibroids can be located; the outer wall of the womb, the middle wall, and inside the womb cavity. Fibroids located inside the womb cavity may adversely affect pregnancy, especially if they are big. Fibroid is largely a disease of Africans or Black people and are 9 times more common in Black women than Caucasians. It is not uncommon to see African women with huge multiple fibroids. Despite this, some do achieve pregnancy but many do present with infertility. Fibroids are like sitting tenants in the womb with more rights of occupancy over the baby. Often, fibroids disallow pregnancy from coexisting. During the assessment period for IVF, the womb cavity is usually carefully appraised to see if the location and size of a fibroid will adversely affect pregnancy. This assessment is commonly done by an ultrasound scan. If it is adjudged to be capable of affecting the chance of pregnancy, the doctor may suggest its removal through an open surgical operation called myomectomy. In some cases, a hysteroscopy, which enables a clear view of the inside of the womb, is carried out and the fibroid removed if necessary.

### 93. What is surrogacy?

The term surrogacy is used in IVF when a woman carries a pregnancy which legally belongs to another couple. This means that the woman has consented to carry the pregnancy on behalf of the couple with the full knowledge that she has no legal right of ownership of the baby after delivery. The carrier woman's eggs are fertilized using the sperm of the man in the laboratory. The embryos generated are then placed in the carrier's womb and she carries the pregnancy on behalf of the couple. The woman who carries the pregnancy is called a surrogate. Sometimes, the embryos are produced using the eggs of the owner or donor egg and sperm of the husband or donor sperm. The embryos are then replaced in the womb of another woman, who carries the pregnancy. In this case, the woman is called a pregnancy carrier. The important difference between a surrogate and a pregnancy carrier is that because the surrogate's eggs are used, it means she has a genetic relationship to the baby. A pregnancy carrier only carries the pregnancy; she has no genetic relationship with the baby. She is only a carrier. A couple may need a carrier or surrogate if the wife has serious medical problems where pregnancy will endanger her life. Other reasons include previous removal of the womb through surgery or a womb filled with multiple large fibroids. It may also be considered in other instances such as repeated failures of IVF, when reasons for the failures are not known. Women who are advanced in age or would rather not go through pregnancy, may also be considered for surrogacy. In all cases, appropriate consents and legal documentation by both parties are mandatory, to forestall future disagreements over ownership of the child.

### 94. Who will a child born through surrogacy resemble?

Generally speaking, a child either resembles the father or mother or a little bit of both. If a donor egg is used with your husband's sperm, the baby has about 50% chance of resembling your husband and an equal 50% chance of resembling the egg donor. If your eggs are used with a donor sperm, there is also a 50% chance that the child will resemble you or the sperm donor. However, if you have embryos produced by donor sperm and donor eggs, the chance that the baby will resemble any of you is theoretically zero. Despite this, surrogacy is still better than adoption. Even where the embryo is a product of a donor egg and donor sperm, surrogacy is likely to bring better parent and child bonding and a greater sense of ownership, since the baby begins life with the parents. These advantages are absent in adoption as bonding and affection depend to a large extent on the age of the child at the time of adoption and the degree of integration with the family. Finally, adoption is about a baby while surrogacy and pregnancy carrier issues are about pregnancy.

### 95. If embryos are frozen, will the babies still be normal?

Yes, embryos, sperm and eggs can be frozen and preserved in a special freezing chamber, to be used when they are needed in the future. Embryos and sperm can be preserved for 5 years and beyond in a good IVF facility. Perhaps the major disadvantage of using frozen embryos is that pregnancy rate is slightly reduced when compared with fresh embryos. However, babies conceived from frozen embryos are just as normal as those from fresh embryos.

### 96. What are the reasons for freezing embryos?

There are several good reasons why embryos may be frozen. These include:
- Excess embryos: More embryos may be produced in the laboratory, than what the doctor can transfer to the woman's womb at once
- Unavoidable delays: Sometimes, during IVF treatment, conditions may develop which either make embryo transfer inadvisable or dangerous, for example, the woman may suddenly become ill. In such cases, embryo transfers are delayed till a more appropriate time
- Cost: In cases where there are an excess number of embryos, the woman may use the frozen embryos at intervals when she desires pregnancy. This is cost effective, as she will not need to undergo

- extensive preparation like she did previously. Sperm and female eggs can also be frozen for future use
- Distance: Where couples live apart, embryos, sperm and female eggs may be frozen, to be used when desired

## 97. I am 48 years old and still menstruate, so why does the doctor suggest that I use donor eggs for my IVF?

Menstruation and ovulation are two different things and some women menstruate but do not ovulate. Since they do not release eggs, they cannot become pregnant. So, the fact that you still menstruate does not mean you ovulate or have good eggs that can be used for IVF. At 48 years of age, you are most likely to have a poor ovarian reserve and donor eggs should be more appropriate for you.

Invitro fertilization treatment is usually commenced after thorough investigations of the couple. During the IVF process, you will undergo tests to see if your ovaries can still produce a sufficient number of good quality eggs. If the investigations show that you have a poor ovarian reserve, then the doctor will most likely advice that higher quality donor eggs be used. These eggs are usually obtained from younger women with very good ovarian reserves. One advantage is that eggs from young women are usually qualitative and quantitative, thus producing a sufficient number of high grade embryos.

## 98. So, what happens when there are excess embryos?

Sometimes during IVF, an excess number of embryos are produced and the question of what to do with them becomes important. The best situation, of course, is to freeze and preserve them, so that the couples can make use of them if the need arises in future. Alternatively, the couple may save the embryos by consenting to donate them to other couples who need them.

## 99. Why is the cost of IVF so exorbitant?

All over the world, the expensive nature of IVF is an issue. This is more so when you consider that conception occurs naturally and freely for about 80% of couples who don't pay a dime! The cost of IVF varies from one part of the world to another, from one clinic to another and from one IVF program to another. The overall cost depends on the type of IVF program and other factors. Routine IVF is the cheapest but when more extensive investigations are carried out or additional procedures are performed, the individual costs of these procedures inflate the final cost. The quality of program, rating of an IVF center and the caliber of personnel are also important contributors. So most times, costs are personalized. Couples should have aa rough estimate of the cost of their intended IVF program from the onset, in order to avoid dropping out due to financial reasons. The general thinking is that costs will drop further in the future, as facilities become more available and equipment and consumables become cheaper.

### 100. Are there ways of reducing the high cost of IVF?

Yes, there are a number of strategies that can be deployed in order to reduce the cost of IVF programs. These strategies can be applied where appropriate, according to the type of program being planned. The strategies are:

- Start your treatment early: There are some key issues that determine the type or combination of an IVF program. Chief among this is the age of the woman. This is important with respect to her ovarian reserve. Many young women have good ovarian reserves and can use their own eggs for the program. This saves the costs of donor eggs or embryos in most cases. So, the decision must be taken as early as possible. The second issue is the cost of drugs. In most cases, older women need higher doses of drugs for longer durations. This invariably adds to the cost of treatment
- Egg sharing: If you must use donor eggs for your IVF procedure, ask your doctor if you can enroll in an egg sharing program with another couple, instead of singlehandedly paying for donor eggs. This may reduce the cost of donor eggs by as much as 50%
- Donor embryos: If your program requires donor eggs and donor sperm, you may also ask your doctor if donor embryos are available
- Frozen embryos: If you have excess embryos from a current cycle, it's a good idea to ask your doctor if you can freeze them, so the frozen embryos can be used in subsequent cycles. This will save you the cost of drugs used for hyper-stimulation, the pain of having to take so many injections as well as not going through the egg retrieval process
- Use of less expensive but effective drugs: Some drugs, especially those used in stimulation are cheaper and less expensive. Ask the doctor if alternative and cheaper drugs or protocols are appropriate for your program
- Sharing of personnel between centers: Key personnel such as embryologists may be shared between centers through cooperation. Also, equipment for cryopreservation and pre-implantation genetic diagnosis may be done at different centers instead of investing in such expensive equipment and underutilizing them. This measure may translate into cheaper costs across many cooperating centers.

### 101. Despite the high cost, why is the success rate of IVF so low?

The success rate of IVF is generally 15 to 35% and depends on many factors. These include the age of the woman, the quality and quantity of eggs, the cause of infertility, the quality of sperm and the quality and number of embryo replaced in the womb. Also, the skills and experience of attending personnel, equipment available and overall program quality at the particular IVF center are important factors. Success rates vary from one center to another but there may be significant differences between IVF batches, even in the same center. Success rates are higher:

- In young women less than 35 years
- In couples with unexplained infertility
- When donor eggs are used
- With donor sperm generated embryos, when the husband's sperm quality is very poor
- When blastocysts are transferred

Where there are repeated IVF failures, it seems that the greater the number of previously failed cycles, the lower the possibility of pregnancy in subsequent treatment cycles, unless the causes of such failures can be identified and corrected ahead of the next IVF treatment.

The chance that a woman will achieve natural pregnancy in any particular month is about 20%. Even if a couple takes their chances on a monthly basis for 12 consecutive months, the highest chance of achieving pregnancy naturally is 80%. It never gets to 100%. Since to some extent, reproduction in human beings is a wasteful process, the success rate of IVF is higher than the chance of achieving pregnancy naturally. The one big difference and disadvantage is the huge financial cost of IVF.

## 102. How soon can one embark on a repeat IVF treatment?

People can access IVF treatment facilities as many times as possible depending on age, level of fitness, results of previous IVF and whether or not you are using donated eggs or donated embryos. It is however very important to give good intervals to rest the body well in between IVF treatment cycles. If repeat cycles are due to previously failed cycles, your doctor will most certainly like to investigate the cause of such failures before embarking on another cycle. Sometimes, a repeat treatment in a different but better equipped center may achieve good results but generally, an interval of 6 months or more is adequate. If you **are** using donor eggs, donor or frozen embryos, you could have repeats as many times as possible, once the doctor confirms that it is appropriate to do so. However, if you are using your own eggs, a repeat of 3 to 4 times is healthy, but the cycles should be well spaced. In situations like this, frozen embryos are more appropriate. This will not only enable you to have repeat IVF cycles at more convenient intervals but also enable you to overcome the effect of drugs and give you more time to completely rest your body. Using frozen embryos for repeat cycles will also cut down on your bills.

103. **The doctor told me to have an X-ray of my tubes but I was discouraged by my friend who said an HSG was a very painful test. Should I still do it?**

I strongly advise you to get it done immediately, so that you can begin your treatment as soon as possible. You may specifically request for pain killers to reduce pain during and after the test but I think the advantages of an HSG outweigh the issue of pain.

104. **The doctor confirmed that my ovaries are not producing eggs even though I am just 35 years old. What is the remedy?**

There are many reasons why a woman may fail to ovulate. The most common is hormonal imbalance. The initial step is that the doctor thoroughly investigates the cause before giving you the appropriate treatment. However, if the problem is due to resistant ovary syndrome or premature ovarian failure, there is not much that can be done other than to wait and monitor your situation. Some women in your situation do resume ovulation spontaneously without treatment, so all hope is not lost. In the event that ovulation fails to resume despite treatment, the doctor may suggest IVF treatment using donor eggs.

105. **Doctor, what is the best way to treat ovulation challenges?**

The treatment depends on the cause, which is usually ascertained by the doctor after thorough examination and investigations. Perhaps the most important step is to restore ovulation. This can be achieved through the correction of hormonal imbalances or stimulation of the ovaries or both. Disturbances caused by hyperprolactinaemia can be corrected by giving bromocriptine for a period of time which may lead to the resumption of ovulation without further treatment. Sometimes, lifestyle modifications like weight reduction, stoppage of tobacco use and alcohol may be beneficial.

106. **My doctor said I have mild endometriosis. Are there any measures that can help me before I get married?**

Combined Oral Contraceptives (COC) are useful in slowing down the development of endometriosis, especially if you are not in a hurry to get pregnant. However, you should consult your doctor for proper diagnosis and management. It is advisable that you start making your family as early as possible because endometriosis may delay pregnancy.

107. **Can IVF successfully treat all cases of infertility?**

In vitro fertilization (IVF) has had tremendously positive impact on the treatment of infertility. However, the success rates in IVF treatment depend largely on several factors:
- The cause of infertility

- Duration of infertility
- Number and quality of embryos available for transfer during IVF
- Age of the woman - this is perhaps the most important factor
- Type of ART or IVF
- Expertise and facilities available at the IVF clinic

**108. I am 30 years old. After conducting a series of tests, the doctor did not find any reason for my inability to achieve pregnancy. What are my chances of having my own baby if I decide on IVF?**

It is usually difficult to give a forecast or probability of success with IVF. The chance of success depends on many factors. These include age, reason for infertility, type of IVF treatment chosen, number of embryos replaced in the womb, previous miscarriages and live births. Where appropriate, use of donor eggs or semen improves result. Success is less with the use of frozen embryos. The level expertise and availability of essential equipment in a particular clinic are also important. The age of a woman at the time of treatment seems to be the most important factor for success. The older a woman is, the poorer the chance. According to the Center for Disease Control and Prevention report of success rates in the USA (2015), the percentage of IVF treatments that resulted in healthy babies at various ages of women are contained in the table below:

| AGE | SUCCESS RATE |
|---|---|
| Less than 35 years | 31% |
| 35-37 years | 24% |
| 38-40 years | 16% |
| 41-42 years | 8% |
| 43-44 years | 3.% |
| More than 44 years | 3% |

The above rates are valid for women in the USA. However, it can serve as a guide to the outcome of IVF treatment with regards to age.

**109. Why is it necessary to have my husband investigated?**

Just like women, men are responsible for 30% of cases of infertility. In another 30% of cases, the fault may be in both partners. Oftentimes, investigations reveal that both the husband and his wife have problems, so it is important for your husband to be counseled and investigated properly, in order to identify the cause of infertility and plan appropriate treatment. The most important test in men is seminal fluid analysis (SFA). Some men may refuse to be tested, giving one excuse or the other. So, do your very best to persuade and encourage your husband to have this important test done.

### 110. I got married 4 years ago and have been pregnant 4 times but I lost all the pregnancies within 3 months. What should I do?

You are most probably experiencing recurrent pregnancy loss (RPL). There are many causes of pregnancy wastage but they may not be applicable in your case. Since the losses happened regularly within 3 months, doctors would most probably call this recurrent abortion. The most essential step is for you to visit your doctor for proper assessment and diagnosis, following which the appropriate treatment can be given.

### 111. What are the causes of recurrent abortion?

There are several causes but the most important ones include:

- Cervical incompetence: The cervix is the neck of the womb and the last barrier holding back the pregnancy, thus preventing it from coming down or being aborted. If the cervix is able to do this and the pregnancy is carried to its 40- week term, the cervix is said to be competent. Sometimes, the cervix is unable to do this and is said to be incompetent. Cervical incompetence may be congenital or acquired. Whatever the cause may be, as the weight of the pregnancy increases, pressure builds on the cervix until it eventually gives way, and abortion occurs. Such abortion episodes are typically painless.

Other womb problems that may be considered in your case include:

- Abnormalities: For example, the womb cavity may be divided into two by a wall
- Scar tissue: This may be present due to long standing infections or previous instrumentations
- Masses: Such as fibroids and polyps in the womb cavity
- Progesterone deficiency - progesterone is the important hormone that sustains pregnancy. When a woman becomes pregnant, while the placenta is developing, the corpus luteum in the ovary begins to produce progesterone in increasing amounts. As the pregnancy advances, the placenta produces progesterone to match up with its demand. The placenta produces far more progesterone than the corpus luteum. The corpus luteum begins to hand over the production of progesterone to the placenta gradually as from the 8th to 9th week of pregnancy. This is called luteo-placental shift. The corpus luteum and placenta work together to produce progesterone such that by the end of the 12th or 13th week of pregnancy, the placenta has totally taken over and is solely responsible for the production of progesterone. In some women, the process described above is

defective; therefore, progesterone production is deficient or inadequate to maintain pregnancy. This ultimately leads to abortion. For this reason, such women are given progesterone during pregnancy. Unfortunately, there is no scientific proof to confirm that this treatment helps.

### 112. Are there postures during sexual intercourse that can facilitate the chance of pregnancy?

There are various suggestions that have been put forward by doctors who believe that some postures during sexual intercourse may promote pregnancy and even increase the probability of getting a particular gender. One view is that having coitus with the man penetrating from the back increases the chance of pregnancy and the probability of a baby boy. The argument is that ejaculation in this position ensures a heavy shower of motile sperm that gain access and travel faster through the womb and fallopian tubes to meet and fertilize the female egg. The faster moving and lighter spermatozoa are supposed to be predominantly Y (boy) sperm cells. The other argument is that this posture ensures deeper penetration and reduces the distance travelled by the sperm cells. Over all, this means that the swimming sperm cells arrive to fertilize the egg earlier, thereby improving the chance of pregnancy.

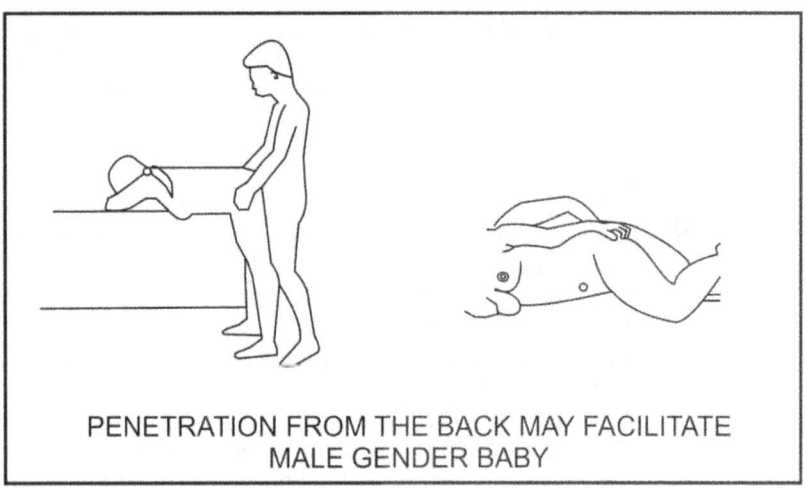

PENETRATION FROM THE BACK MAY FACILITATE MALE GENDER BABY

### 113. Is dilatation and curettage (D & C) or "washing of the womb" a strategy for getting pregnant?

It is important for women to recognize that D&C can lead to infertility and is not a treatment except it is recommended by the doctor. However, many infertile women and quacks do this in the hope that cleaning the womb will facilitate pregnancy. In developing countries, because of the crude methods deployed and the use of unsterilized instruments, serious complications like perforation of the womb, excessive scraping of the important inner lining and severe infections may occur. One of the very important consequences is tubal blockage which makes the situation worse.

### 114. During sexual intercourse, I do not experience orgasm but my husband regularly does. Can this be the cause of my infertility?

No, women don't have to experience orgasm for pregnancy to occur. Orgasm is only necessary for the ejaculation of sperm to occur in males. This is necessary so that the semen can be deposited deep in the vagina. Such ejaculation does not need to occur in women. It is true that many women experience orgasm but only few experience "squirting orgasm" during sexual intercourse.

### 115. Why is it that men are able to participate longer in the reproductive process than women?

In males, when puberty is attained, sperm production begins and this process is continued throughout life. In women, egg production and menstruation stop at the time of menopause. This means that they can no longer become pregnant naturally. There is no age limitation for a man as long as he is healthy enough to partake in sexual intercourse. I must however add that after 60 years of age, the fertility potential, that is, the quantity, quality and vitality of sperm, may be reduced in men due to ageing.

### 116. My husband has low sperm count, what is the solution?

There are various reasons why a man may have low sperm count. The first step is for you to see a doctor, preferably a gynecologist or urologist. The diagnosis of low sperm count is usually not made unless the sperm count in 2 consecutive seminal fluid analyses (SFA) turn out to be low and both tests must be performed within 2 or 3 weeks. After confirmation, investigations and treatment can begin. These may include treatment of infections, correction of hormonal imbalance or use of drugs that stimulate the production of sperm by the testes. Sometimes, surgical interventions such as removal of dilated veins in the scrotum may be required. However, there is no convincing evidence that this type of operation improves sperm count. If as in some cases, no reason can be found for the low sperm count, drugs like clomiphene which stimulates sperm production may be helpful. Where drug treatment is not successful, other treatments like intra-cytoplasmic sperm injection (ICSI) and in vitro fertilization (IVF) may achieve pregnancy.

### 117. Now that we know that my husband has low sperm count, what tips or self-help measures can you suggest for him?

The most important step is to see a doctor as soon as he can and avoid using drugs that have not been properly prescribed by the doctor. Drugs suggested by friends and relations, who may innocently and genuinely wish to help, may worsen the situation. Modification of life styles, like stoppage of smoking and alcohol may help. Prolonged exposure to insecticides, dyes and other obnoxious chemicals should be avoided. He should exercise regularly to keep fit and it is advisable for him to keep to a single sexual partner, in order to reduce the risk of sexually transmitted infections. Changing from occupations that lower the production of sperm cells like baking, fish mongering or being a chef, to other less hazardous occupations may be beneficial.

### 118. The doctor diagnosed that my husband does not have sperm at all, what is your advice on the way forward?

When a man has no spermatozoon in his seminal fluid, the condition is called azoospermia. In simple terms, this means that sperm cells do not appear in the semen when the man ejaculates. In some cases, this is inherited and other family members may have the same condition. Azoospermia may arise as a result of illnesses during childhood, adolescence or adulthood. In parts of the world like Africa where the quality of the environment is poor, infection is an important cause. Sperm cells are produced in the testes and conveyed by a system of pipes. During the journey through these pipes, some fluids or secretions are added, such that, by the time it is ejaculated, the semen has a typical grayish white appearance. The sperm cells swim inside this fluid like tadpoles but cannot be seen with the naked eyes. Now, due to some diseases, the pipes may be blocked at any point, so even though sperm cells are produced, laboratory tests will show that there are none in the semen. This type of condition is called obstructive azoospermia, as opposed to non-obstructive azoospermia, where the man truly does not have the ability to produce sperm cells. When obstructive azoospermia is operated on and the obstruction removed, sperm cells will begin to appear in the semen. Sometimes too, sperm cells are produced in the testes but do not swim out into the fluid and may need to be extracted through minor operations such as:

TESE - is an acronym for Testicular Sperm Extraction. During this procedure, an incision is made on the skin of the scrotum and the dissection is carried on to the testes. Samples of testicular tissues are taken at designated points, and examined in the laboratory immediately for the presence of viable sperm cells.

PESA - is an acronym for Percutaneous Epididymal Sperm Aspiration. During PESA, the epididymis is accessed through the skin and a needle is used to aspirate the content. The aspirate is examined for sperm cells very quickly. In either of these two procedures, if viable sperm cells are obtained, they are further processed and injected into the female eggs through ICSI.

It is important that you and your husband visit a good fertility clinic for proper diagnosis of the cause and type of azoospermia before appropriate infertility treatment is begun. If after thorough investigation of the testes and its surrounding structures, no sperm cells are found, then your husband is truly azoospermic. The solution to non-obstructive azoospermia is donor sperm, which can be used for intra uterine insemination (IUI) or IVF.

**119. I am now 28 years old. My womb was removed during the delivery of my first baby due to uncontrollable bleeding. Unfortunately, the baby also died. How can I ever get pregnant?**

Unfortunately, since your womb has been removed, it is impossible for you to carry another pregnancy except through what doctors call a womb transplant. Womb transplants are still new and the expertise is not widely available. However, since your ovaries were not removed, and at your age, I guess you still have good eggs, your eggs can be combined with your husband's sperm during IVF. Since the major role of the womb is to house the baby during pregnancy, another woman will have to carry the pregnancy on your behalf. The baby is yours in every sense, genetically and legally. The only difference is that you did not carry the pregnancy yourself.

**120. The doctor said I have a retroverted womb. What does this mean? Is it the reason why I have difficulty in getting pregnant?**

Wombs in most women are bent forward and are said to be anteverted. In the past, this is the position that doctors regarded as normal. However, in about 20% of women, the body of the womb is bent backwards or retroverted. In the past, a retroverted womb was considered to be associated with some problems including low back pain and infertility. Currently, doctors believe that retroverted wombs do not cause infertility or difficulty in getting pregnant. It should also not cause back pain unless there are other problems in the waist region. You need to see a gynecologist for proper diagnosis and treatment.

# CHAPTER 11
# ECTOPIC PREGNANCY

*"An angel in the book of life, wrote down my baby's birth....Then whispered as she closed the book... Too beautiful for earth."*
– ANONYMOUS

**1.    What does ectopic pregnancy mean?**

The natural place for the development of pregnancy is the womb cavity. Any pregnancy that develops outside the womb cavity is called an ectopic pregnancy.

**2.    How common is an ectopic pregnancy?**

The occurrence of an ectopic pregnancy varies from one place to another. Globally, ectopic pregnancy is most common in West Africa because of the high incidence of pelvic inflammatory disease. In Nigeria, it is a common problem mainly because of pelvic infection. It is more common in Southern Nigeria where about 1 out of every 20 pregnancies is ectopic.

**3.    Where are the common sites of ectopic pregnancy?**

About 95% of ectopic pregnancy occurs in the fallopian tubes (tubal pregnancy). Other sites are the ovaries, cervix, broad ligament, angles of the womb and the abdominal cavity (abdominal pregnancy).

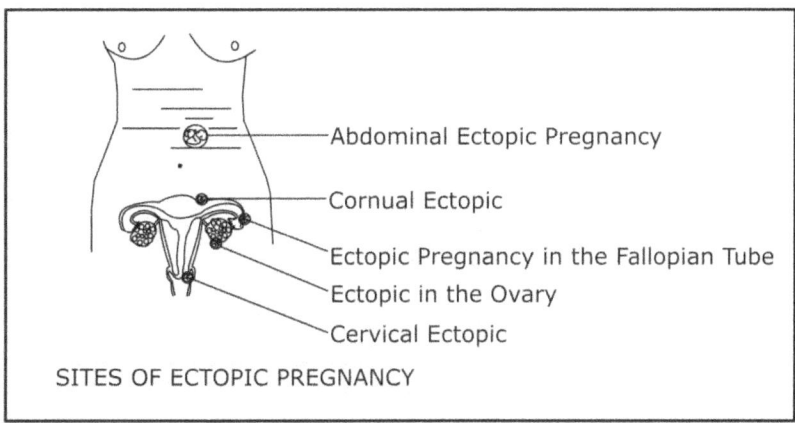

SITES OF ECTOPIC PREGNANCY

### 4. What do you mean by abdominal pregnancy?

Ectopic pregnancy may be located in the abdominal cavity, right among the bowel loops. In some cases, the pregnancy may grow for a reasonable length of time, sometimes for 20 weeks or more. The baby and the placenta are usually attached to the bowels. Women with abdominal ectopic pregnancy experience severe abdominal pain and prolonged vomiting. The abdomen is usually large and out of proportion to the age of pregnancy since the baby, placenta and birth water are not contained in the womb as in normal pregnancy. On a few occasions, it is possible to open up the abdomen surgically and deliver the baby alive. However, in most cases, the babies die in the tummy even before diagnosis is made by the doctor through an abdominal ultrasound scan. Whether the baby is alive or dead, an operation must be performed to deliver the baby, bring out the placenta, and clean up the site of pregnancy inside the tummy.

### 5. How can ectopic pregnancy be prevented?

In developing countries, most cases of ectopic pregnancy are due to pelvic inflammatory disease, following episodes of poorly treated sexually transmitted infections (STIs). Therefore, the best way to prevent ectopic pregnancy is through prevention of sexually transmitted infections. Women should stick to one uninfected sexual partner and use condoms if they must engage in casual sex. It is also important to treat all established cases of STIs adequately by a qualified healthcare giver.

### 6. What are the causes of ectopic pregnancy?

Pelvic infections are the most common cause. Sexually transmitted infections (STI), septic abortions, infections of the appendix and infections after surgical operations are associated with ectopic pregnancy. Other causes include hormonal imbalance, especially high progesterone, presence of intrauterine contraceptive devices (IUCD) and structural abnormalities of the fallopian tubes.

### 7. What should I look out for if I suspect that I have an ectopic pregnancy?

The first thing is that you would have missed your period, usually for about 6-8 weeks. You may experience pain in the lower abdomen. The pain may be felt more on one side, right or left, followed by spotting or vaginal bleeding. Some women in developing countries often delay seeking medical attention until they start to feel dizzy and are rushed to the hospital on the verge of collapse. This happens when the ectopic pregnancy ruptures and there is internal bleeding. Typically, in developing countries, most women with ectopic pregnancy rapidly go into shock. They look pale and their feet and hands become cold. This is a serious emergency, which necessitates urgent medical attention.

### 8. What other symptoms indicate ectopic pregnancy?

Some ectopic gestations may not rupture. Instead, they leak blood into the abdominal cavity slowly (known as a leaking ectopic pregnancy). In this situation, weakness and pain progresses more slowly, while the pale complexion also develops gradually, becoming noticeable with time. The woman may stop feeling pregnant, when the fetus eventually dies. If any woman believes she is pregnant and exhibits any of these symptoms, she should go to the hospital immediately, to forestall imminent collapse.

### 9. What conditions may be confused with ectopic pregnancy?

Conditions that are associated with low abdominal pain and vaginal bleeding in women can be confused with ectopic pregnancy. These conditions should be taken seriously and reported to the doctor as soon as possible. They include:

- Acute appendicitis: This is a major Infection of the appendix that causes severe pain or discomfort. There may be fever, vomiting, and headache. The appendix is usually on the right side of the lower tummy, so experiencing pain in the same location, could be confused with an ectopic pregnancy in the right fallopian tube
- Abortion: Septic abortion is common in the developing countries. A woman may also abort early in pregnancy without any apparent cause. It could be mistaken for an ectopic pregnancy because of amenorrhea, lower abdominal pain and vaginal bleeding. Also, confusion may arise in cases of threatened abortion and natural, spontaneous abortions in early pregnancy. In both situations, pain or lower abdominal discomfort and bleeding may be present
- Pelvic inflammatory disease: Acute Pelvic Inflammatory Disease (PID) may easily be mistaken for an ectopic pregnancy

- Torsion or rupture of an ovarian cyst: This is another emergency that may easily be confused with ectopic pregnancy

**10. If am afraid that my pregnancy is ectopic, what test can I take?**

You must have missed your period. The first thing is to confirm whether you are pregnant or not because there are other reasons why you may miss your period. If urine or blood pregnancy tests confirm that you are pregnant, an ultrasound scan test should be done to confirm the location of the pregnancy. Ultrasound scan examinations done through the vagina are more accurate than those done on the abdomen. They are also painless and affordable.

**11. Are there groups of women who run a higher risk of having ectopic pregnancy?**

Yes, there are certain groups of women and they include:
- Women with a previous history of PID
- Women who have had abdominal surgery, especially appendectomy
- Women who have had previous operations on their tubes, e.g. for sterilization
- Women who use family planning coils
- Women using POP family planning
- Women who are undergoing IVF
- Women who have previously had an ectopic pregnancy

**12. Are women who smoke high risk candidates for ectopic pregnancy?**

Yes, smoking at the time of pregnancy is associated with increased risk of ectopic pregnancy. As usual, there is no real medical benefit derivable from smoking, which incidentally, is also associated with other adverse effects in pregnancy.

**13. What should be done if a woman with an ectopic pregnancy collapses due to excessive internal bleeding?**

If such an emergency arises, no time should be lost. Guide the patient's fall, lay her flat on the ground and hold her legs up. This action diverts the remaining blood to the important parts of the body like the brain, heart, lungs and keeps the patient alive. At this point, immediate arrangements must be made to take her to the nearest hospital for proper attention. Unfortunately, in developing countries, the common practice is to keep the patient upright, instead of laying her flat, because of the belief that she may die if she is allowed to lie down. This practice is totally wrong and is likely to worsen her situation.

**14. Is there a relationship between ectopic pregnancy and infertility?**

The tubes are responsible for transporting sperm cells to the female egg. So about 50% of those who have had an ectopic pregnancy, also have infertility issues. After fertilization, the zygote or fertilized egg also passes through the tube on its way to implant or nest in the womb cavity but with a tubal ectopic pregnancy, that particular fallopian tube is usually damaged. Consequently, the sperm and female egg cannot meet, fertilization is frustrated and pregnancy cannot take place naturally. Since a woman has 2 fallopian tubes, if one tube is blocked, the natural chance of pregnancy is reduced by 50% and where both tubes are blocked, the theoretical chance of natural pregnancy is zero.

**15. What is the immediate danger in ectopic pregnancy?**

The immediate danger is rupturing. When the ectopic gestation bursts, there is severe internal bleeding. If medical intervention is not quick, the patient may collapse, go into shock and die. It is therefore vital to go to hospital, where blood replacement and surgery can be done early.

**16. What is the long term consequence of ectopic gestation?**

The most important long term consequence of ectopic gestation is infertility. When both fallopian tubes have been damaged or operated upon because of ectopic gestations, it is impossible for the woman to get pregnant naturally. The only means of achieving pregnancy is through in-vitro fertilization (IVF). In times past, attempts were made to repair such tubes or to force them open but the outcomes were poor. These practices are much less common now.

**17. What important steps must a woman who has had a previous ectopic pregnancy take whenever she becomes pregnant again?**

It is absolutely vital to consult a doctor immediately, so that an ultrasound scan examination is carried out to locate the pregnancy and confirm that it is inside the womb. If the pregnancy is outside the womb, urgent treatment is required to ensure that the ectopic pregnancy does not rupture.

**18. Is it true that a woman can simultaneously carry one pregnancy inside the womb while another is outside?**

Yes, this is called heterotopic pregnancy. It was very rare in the past but it is now becoming more common in women who achieve pregnancy through IVF.

# DEAR DOCTOR:

**19. Doctor, if my pregnancy is not in my womb, why am I still bleeding from my vagina?**

When a woman is pregnant, some hormones are produced in the body, acting on the inner lining of the womb to cause decidualization. Decidualization is a necessary preparation for pregnancy but if pregnancy does not occur, the decidualized womb must shed its lining, just as it does during menstruation. The production of these hormones does not depend on the location of pregnancy. In other words, decidulization will occur regardless of whether the pregnancy is inside the womb or ectopic. However, in ectopic gestations, the levels of the hormones are usually lower than when the pregnancy is located inside the womb cavity. As a result of these lower levels, the decidualized inner lining of the non-pregnant womb breaks down. So, vaginal bleeding in ectopic pregnancy is still from the womb.

**20. If I had one tubal ectopic pregnancy, what is my future risk of having another ectopic pregnancy?**

Once you have had an episode of ruptured tubal ectopic pregnancy, you run a 25% risk of having another one. The risk becomes much higher after the 2nd pregnancy and the chance of a 3rd ectopic episode is about 40%. My advice to you is that if you become pregnant after going through a previous ectopic experience, you need to have a scan very early. Please ensure that you locate the pregnancy and confirm that it is indeed properly positioned in your womb.

**21. What if my tube was preserved after my first ectopic pregnancy?**

If your tube was preserved, the chance of having another ectopic episode is 15%. So, generally speaking, people who have had previous ectopic gestation are at higher risk of experiencing ectopic pregnancy than those who have not.

**22. After an operation on one of my tubes due to an ectopic pregnancy, what is my chance of getting pregnant again?**

You can get pregnant again, although your chance may be reduced by 50%. You need to understand that eggs from the ovary on the side of the bad fallopian tube can't be fertilized because the egg and sperm are no longer able to come into contact. Consequently, every month, your chance of getting pregnant rests squarely on the other ovary and normal tube.

**23. If both my tubes are damaged due to previous ectopic pregnancies, can IVF help me?**

IVF is the perfect solution for bilateral tubal blockage. There is no way natural fertilization can occur where both tubes have been damaged. The only way to achieve pregnancy is through in-vitro fertilization (IVF) and interestingly, IVF was purposely devised to help women with bilateral tubal blockage.

# CHAPTER 12
# Pregnancy

*"Whether your baby was meticulously planned, medically coaxed, or happened by surprise, one thing is certain – your life will never be the same."*
– CATHERINE JONES

### 1. What is the best time to achieve pregnancy during the menstrual cycle?

The best time to achieve pregnancy is usually at about the middle of the cycle. This coincides with the ovulation or fertile period in most women who have regular menstruations. For example, if your cycle length is 28 days, 14 days will be mid cycle, so a period between days 12 and 16 will be an appropriate window for the woman to get pregnant. However, note that the female egg can only survive for about 24 hours after ovulation, while the male sperm can survive up to 3 days or more. For this reason, it is advisable for couples to have sexual intercourse within 1 day of ovulation for pregnancy to occur.

### 2. Why is a woman's age important in pregnancy?

The age of a woman at the time of pregnancy is an important factor with respect to the outcome of pregnancy. From a medical viewpoint, for women below the age of 18 years and those above the age of 35 years, pregnancy is more dangerous because of the various complications that may arise during pregnancy and labor, for both the mother and the baby. For example, in women below 18 years or in teenagers, the pelvis or birth canal is small and not fully developed, so complications such as fetal-pelvic disproportion, obstructed labor and its consequences, (including maternal and fetal deaths), infections and fistula formation, are more common. This situation is worsened by typical teenage or adolescent behaviors. Teenagers are known not to attend antenatal clinics regularly, consequently, labor in teenagers and adolescents is more problematic.

On the other hand, for women over 35 years, the strength and stamina to carry a successful pregnancy is much less. Also, it is possible that many women over 35 years have probably had multiple pregnancies and deliveries at short intervals in the past, so, body systems and organs, including the womb, are weak and depleted. There is also increased risk of operations and complications like severe bleeding during pregnancy and labor. In addition, the probability of having babies with congenital abnormalities especially Down's syndrome is higher in women above 35 years. Therefore, pregnancy in teenagers and women over 35 years should be avoided through family planning. However, if pregnancy happens, antenatal care in a good hospital, supervised by an obstetrician, is advised.

### 3. What is the duration of a normal Pregnancy?

A pregnant woman is supposed to carry her pregnancy for about 280 days which is equivalent to 40 weeks. The count starts from day 1 of the last normal menstrual period. It is simpler to make straight counts of 4 weeks per month. In this way, 280 days will be equal to 10 months or 40 weeks.

### 4. What substance is being tested in the blood or urine during a pregnancy test?

In blood and urine pregnancy tests, the presence of human Chorionic Gonadotrophin (hCG) hormone is determined. hCG is produced by the pregnancy and appears in the blood or urine in increasing quantities as pregnancy progresses.

### 5. Which pregnancy test is superior, blood or urine?

A blood pregnancy test is more sensitive than a urine test. It can also be done earlier than a urine test, however, urine pregnancy tests are cheaper and more commonly performed. To make it more accurate, the first early morning urine is tested, whereas blood sample pregnancy tests, can be done at any time of the day.

### 6. Why is early morning urine preferred?

Early morning urine is mainly the urine made overnight, so it is usually more concentrated and has higher levels of substances including hCG, the substance that confirms pregnancy. At any other time of the day, women are likely to have had water or other drinks which will make their urine lighter. Consequently, the amount of hCG will be less, leading to difficulty in interpreting test results correctly.

**7. If a urine or blood pregnancy test is positive, is it 100% correct that a woman is truly carrying a baby?**

No. It is never 100% sure. Sometimes, diseases, human errors and drugs are among other reasons that indicate positive test results, even though there is no pregnancy. In such situations, the test is said to be false positive.

**8. What are the causes of false positive pregnancy tests?**

Pregnancy tests may be positive in some instances even though a woman is not truly pregnant. This could be because of the presence of hCG, the substance being tested for in urine or blood to confirm pregnancy. It is rare but when it happens, it could be a source of confusion for women and doctors. The causes include:

- Human errors
  - Wrong labeling of samples
  - Substitution of one sample for another
  - Human observer errors
  - Typing and documentation errors
- Contaminants which are not hCG (but behaves like hCG)
- hLH and beta-subunit of human LH
- hCG injection; if you have been given recently
- Pituitary hCG-like substance
- hCG secreting tumors

In all cases of false positive pregnancy tests where an ultrasound has confirmed that there is no pregnancy inside the womb, most doctors will make efforts to search for an ectopic pregnancy outside the womb cavity, using ultrasound scans. Perhaps the most common reasons for false pregnancy tests are human errors and wrong labeling of blood or urine samples.

**9. What are the conditions that may make women look pregnant, whereas they are not?**

Some conditions may cause the tummy to be enlarged, thereby confusing it with pregnancy. This may be more puzzling if the woman is also not menstruating. These conditions include:

- Presence of fibroids
- Ovarian cysts and other masses
- Pelvic collections
- Pseudo cyesis
- Conditions that cause prolonged nausea and vomiting

### 10. What is the best way of confirming pregnancy?

Currently, the best way to confirm pregnancy is through an ultrasound scan. This can show the gestational sac of the baby as early as 5 weeks, especially with a trans-vaginal scan. It also demonstrates the little fetus and activity of the heart. If the scan is done too early, the pregnancy may not be detected. In such a situation, a repeat scan 2 weeks later, will usually confirm the presence or absence of pregnancy.

### 11. What are the signs that may suggest that I am about to ovulate?

With experience, it is possible for a woman to guess the time of her ovulation with good accuracy. At about the time of ovulation, the vaginal discharge is more copious, watery and draws or becomes stretchable. So the woman feels wet. Also, the body temperature may be slightly increased. The woman and her partner may notice this. In Africa, where infection and febrile illnesses like malaria are common, using your temperature to monitor your ovulation time may be less reliable. Some women may also feel a mild to moderate dull pain on the side of the ovary where ovulation is taking place. This is called ovulation pain. All these signs are subjective and not 100% accurate. You may also monitor your ovulation by testing your urine early in the morning, during your fertile period using a dipstick. A urine test is better than body signs; however, the surest evidence that you indeed ovulated is when you become pregnant.

### 12. How is the sex of a baby determined during fertilization?

The eggs produced by all women have only XX chromosome pair. The male sperm has XY. The Y sperm is the "boy" sperm while the X sperm is the "girl" sperm. At fertilization the X and Y chromosomes combine at random. The X and Y chromosomes from the man have roughly equal chance of fertilizing any of the X chromosomes of the woman's egg. If a woman's X chromosome combines with a man's X chromosome, the combination is XX and the baby will be a girl. If a woman's X chromosome combines with a man's Y chromosome, the combination is XY and the baby will be a boy. This means that it is the man's Y chromosome that determines whether a baby boy is formed or not. We can now see that women are not to blame for having all or preponderantly girl children. The partner is responsible!

### 13. Why do some couples want to choose the sex of their baby?

Sex selection is a form of discrimination. Most people who desire sex selection do so to select the male gender and exclude giving birth to girls. This practice is unacceptable and in some countries it is forbidden.

However, sex selection is done for 3 main reasons:
- Medical - Sex selection can be done for medical reasons. One of the most important medical reasons is to prevent the birth of a child with

an inherited X- linked disease. To do this, tests are carried out on the unborn baby very early in pregnancy. If it happens that the baby is a boy and is carrying a sex - linked disease, the doctor may counsel that the pregnancy be terminated, subject to the consent of the couple
- Gender balancing - The second reason for sex selection is gender balancing. Some couples have a predominance of female or male gender siblings and may decide to balance the number of boys and girls in the family. This issue is somehow discriminatory but may be understandable if the couple does not have one of the genders at all, that is, all the children are either boys or girls
- Cultural - In some communities, great emphasis is placed on male children. This may be in order to preserve the family lineage or for the purpose of inheritance. In some parts of the world, especially Africa, the inheritance of property is the exclusive right of male siblings. Some men also regard women who cannot bear male children with little or no respect and may not mind taking more wives because of this. Obviously, this is one of the worst instances of gender discrimination against females.

## 14. Doctor, I need a boy child. Please how can I choose the sex of my baby?

There are so many suggestions about conceiving boys or girls, however, the only sure method of choosing the sex of a baby before conception is through DNA analysis of the sex chromosomes of the embryo. All other methods are not reliable.

DNA analysis can be done in 2 ways:
- Before pregnancy - This is done during In Vitro Fertilization (IVF). When a patient undergoes IVF, a one-cell embryo, called a zygote, is generated. The zygote divides to form 2 cells and then 4, 6 etc. Roughly speaking, 2 cells are formed per day such that by day 3, the embryo has 6-8 cells. Now, each of these cells is identical in genetic composition and contains the sex chromosomes of the embryo concerned. To determine the sex of a particular embryo, one cell out of the 6-8 cells is selected and subjected to DNA analysis. Through this procedure, the sex is ascertained. If it is XY, then it is a boy, an XX means it is a girl. Having ascertained the sex, the embryos with the desired sex can be transferred into the patient's womb. The transfer of such embryos is done on days 5 or 6 in the IVF laboratory. This method is 100% accurate and is the most reliable method of determining the sex of a baby before pregnancy. The advantage of this method is that the sex of the baby is already known before pregnancy because only embryos of the desired sex are transferred into the womb
- During early pregnancy - This is another method whereby the DNA of the baby can be analyzed to determine sex. In this case, cells from the placenta or the birth water are obtained by doctors and analyzed

to ascertain whether the baby is a boy or a girl. This test is usually done between weeks 9 and 14 of pregnancy. The disadvantage is that, since the woman is already pregnant, if she does not desire the baby because it is not of the preferred sex, it becomes a dilemma as to what to do with the ongoing pregnancy.

In summary, these are the only methods that can increase your chance of having either a baby boy or girl.

### 15. What is the relationship between orgasm and sex selection?

It is an on-going myth in gender selection that boys are more likely to be conceived from sexual intercourse during which the woman experiences orgasm alone or when both partners achieve orgasm simultaneously. It is said that if the woman does not experience orgasm, the result is more likely to be a girl but again, there is no scientific proof of this.

### 16. Does the degree of penetration by the man during sexual intercourse have any relationship to the sex of the baby?

Although there is no proof, it has been suggested that when penetration is deep during sexual intercourse, the chance of a baby boy is increased, while with shallow penetration, a baby girl is more likely.

### 17. I already have 3 girls. I need a boy now. My friend advised that penetration from the back can increase my chance. Doctor, is this true?

Some women believe so, but it has not been proven. The thinking is that penetration from the back by the man will increase the chance of depositing the semen deep in the cervix or neck of the womb. This is supposed to facilitate the movement of sperm quickly to meet the female egg for fertilization. It may work with some people. You may need to try it out. It is also believed by some people that face to face intercourse enhances the chance of giving birth to a girl.

### 18. Does the personality or physical build of a woman influence the sex of her baby?

Yes, there is also the suggestion that women's personalities may influence the gender of their babies and that woman with strong or domineering personalities, are more likely to have baby boys than those that are less domineering.

### 19. What is considered to be a high risk pregnancy?

In pregnancy, there are various situations that may pose increased dangers to a woman, her baby or both. The problems may be due to simple factors

like age, parity or serious medical conditions in the woman or her baby. Situations that constitute high risk pregnancy include:
- Age: Pregnancy in women above 35 years of age
- Elderly Primips: These are women carrying pregnancy for the first time at the age of 35 years and above
- Grand Multips: Women who have delivered 5 times or more irrespective of whether the children are alive or not
- Height: Short women less than 5 ft. (1.53m) are at higher risk of obstructed labor
- Weight: Obese women tend to have big babies and many other complications which make labor difficult
- Issues in previous pregnancy
  - Deformity of the bony cage of the pelvis
  - Unsuccessful labor resulting in an operation
  - Caesarean section especially classical CS performed for problems that are likely to happen again during another pregnancy
  - Delivery before term
  - Intra uterine growth restriction
- Hypertension, preeclampsia and eclampsia
- Rhesus ISO immunization
- Bleeding after delivery
- Placenta abruption and placenta previa
- Thromboembolism
- Bad outcomes of pregnancy: Still birth, recurrent pregnancy loss, deformed baby etc.
- Psychiatric illness
- Medical problems in current pregnancy
- Chronic heart disease
- Uncontrolled hypertension
- Chronic kidney disease
- Uncontrolled Diabetes
- Epilepsy
- Thyroid disease
- Thromboembolism
- Chronic respiratory disease:
  - Asthma
  - Tuberculosis
  - Chronic Obstructive airway diseases
- Anemia in pregnancy
- Mental illness in current pregnancy
- Others include:
  - Multiple pregnancy
  - Malpresentation of the baby inside the womb close to time of delivery

**20. Apart from pregnancy tests on my urine or blood, what are the symptoms that I may experience?**

There is no sure way to confirm pregnancy apart from laboratory tests or ultrasound scan. However, you may suspect that you are pregnant if you miss your period, especially if your periods have been regular. Also, you may have breast tenderness, tiredness and sleepiness. Some early symptoms that you may experience include nausea, excessive salivation and frequent vomiting. Some women develop an aversion to certain accustomed food items, some eat more while others eat less, once they become pregnant. These are all suspicious symptoms and complaints which require confirmation of pregnancy.

**21. What is morning sickness?**

This term refers to the feelings of increased nausea and vomiting which commonly occur in pregnancy. They are called morning sickness because they occur more in the mornings. However, the symptoms can occur at other times of the day, including nights.

**22. What is the cause of excessive nausea and vomiting during pregnancy?**

Doctors do not know the exact cause of this condition. However, it is suspected to be due to the excessive production of human chorionic gonadotropin (hCG), which is a pregnancy hormone produced by the placenta. Some doctors believe that it may be due to the high estrogen level in pregnancy, although the nausea and vomiting are usually initiated by the smell of food, kitchen odors and the sight or taste of certain food items. Vomit may also well-up in a woman suddenly without any cause.

**23. Is this the same as excessive salivation?**

No. Excessive salivation is called ptyalism in medical parlance. Ptyalism in pregnancy is most probably due to a high turnover of the enzyme ptyalin in the mouth. The relationship to nausea is that because some pregnant women salivate excessively, they also feel easily nauseated or irritated and are therefore more likely to vomit.

**24. Why is excessive vomiting dangerous during pregnancy?**

If a pregnant woman vomits excessively for a considerable length of time, she becomes dehydrated and weak through the loss of water and body salts. This is dangerous for her and her baby and it is absolutely necessary that she goes to hospital for treatment.

## 25. What is hyperemesis gravidarum?

Hyperemesis gravidarum can be regarded as an exaggerated or extreme form of morning sickness. Some women experience aggravated episodes of vomiting and feel extremely nauseated in pregnancy. This is very stressful, because they lose so much body salts and water and cannot tolerate food at all. Such women become weak, tired and dehydrated. This condition is also suspected to be due to excessive HCG or estrogen hormones in pregnancy. It happens more commonly in multiple pregnancy or molar pregnancy. In order to prevent the consequences of severe dehydration, it is important to report to hospital for treatment as early as possible. Treatment usually requires the supervised replacement of body water and salts through drips.

## 26. Why do some women have mouth odor during pregnancy?

Some pregnant women retain saliva in their mouths. This allows more time for the enzyme ptyalin to act on the contents of the mouth which include food particles, bacteria products (infection) and saliva. The copious saliva secretion results in the strong smell of ptyalin. When the mouth retains saliva, there is a constant urge to spit and many women are often embarrassed by their inability to keep the saliva in their mouths. Some women are forced keep sputum cups or mugs by their sides, when they are pregnant.

## 27. How long does it take for vomiting, nausea and spitting to subside?

Most cases of vomiting or nausea should subside by the 16$^{th}$ week of pregnancy. Since they may be provoked by the sight and smell of food, certain drugs, perfumes, kitchen odors etc. these should be avoided as much as possible. Oily foods are notorious for causing this type of vomiting, so sometimes it helps to keep dry foods and snacks like biscuits, handy. There are also drugs that may reduce vomiting, so that the resultant dehydration does not also affect the baby in the womb. However, they must be prescribed and administered by a doctor. For women who suffer from hyperenmesis gravidarum, admission is usually necessary.

## 28. Is it normal for women to have increased vaginal discharge during pregnancy?

A mild to moderate, non-offensive, vaginal discharge is normal in pregnancy. Where the woman experiences unusual, copious, foul-smelling vaginal discharge or blood stained vaginal discharge, she must seek medical advice immediately. In particular, any blood stained vaginal discharge must be taken seriously and reported to the doctor for effective diagnosis and treatment.

### 29. Is slight bleeding in pregnancy a normal occurrence?

Bleeding during pregnancy is not normal, so whenever a woman bleeds in pregnancy, she must report such to her doctor. However, harmless spotting may occur early in pregnancy as the embryo tries to attach to the womb and it may continue at intervals, sometimes up to the 12th week. Apart from this and until labor begins, bleeding in pregnancy is regarded as a bad sign. Since there is no sure way of differentiating implantation bleeding described above, from harmful bleeding, all episodes of bleeding in pregnancy should be brought to the attention of the doctor.

### 30. What is threatened abortion?

This is the near painless bleeding that occurs around 24 weeks of pregnancy in developed counties like the USA or 28 weeks in developing countries. There may only be mild discomfort, which may make the patient believe that all is well but it is safer to consult your doctor in all cases of bleeding. If the hospital is out of reach, bed rest should be immediate, until a hospital visit is possible.

### 31. Sometimes the legs and feet get swollen in pregnancy, is this as a result drinking too much water?

No. During pregnancy, the enlarged womb sits and compresses the blood pipes of the legs. These pipes normally return blood from the legs to the heart. Because of the compression, blood flow is slower in the legs and not all the blood is returned to the heart, making the water in the blood to pass into the tissues around the ankles, feet and front of the legs. At night time, when the woman lies down on the bed, the pressure on the pipes is reduced and blood flow is improved. The water then leaves the tissue and re-enters the blood stream and swelling is reduced. This is why swollen legs are less frequent in the mornings. During the day, when the woman walks about in the upright posture or sits, the compression by the womb is more prolonged, therefore swollen legs are experienced more in the evenings. Pregnant women should lie or sit down with their legs raised on pillows, where possible. This improves blood flow away from the legs towards the heart.

### 32. Why do pregnant women urinate more frequently?

The pregnant womb and urinary bladder are located in the pelvic cavity next to each other. The enlarging womb may compress the bladder, especially within the first 3 months and in late pregnancy. This reduces the capacity of the bladder to hold urine until it is full as usual. However, during pregnancy it fills up more quickly, causing frequent urination. It is important to note that frequent urination, especially if it is also painful, can be as a result of disease conditions, more often urinary tract infections (UTI) or pyelonephritis. These diseases are dangerous and should be reported to the doctor for immediate treatment.

**33. Why do some women experience profound changes in facial and general physical appearances when they become pregnant?**

The face, nose and ears usually retain their ability to enlarge almost throughout life. During pregnancy, the placenta produces a hormone called human placenta lactogen (hPL), which has a similar chemical structure to human growth hormone (hGH). It is also called the "Growth hormone of pregnancy." During pregnancy, hPL may act on the body, causing structures like the ears and nose to enlarge. Some women may become uglier while others look more beautiful with the change in facial appearance. The effect is practically reversed after childbirth. It should not be a source of undue worry to pregnant women.

**34. Do women have more facial pimples when they are pregnant?**

In pregnancy, most body secretions tend to increase generally. The increase in sebaceous secretions may lead to increased pimples formation. In a similar manner, many women experience increased skin pigmentation, with some becoming darker in complexion. There may also be dark patches on the face which are harmless. This type of facial pigmentation is called chloasma.

**35. What about excessive sweating?**

In pregnancy, the blood volume is increased by up to 40%. The heart also pumps more blood round the body. The body's metabolic activities also increase, most of which lead to the generation of heat. In addition, the main hormone in pregnancy called progesterone, which is responsible for maintaining the pregnancy, is thermogenic, that is, it produces heat. Such excessive heat is not good for the well-being of the pregnant woman and must be expelled. Consequently, the veins under the skin dilate and the increased blood supply, conveys the additional heat to the skin's surface. The sweat glands also become more active. The sweat dries off, changing from liquid to air. This process involves the loss of heat from the skin's surface. Consequently, the skin temperature falls. Sweating in pregnancy is therefore not a disease; rather, it serves to cool the body.

**36. Why do pregnant women feel warm when touched?**

There are many reasons for this. Firstly, after ovulation and during pregnancy the hormone called progesterone is produced. This is the main hormone of pregnancy and one of its properties is that it produces heat in the body. Also in pregnancy, the blood volume is increased by about 40% and blood carries heat around the body, bringing more heat to the skin surface. For these reasons, pregnant women feel warm when they are touched.

### 37. Why is heart burn more common in pregnancy?

The stomach produces acid in a normal individual which is needed for the digestion of food. During pregnancy, the enlarged uterus pushes the stomach up as it compresses it. The acidic contents of the stomach sometimes flow back into the esophagus which connects the stomach to the back of the mouth. The acidic content of the stomach is responsible for the burning sensation or heart burn.

This may cause distress but there are many drugs that effectively neutralize the acid and relieve the burning sensation.

### 38. Why do some pregnant women experience "fainting attacks" or dizziness when they lie down?

As pregnancy progresses and the uterus becomes bigger, it sometimes rests on and compresses the major blood pipes in the waist and lower abdomen, especially the aorta and vena cava, which are the largest blood vessels in the body. The compression reduces the flow of blood to the legs and the volume of blood returning from the legs to the heart. This causes a reduction in the amount of blood available to be pumped to all parts of the body, including the brain. The blood pressure falls and there is reduction of oxygen delivery to the brain. The woman therefore suffers dizzy spells or fainting attacks. This happens in about 10% of women. Dizzy spells are more common when a pregnant woman lies on her back. It is called postural hypotension. Postural hypotension is more common and more severe in multiple pregnancy. To prevent this situation, pregnant women are advised to lie on their sides when in bed.

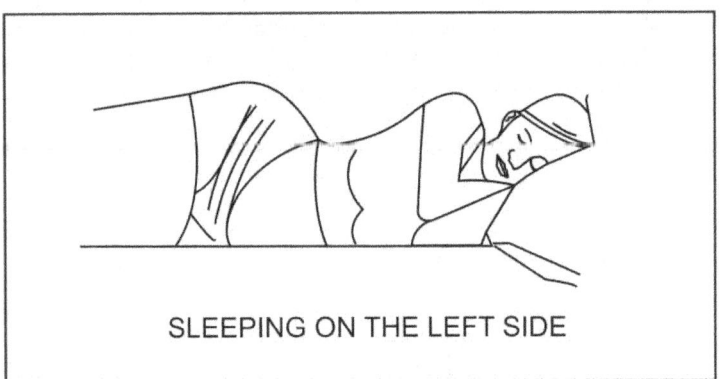

SLEEPING ON THE LEFT SIDE

### 39. How does pregnancy affect breathing?

With pregnancy and the presence of the growing womb, women tend to breathe faster and shallower. This becomes more noticeable with multiple pregnancy, especially when the woman is engaged in activities, including walking. When pregnancy is more advanced, the enlarged womb may push up the diaphragm and disturb its movements and rhythm. This may result in slight difficulty in breathing. All these are temporary and normally disappear after delivery.

### 40. How does pregnancy affect bowel movement?

Pregnancy slows down bowel movement, probably because of some of the hormones produced by the placenta during pregnancy, especially progesterone. Progesterone relaxes the bowel and slows down the movement and passage of stool. The enlarged womb also compresses the bowel and impedes the passage of stool. So, for many women, pregnancy is associated with constipation.

### 41. Why do blood vessels become more prominent in some women during pregnancy?

With the enlargement of the womb during pregnancy, the veins of the legs are partially compressed by the womb; such that blood accumulates inside the vessels, causing them to dilate. This makes the veins sometimes look ugly and more pronounced. This is also the reason why the legs, ankles and feet become swollen.

### 42. What is normal weight gain in pregnancy?

During pregnancy, it is logical for a pregnant woman to gain weight. On the average, weight gain of around 27.5 lbs is normal but it could increase if she is carrying twins or more. However, excessive or rapid weight gain may be an indication that all is not well with the pregnancy. This could be due to multiple pregnancy, big babies, excessive birth water or liquor and diseases such as diabetes, heart and kidney failure. These make pregnancy more dangerous. When noticed, abnormal weight gain should be reported to the doctor as soon as possible.

### 43. What about weight loss?

This is less common than weight gain, nevertheless, weight loss is an important issue in pregnancy. Ordinarily, if a pregnant woman enjoys good health, eats well and rests well, she should gain weight. Therefore, rapid weight loss or poor weight gain is an ominous sign. It may suggest that the woman is not eating well or she is ill, even though she may look well. In the developing countries, malaria is notorious for poor weight gain in pregnancy. When one considers that a pregnant woman has to eat for two people: herself and her baby, if the mother loses weight or gains weight poorly, the unborn baby also does not gain the needed weight. Doctors call this intra - uterine growth restriction (IUGR), which may cause death, in very severe cases.

## 44. What causes poor weight gain in pregnancy?

There are many reasons but the most common cause is poor intake. This is closely linked with high levels of poverty, unplanned pregnancies and large families. Some women also do not have access to food in war torn countries, where livelihoods have been destroyed and security concerns hamper free movement. Other pregnant women also suffer from poor appetite, unusual cravings or unrelenting nausea and vomiting.

Diseases and other conditions such as malaria, typhoid, diarrhea, tuberculosis, stress, social and financial insecurity may lead to profound weight loss. All these situations have adverse effects on the outcome of pregnancy.

## 45. Is it safe to work and exercise during pregnancy?

Yes. Women can work during pregnancy but highly demanding, stressful and unaccustomed work is not advisable. Every day, adequate rest and sleep are essential for the good health and well-being of expectant mothers and their babies. However, light to moderate exercise is also advisable; about 50% less intensive than before pregnancy. If walking or aerobics has been part of a regular routine, that may be continued but energy sapping or body bouncing exercises like jogging or running, may not be appropriate and could actually threaten the pregnancy. Should there be any alarming danger signs like dizziness, headache, increased heart rate or breathlessness, the exercise should be discontinued and the body rested. If bleeding occurs, the doctor should be contacted immediately.

## 46. What are the dangers of smoking in pregnancy?

Smoking in pregnancy has many adverse effects. Smoking is associated with high risks of the following:
- Small baby (low birth weight)
- Increased risk of diseases
- Abortion
- Placenta abruptio, which may lead to fetal death in the womb

## 47. Is it safe to drink alcohol during pregnancy?

Alcohol should be regarded as an un-prescribed drug and it is advisable to abstain from alcohol as much as possible, during pregnancy. It is particularly unsafe to drink alcohol while pregnant, if it has never been tried before. The problem of alcoholism in pregnancy is more common in developed countries and it has adverse effects on the baby. There is a well-known combination of features in babies born to alcoholic women, called fetal alcohol syndrome.

## 48. What is fetal alcohol syndrome?

This term is used to describe the combination of physical birth deformities and mental problems that occur in children of alcoholic pregnant women. They are congenital. These features include:
- Growth retardation
- Heart deformities
- Small head
- Flabby muscle tone
- Deformed face
- Facial features of an imbecile

It has been ascertained that when pregnant women drink alcohol heavily, the fetus is also exposed to alcohol ("baby also drinks") too. It is believed that alcohol is liable for the deformities and the features seen in such babies.

## 49. What level of alcohol is safe during pregnancy?

It is difficult to determine the amount of alcohol that is safe during pregnancy, but it is certain that alcohol has adverse effects on the unborn child. Since no one is sure of what level of alcohol consumption can cause fetal alcohol syndrome and other problems, it is advisable for pregnant women to abstain from or minimize alcohol intake.

## 50. How safe is travel during pregnancy?

In most cases, it is safe to travel during pregnancy but if a woman suffers from motion sickness before pregnancy, it is advisable to minimize such journeys. Long journeys on bad, bumpy roads should also be avoided. It is not usually safe to travel at speed on motorbikes, especially without wearing safety kits to protect you from the harsh impact of falls and accidents. Women who have pregnancy complications like bleeding should avoid or minimize travelling as much as possible. For air travel, it is necessary to be assessed and advised by your doctor before embarking on such journeys. Travel regulations may not permit heavily pregnant women to embark on long distance journeys by air, especially, during the last 4 weeks before their due dates.

## 51. Is sexual intercourse safe during pregnancy?

Generally, sexual intercourse is best avoided very early in pregnancy but gentle sexual intercourse may be resumed after the first 3 months, if there are no complications and the woman is fit. It should be noted that semen contains a substance called prostaglandin. This may cause uterine cramps or low abdominal pain during or after intercourse. In women with complications such as bleeding, threatened abortion, lower abdominal pain, previous premature labor or delivery, sexual intercourse should be avoided until the problems are well over. This decision should be taken after due consultation with the doctor.

## 52. Why is it important to take my routine drugs in pregnancy?

In developing countries, malaria and anemia are two major health issues in pregnancy, which should be prevented. Therefore, in many parts of the world, pregnant women are usually given preventive doses of anti-malaria drugs, iron, folic acid and vitamin B complex supplements to ensure general wellbeing.

## 53. Which common drugs should be avoided during pregnancy?

The first 56 days of pregnancy are critical. Only drugs prescribed by the doctor should be used because some drugs have been found to adversely affect pregnancy. During the critical period when the baby is being formed (i.e. during formation of the heart, eyes, legs, etc.), it is important that the sequence of events in the formation of the baby is as orderly as possible. If it is disturbed or disorganized, the formation process may stop or slow down or there may be wrong formation leading to congenital deformities.

## 54. Which drugs are safe to use during pregnancy?

Drugs that don't have serious harmful effects on the mother or the baby include:

- Simple analgesics like paracetamol
- A few antibiotics like:
  - Ampicilin
  - Cephalosporins
- Sedatives - diazepam
- Drugs used against vomiting:
  - Promethazine
  - Antihistamines
- Antimicrobials

Most drug packages contain instructions on the uses, doses and side effects but it is not advisable for any pregnant woman to use drugs that are not prescribed by the doctor. Spending a few minutes to read and understand instructions on a drug package may save wrong usage, harmful effects and unfortunate regrets.

## 55. What types of food are advisable for pregnant women?

Most conventional foods are still good for pregnancy. The important thing is to eat a balanced diet: adequate carbohydrates, proteins, minerals, vitamins and water. Special attention should be paid to vegetables, high fiber diets and fruits because they help to move the bowels and supply many of the needed vitamins. In developing countries, because of malaria, iron, folic acid, and vitamin supplements are usually given to pregnant women to prevent anemia and for the well-being of the pregnant woman and her unborn baby.

## 56. What are the causes of pain during pregnancy?

Within the first six months, abdominal and back pain may be a consequence of stretching the support of the ligaments of the womb. Infections, abortion, premature contractions, labor and other illnesses that cause abdominal pain but are not peculiar to pregnancy, are important considerations. In Africa, where fibroids are very common in many women, problems such as degeneration in fibroids may cause serious pain. Towards the end of pregnancy, (during the last three months), pain may be due to placental problems such as abruptio. The baby may be lying in an awkward position, such as across the mother's abdomen, which may equally cause pain. For women who have had previous operations on the womb, severe pain may result if there is a rupture of the scar in the womb. This is a very serious problem and warrants quick medical intervention. Of course, premature labor is expectedly painful.

## 57. Why do many women support their backs when they are pregnant?

Some women experience low back and waist pain while some are unable to walk normally. This situation is due to a number of reasons. First, the weight of the pregnant womb, especially in multiple pregnancy, shifts the center of gravity of the body from the normal vertical direction to a slanting position in front and below the waist. This increases the curvature of the lower back, so some women must pull along this weight at a more difficult angle when they walk. Secondly, there are some hormones secreted in pregnancy, especially progesterone that softens the ligaments which hold the pelvic and lower limb joints together. Thus the joints become weaker and loose, leading to discomfort and improper co-ordination. The hips and lower back are mostly affected. For these reasons, many pregnant women usually support their backs with their hands while standing. This posture has been aptly called "the pride of pregnancy." Within 6 weeks after delivery, many of these changes tend to reverse to normal and the woman is able to walk straight and smartly again.

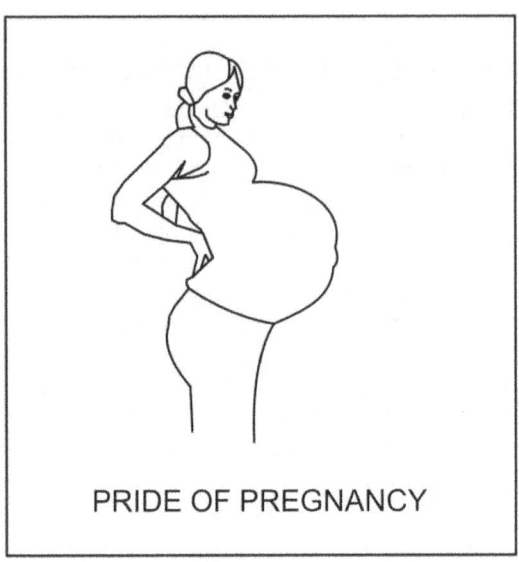

PRIDE OF PREGNANCY

## 58. What may be the cause of the sharp pain that I feel in my lower abdomen? Will it affect my baby?

Pain in the lower abdomen in pregnancy, due to any cause, should be reported to the doctor, especially if it is persistent or it escalates. Such pains may be because of:

- Ovarian Cysts:
    - Corpus luteum of pregnancy - may be responsible for pain in the first 3 months of pregnancy
    - Other functional and non-functional cysts co-existing with pregnancy
    - Torsioned ovarian cyst
    - Bleeding into an ovarian cyst
    - Ruptured ovarian cyst
- Infection:
    - Sexually transmitted infections
    - PID is less common in pregnancy
    - Pelvic abscess
- Appendix problems:
    - Appendicitis
    - Appendix abscess
    - Ruptured appendix
- Kidney diseases:
    - Urinary tract infection
    - Hydronephritis
    - Hydronephrosis

- - Stones in the kidney and ureter
- Pelvic masses: e.g. fibroids
- Constipation
- Pregnancy related problems:
  - Threatened abortion
  - Incomplete abortion
  - Premature labor
  - Ectopic pregnancy
  - Abruptio placenta
  - Acute retention of urine in pregnancy

In all cases of sustained lower abdominal pain in pregnancy, the woman should see her doctor for treatment as early as possible. An urgent visit to the hospital becomes compulsory if vaginal bleeding is also present.

## 59. When should Prenatal Care (PNC) begin?

The timing of PNC depends on whether the patient is considered to be a low or high risk pregnancy. Low risk pregnancy means that the pregnancy is normal and the doctor does not expect serious problems to develop. For such women, PNC can be commenced within 3 - 4 months of pregnancy. For high risk pregnancy, PNC booking should be commenced as soon as the woman discovers that she is pregnant. High risk pregnancy should be looked after by specialist obstetricians in well-equipped hospitals.

## 60. What are the common examples of high risk pregnancy?

High risk pregnancy includes the following:
- Multiple pregnancy e.g. twins, triplets etc.
- Pregnancy with diabetes
- Pregnancy with hypertension
- Women with heart diseases
- Women with kidney diseases
- Women with thyroid diseases
- Women who have had previous operations on the womb, e.g. CS, fibroid operations
- Women with sickle cell anemia

## 61. What is gestational age?

Doctors use this term to refer to the duration of pregnancy. In other words, gestational age means the age of the baby inside the womb. For example, a gestational age of 10 weeks means that the pregnancy is 10 weeks old.

## 62. When should pregnant women feel the movement of their babies in the womb?

Just like adults, babies move or swim about in the womb. Experience has a role to play in the timing of fetal kicks. If a woman has been pregnant before fetal kicks, are usually felt from the 16th week of pregnancy. For those who are in their first pregnancies, such movements may not be recognized until the 18th week. Once the kicks are felt, pregnant women should always note them and even record the number of times per day. It is a good, cost effective way of monitoring the baby's progress. If the movements reduce or fail to occur for a period of time, it may be an indication of a problem and the doctor should be consulted immediately.

## 63. What should I do if I feel reduced fetal kicks?

Just like children, babies swim and move about in the birth water. In the process, they exercise themselves just like healthy adults do. If children are sick, they may prefer to sleep or lie down, instead of playing. The same thing is applicable to babies in the womb. When they are sick, their movements reduce gradually before they finally stop moving. Then they stay in one location inside the womb which probably helps them to conserve energy. So, fetal kicks serve as a measure of the general health of the fetus and 5 – 6 times or more per day is regarded as normal. A reduced number of fetal kicks may suggest that the baby is sick. Under such circumstances, the doctor should be consulted immediately.

## 64. What is the meaning of fetal presentation?

During pregnancy, the baby swims about in the birth water inside the womb. As pregnancy advances, especially from 36 weeks and above, the baby tends to settle down and swim about or change position less frequently. The word presentation is used to indicate how the baby is likely to come out during delivery. It could be head first, bottom first or with any other part of the body. If the head is in the mother's pelvis the baby is likely to present head first. Such presentations are said to be cephalic; however, if it is buttocks first, presentation is said to be breech. Babies can come with the head, buttocks, legs, hands or shoulder, but the safest and most common presentation is cephalic. Other types of presentation are more problematic for both mother and baby.

## 65. How often are babies born head first?

Babies start to settle down and move less frequently from about 36 weeks of pregnancy and in about 96% of cases, they are born head first. However, breech presentation, when the baby comes through the birth canal with the buttocks instead of the head, occurs in about 2-3% of babies during delivery. This is the second most common type of fetal presentation at term. Some babies may lie across the mothers' womb and come with their shoulders or hands. These are far less common presentations but more dangerous.

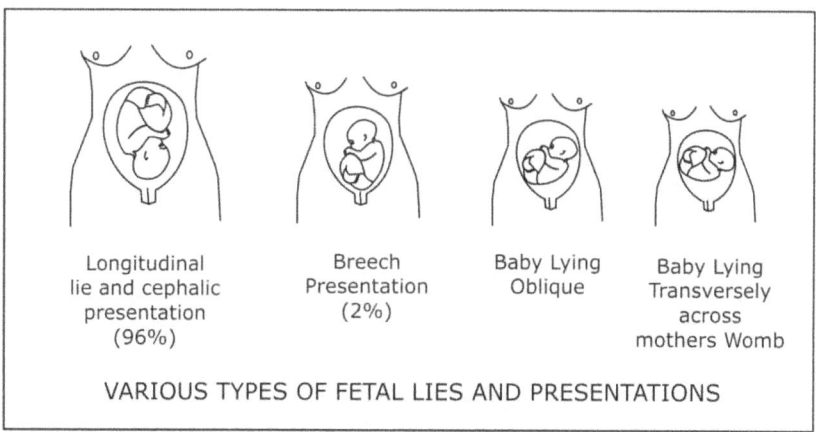

Longitudinal lie and cephalic presentation (96%)  |  Breech Presentation (2%)  |  Baby Lying Oblique  |  Baby Lying Transversely across mothers Womb

VARIOUS TYPES OF FETAL LIES AND PRESENTATIONS

## 66. How do breech pregnancies occur?

Breech presentation is more common during early pregnancy, because that is when at this time, the birth water is sufficient for the baby to swim around freely in the womb. The occurrence of breech presentation early in pregnancy is up to 25%. Late in pregnancy, at about 36 weeks, the volume of liquor is greatly reduced and babies tend to settle down more permanently, instead of swimming and jumping around in the womb. Nevertheless, from the 37th week to the time of delivery, the occurrence of breech is about 2 - 3% but despite this small percentage, breech presentations are high risk.

## 67. What are the causes of breech presentation?

Breech presentation is associated with various situations in pregnancy, although oftentimes, it cannot be pinned down to specific conditions. Sometimes it is associated with the following circumstances:

- Primigravidity: Breech presentation is more common in women experiencing their first pregnancy
- Multiple pregnancy: There is a higher occurrence of breech and other abnormal presentations in multiple pregnancy
- Placenta problems: When the placenta obstructs the free movement of the baby, because they are located very low in the womb, babies may present more with the breech
- Excess Amniotic Fluid: Excess amniotic fluid is called polyhydramnios. It allows the baby to swim and change positions continually throughout pregnancy. This situation is called unstable lie, if at about 36 weeks of pregnancy, the baby's lie keeps changing in the womb

- Womb abnormalities: This may be because of abnormal structures in the womb or masses like fibroids which may hinder the baby's head from descending into the birth canal
- Prematurity: Premature babies are more likely to come out with the breech at term, than mature babies
- Congenital abnormalities: This is also associated with increased occurrence of breech presentation

## 68. Are there any other abnormal birth presentations?

At term, about 96% of babies in singleton pregnancy will present head first but apart from breech presentation there are other types of abnormal presentations. These include:

- Oblique lie: this suggests that the part of the baby that first appears, is not well aligned with the mother's abdomen. For example, if the baby's head is tilted to one side, it is called oblique cephalic (cephalic means head). In the same vein, it may be oblique breech
- Transverse lie: this is when the baby lies across the mother's womb
- Face and brow presentations: the baby may also present with the face or brow. These abnormal presentations, though less common during delivery, present difficult situations

## 69. Is it true that a fetus may start as a twin pregnancy and end up as a single pregnancy?

Yes, because it is possible for one of the fetus to die in the womb unnoticed. Sometimes, the remains of the dead fetus are absorbed into the mother's body and disappear, if the death occurred early in pregnancy. This phenomenon is called the vanishing twin in medical parlance. However, if the death occurs later in pregnancy, the dead baby may be compressed and becomes hardened with time. The other living baby may still be delivered alive and healthy, especially if the twins are in different sacs. In some instances, the death of one of the twins may initiate contractions of the womb, which may result in the abortion of both the living and dead babies. If the mother carries the pregnancy to term, during labor, the living baby is usually delivered first, followed by the expulsion of the dead baby.

## 70. When is the baby said to be engaged?

In simple terms, the baby is said to be engaged when the head is deep and fixed in the birth canal. In most cases, this may imply that labor is either imminent or in progress. In such a situation, the baby cannot move about any more and the only possible movement is to descend through the birth canal.

## 71. What is obstetric height?

Some women appear too short in stature to bear babies without complications. Women who are shorter than 5ft are at higher risk of difficult delivery, because their birth canals are usually too narrow to allow safe passage of the baby during labor. Cesarean section operations are therefore performed more frequently in this group of women. Short and stocky women also experience hypertension and its attendant complications, so in obstetrics, the mother's height is important.

## 72. What are the factors that may hinder successful pregnancy and delivery?

There are some factors or conditions that may indicate poor outcomes in pregnancy. This means that complications are more likely to arise during pregnancy, labor, or delivery. These factors include:

- Age: Girls younger than 16 years or women older than 35 years
- Parity: Parity refers to the number of previous deliveries. Those who have delivered 5 times or more have poorer pregnancy outcomes. They commonly develop problems in pregnancy and childbirth
- Short stature: Women who are shorter than 5ft may have difficult delivery because of narrow birth canals; Cesarean section operation rates are higher in these women
- Bad obstetric history: Bad obstetric history refers to women who have had episodes of bad occurrences in their previous pregnancies. Such occurrences include:
  - Recurrent abortion
  - Premature labor
  - Still births
  - Death of the baby soon after birth
  - Difficult delivery or Caesarean sections
  - Episodes of significant bleeding during pregnancy, labor or after delivery
- Disease conditions like
  - Hypertension
  - Diabetes mellitus
  - Heart problems
  - Kidney problems
  - Obesity
  - Rhesus iso-immunisation
- Mother's life style: Smoking and drugs e.g. heroin and alcohol are associated with problems in pregnancy

## 73. What is Hemorrhage?

The word hemorrhage means bleeding. In developed countries, Antepartum hemorrhage (APH) means bleeding from the birth canal or vagina in a pregnant woman after 24 weeks of pregnancy. In developing countries, bleeding after 28 weeks is regarded as APH.

## 74. What are the causes of Ante Partum Hemorrhage?

There are many causes of bleeding in pregnancy but most of the time, when a pregnant woman bleeds, it is safe to assume that the problem is from the placenta. Hence the common causes of APH are:

- Placenta previa
- Placenta abruptio
- Abnormal placenta forms
- Infections: This may be infection of the womb, placenta and its covering membranes
- Trauma or injury to the tummy or womb: e.g. a woman falling on her tummy or being involved in a road traffic accident. This is less common
- Masses in the womb: especially co-existing uterine fibroids or polyps. Fibroids are rampant in many developing countries, and when a woman with fibroids becomes pregnant, some of the risks she bears includes bleeding and pain in pregnancy
- Premature labor

Other reasons why a woman may bleed in pregnancy are usually considered by the doctor after excluding the common ones stated above. In about 20 - 30% of cases, the reasons may not be apparent. However, it is still of utmost importance that a pregnant woman regards bleeding in pregnancy from whatever cause as an urgent reason to see her doctor. Delay in treatment may endanger her life and that of her baby.

## 75. What is placenta previa?

Placenta previa is a term used by doctors when the placenta is located around the neck of the womb, when pregnancy has attained the age of viability. An ultrasound scan is used to locate the position of the placenta. The 2 main consequences are that it may cause dangerous episodes of bleeding during pregnancy or block the baby from coming out during delivery. If the blockage of the womb is total, such that it is not possible for the baby to come out, a Cesarean section operation is performed to deliver the baby.

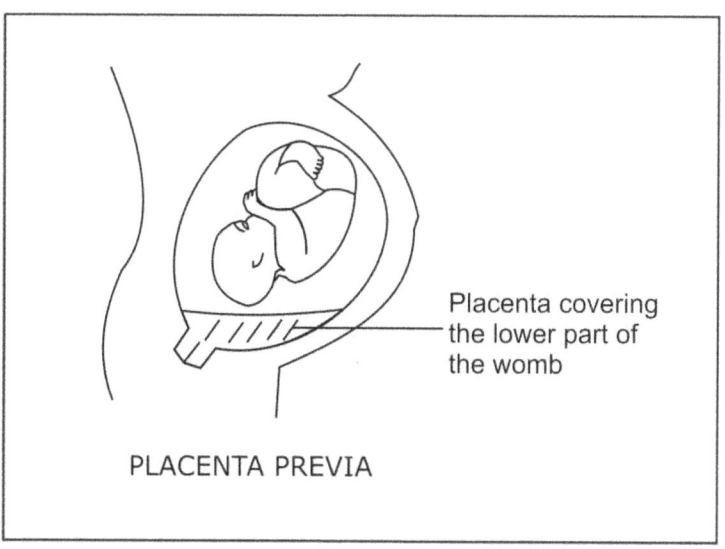

PLACENTA PREVIA

## 76. Who are those at risk of placenta previa?

Those at the risk include:
- Women of high parity
- Older women, 35 and above
- Women with multiple pregnancy
- Women with previous womb surgery
- Women with previous bad obstetric history
- Infection in pregnancy
- Women with deformed wombs
- Women carrying abnormal babies
- Women with systemic illnesses such as diabetes and hypertension
- Women with folate deficiency

## 77. What is placenta abruptio?

Abruptio placenta usually happens in the latter part of pregnancy. In plain language this means a break, tear or separation in the placenta tissue from its point of attachment to the womb. This results in bleeding. Sometimes, this bleeding may not be noticeable for some time while blood accumulates behind the placenta. It becomes obvious when the woman begins to experience bleeding from the vagina. It is usually associated with abdominal pain. The woman may notice reduction in the baby's movement inside her womb. Abruptio placenta is more dangerous but less common than placenta previa. If the abruption is severe, the baby usually dies before the woman has had time to get to a hospital. The other features include:
- Nausea and vomiting
- Tenderness over the abdomen
- Tenderness over the womb itself

- Low back pain
- Paleness due to bleeding
- Restlessness
- Shock
- High probability of death of the baby inside the womb

## 78. Who are those at risk of placenta abruption?

Some women are more at risk of experiencing placenta abruption in pregnancy. The risk factors include:
- Being above 35 years old at the time of pregnancy
- Age of gestation: commonly from 28 to 40 weeks
- Women with hypertension
- Women with diabetes
- Women with womb infections
- Women with blood clotting disorders
- Presence of masses like fibroids in the womb
- Multiple pregnancy
- Women who have ruptured membranes or premature draining of liquor (before 37 weeks)
- Women whose babies have short umbilical cords
- Women with previous history of abruption
- Pregnant women with physical injuries such as falling on the tummy
- Women with previous surgery including cesarean sections
- Women who smoke or drink heavily
- Drug abuse: Placenta abruption is more common in women with substance abuse

## 79. What is regarded as the normal blood pressure in pregnancy?

The generally quoted normal blood pressure is 120/80 mmHg. The general trend is that blood pressure goes down slightly when a woman is pregnant. However, a woman is said to be hypertensive if there is an increase of 30mm or more in systolic blood pressure (the figure on top) or 10mmHg or more in the diastolic blood pressure (the figure below), over the booking blood pressure at the beginning of antenatal care. Most doctors will regard hypertension as from 140/90 mmHg.

## 80. What are the effects of hypertension on pregnancy?

When a pregnant woman is hypertensive, the condition has some adverse effects on the baby. However, mild hypertension or controlled hypertension may not be harmful to pregnancy. The major effects of severe or uncontrolled hypertension in pregnancy include:
- Abortion - Uncontrolled hypertension is associated with increased risk of abortion, premature labor and delivery
- Small Baby - Severe hypertension leads to poor growth of the baby in the womb. This is because the baby does not get adequate

nutrition and support in the womb, so it does not grow or gain weight normally. Doctors call this intra uterine growth restriction (IUGR). When the weight of a newborn is less than 5 pounds, 8 ounces (2,500g), the baby is said to have Low Birth Weight (LBW). In many cases of uncontrolled hypertension, the weights of new born babies are less than 5 pounds, 8 ounces. Over 8% of newborn babies in the USA have low birth weight.

- Scanty birth water: Birth water is called liquor. The function of birth water is to enable the baby to move about by swimming freely in the womb. In many cases of uncontrolled hypertension, the birth water is scanty, so the baby's movement is hindered. This may make the baby remain in one place and maintain the same posture for a long time. If for instance, the baby maintains a squatting position for weeks or months, his/her legs or feet will end up by being bent and deformed. This type of deformity is called Talipes. So, uncontrolled hypertension is associated with congenital deformities
- Death: There is a higher risk of the baby dying in the mother's womb because of some of the problems mentioned above, including the side effects of the drugs used by the mother
- Operations: More operations are carries out to ensure the safety of mother and baby. In many cases, once the baby is out of the womb, the mother's condition will improve as the blood pressure is likely to fall
- Abruption: Severe hypertension is associated with increased risks of abruption. Depending on the severity, abruption may result in the death of the baby inside the womb
- Eclampsia: Uncontrolled hypertension may progress in pregnancy. When protein begins to appear in the urine, the woman is said to have pre-eclampsia. The combination of hypertension, protein in the urine and fits or seizures is called eclampsia. It affects both mother and child adversely. In extreme cases, the lives of both the mother and the baby may be lost unless the condition is aggressively managed by the doctor

## 81. What is Pre-eclampsia?

Some women develop hypertension in pregnancy. In some cases, apart from high blood pressure, the urine also contains protein. The appearance of protein in urine is called proteinuria and it is regarded as a bad sign which may indicate mal-functioning kidneys. The occurrence of hypertension and protienuria in a pregnant woman is called pre-eclampsia. Unless the hypertension is controlled, the condition may deteriorate to the point where it affects other organs of the body. In particular, the woman may experience convulsions or fits. Once she begins to experience convulsions, a pregnant woman who has hypertension and proteinuria is said to have eclampsia. Eclampsia is dangerous to both the woman and her unborn baby. It is one of the leading causes of death in pregnancy in developing countries.

## 82. What are the symptoms that may suggest impending eclampsia?

Pregnant women may manifest several features that indicate imminent eclampsia. These include:
- Rapid rise in blood pressure
- Persistent headache, especially, if it is associated with disturbance of vision
- Restlessness
- Hyper-reflexia or excessive irritability
- Pain around the stomach area and vomiting
- Oliguria or the production of very scanty urine
- Generalized edema or puffiness

These are bad signs which require quick medical intervention to lower the blood pressure and prevent fatalities to mother and baby.

## 83. What is diabetes and how does it affect pregnancy?

Diabetes is a condition where there is excessive sugar in the body system.

The main features are:
- Elevated blood sugar level
- High appetite and excessive eating
- Excessive hunger
- Excessive thirst
- Excessive and frequent urination
- Many diabetics are overweight

Since diabetes is frequently associated with other diseases, especially hypertension, and infections, it makes pregnancy risky. It is important for the diabetes to be properly controlled. As much as possible, the blood sugar should be maintained at normal levels because when blood sugar is poorly controlled, there may be serious adverse effects on the woman and her baby. These include:
- Big babies - most of these babies are big but not mature. For example, the lungs and other important organs are not mature and create problems for the survival of the baby. Also the big size makes the passage through the birth canal unsafe and complicated during delivery. Some may die because of difficult delivery
- Excessive birth water - many diabetic pregnancies are associated with excessive birth water. This means that the woman carries excessive weight in pregnancy and the baby also swims about rapidly even until labor starts. In other words, the position of the baby is not stable. It is difficult for doctors to monitor or feel the baby during examinations because the excess water shields the baby, making it difficult to collect important information about the baby

- Still birth: Uncontrolled diabetes in pregnancy is associated with increased risk of the baby dying in the womb, higher rate of infections, jaundice, and congenital abnormality at birth
- Immediately after delivery, babies of diabetic mothers run the risk of having abnormally low blood sugar which may result in death, unless it is quickly recognized and corrected by the midwife or doctor

## 84. What are the effects of asthma on pregnancy?

It is difficult to predict the rate of asthmatic attacks and its severity during pregnancy but interestingly, thirty percent of asthmatic women experience a reduction in the rate of attacks, while pregnant. However, 30% experience an increase in asthmatic attacks, while another 30% of pregnant women record no change in rate or severity. The experience or pattern in one pregnancy may serve as a guide as to what will happen in subsequent pregnancies. The important thing is to book early for antenatal care, under a doctor that is familiar with the pattern of the woman's attacks. It is advisable for asthmatic women to have their drugs very handy, especially inhalers, in case of acute attacks.

## 85. What are the major causes of death in pregnant women in the USA?

The USA has a high death rate of mothers during pregnancy and childbirth. This type of death is called maternal mortality. It is usually recorded as the number of deaths of women due to pregnancy and related complications per 100,000 live births. According to related data from the Center for Disease Control and Prevention (CDC), the maternal mortality rate for the USA for the period 2011-2013 was 18.5 deaths per 100,000 live births. This is extremely high when compared with countries like Germany, Britain, and Japan with maternal mortalities of about 6 per 100,000.

One of the main reasons for this high death rate in the USA is that most women enter pregnancy with various pre-existing health conditions. Of all the racial groups, African American women have the highest risk of death from pregnancy and related causes. The major reasons for the high mortality rate in the USA are:

- Cardiomyopathy: 11%
- Thrombo-embolism: 9.2%
- Other medical non-cardiovascular disorders: 14.5%
- Cardio-vascular disorders: 15.5%
- Infections: 12.7%
- Hemorrhage: 11.4%
- Hypertensive disorders of pregnancy: 7.4%

**86. I have been told I can only marry a man with the same blood group like me. Can you educate me better on this?**

This is a very important issue that young women and men who intend to get married need to understand and carefully consider. Regarding blood group and marriage, there are 3 important issues. These are:

- 1. Blood groups - A, B, AB, O
- 2. Rhesus factor - Positive or Negative
- 3. Blood hemoglobin genotype - Hb AA, Hb SS, Hb AS

There is usually no problem with the blood groups in category 1, so we will concentrate on Rhesus factor and genotype.

- Rhesus factor - An individual is either rhesus positive or rhesus negative e.g. A+, B-. The positive sign (+) means that a person exhibits the rhesus antigen while negative (–) means he does not. When a woman is blood group O and rhesus negative (O-), ordinarily she does not have antibodies to the rhesus antigen in her blood, unless she has been previously sensitized or exposed. If a woman is O- and her unborn baby is rhesus + and there is bleeding in pregnancy, the blood cells of the baby may cross the placenta and become mixed with the mother's blood. The mother then produces antibodies to the baby's cells, which pass back to the blood circulation of the unborn baby through the placenta circulation. This leads to destruction of the baby's red blood cells. Depending on the severity of cell destruction, the baby may be born with jaundice, may become very sick or may die inside the womb. Women who are in this situation are usually given an injection called "Rhogam" soon after delivery or following bleeding episodes during pregnancy, so it is important for RHESUS NEGATIVE WOMEN to AVOID getting married to RHESUS POSITIVE MEN if possible. If they cannot, then they should pass information regarding their rhesus status to their doctor, once they become pregnant

- Blood genotype – The normal hemoglobin genotype is AA. About 10-15% of Sub Saharan Africans have the S hemoglobin, so it is fairly common. Hemoglobin SS is called sickle cell anemia. Sometimes, people have the incomplete types e.g. AS which is called sickle cell trait. The problem is that, unlike hemoglobin A, hemoglobin S cannot withstand low oxygen tension. It is also more easily destroyed. People with sickle cell anemia usually fall sick frequently, suffer frequent body and bone pains, jaundice, poor life quality and shorter life spans, unless they are managed properly. To sicklers, as they are called, pregnancy constitutes a big stress, therefore sicklers should avoid getting married to fellow sicklers, to reduce complications during pregnancy which may lead to the death of both mother and baby. When sicklers marry each other, the possibility of giving birth to a sickler is 100%. This is depicted in the table below:

Father:

|  |  |  | MOTHER | |
|---|---|---|---|---|
|  |  |  | S | S |
|  |  | X |  |  |
| FATHER | S |  | SS | SS |
| FATHER | S |  | SS | SS |
|  |  |  | CHILDREN | |

Baby: Thus – All the babies will be sicklers (SS)

## 87. Can a sickler (SS) get married to somebody with a sickle cell trait (AS)?

Yes, even though it should be avoided if possible, there is a chance that they may have at least 2 Sicklers out of every 4 children (50%). In real life experiences, they have one or more sicklers. This is depicted below.

Father:

|  |  |  | MOTHER | |
|---|---|---|---|---|
|  |  |  | A | S |
|  |  | X |  |  |
| FATHER | S |  | AS | SS |
| FATHER | S |  | AS | SS |
|  |  |  | CHILDREN | |

50% of the children will have sickle cell traits = 2 children

Equally, 50% will be Sicklers = 2 children

## 88. What happens when two people with sickle cell trait get married to each other?

They have the possibility of having one sickler out of every 4 children (25%). In real life experiences, it may be more.

Father:

|  |  | MOTHER | |
|---|---|---|---|
|  |  | A | S |
|  | X |  |  |
| FATHER  A | | AA | AS |
| FATHER  S | | AS | SS |
|  |  | CHILDREN | |

Thus they have:  AA = 1 child (normal)
AS = 2 children (sickle cell traits)
SS = 1 child (sickler)

## 89. What are the effects of sickle cell on the mother in pregnancy?

Pregnancy in a sickle cell anemia woman is high risk, and it is fraught with so many problems. These include:

- Frequent crisis (bone pain)
- Anemia or shortage of blood due to frequent blood destruction
- Jaundice
- Increased episodes of illness: malaria, infection, tiredness and poor general health
- Cost – there is increased number of visits to hospital due to frequent crisis or sickness
- Premature labor
- Death

## 90. What are the effects of sickle cell on the unborn baby?

This depends on the severity, type of crises, and the level of care received by the woman during pregnancy. The important effects include:

- Small babies, due to poor growth in the womb
- Premature labor and delivery
- Recurrent abortion
- Stillbirth
- Inheritance of the sickle cell gene (HbSS)

## 91. Is it an advantage to bear twins?

No, it is not an advantage. The best situation is to carry one single, healthy baby although in developing countries, twins or multiples are regarded as multiple blessings from God. Medically speaking, multiple pregnancy carries risks and complications to the mother and the babies. These include increased rate and severity of most pregnancy related diseases like hypertension, diabetes, premature labor, premature delivery and fetal death. Others include higher risk of bleeding, or operative delivery, with the attendant dangers or injury and death of the mother.

### 92. How many types of twins are there?

There are two types:
- Those produced by the division of a single embryo into two equal halves are called identical twins
- Those produced when two different eggs are separately fertilized by two different spermatozoa are called non-identical twins

Globally non-identical twins are more common than identical twins but the rate of non-identical twins varies from one community to another.

### 93. So what are the factors that predispose to twin pregnancy?

There is no sure way of ensuring that a woman will have twins or multiple pregnancy. However, there are some factors that may predispose a woman to twin pregnancy:
- Familial - It is a known fact that twinning runs in some families, therefore a history of twins may predispose women to having twins or multiple pregnancy
- Assisted Reproductive Techniques - Multiple pregnancy is more common with assisted reproductive techniques (IVF). Up to 20% of women who become pregnant through IVF may bear twins or higher order multiple pregnancy
- Other factors include:
- Race - twin pregnancy is most common in the Black race
- Age - twin pregnancy is more common in older women
- Parity – the more the number of childbirths, the higher the possibility of twin pregnancy
- Genetic – Some families within a community may have more twins than other families for reasons that are not totally clear
- Physical appearance – It has been suggested by some doctors, that tall and heavily built women are more likely to have twins than women of average statures
- Diet - Some experts found that twins are more common in communities where women eat yam and yam flour based meals as staple diets. One of such communities is Ijesha land in the South Western part of Nigeria, where the rate of twinning is one of the highest in the world. Further research has shown that yam contains a clomiphene-like substance and clomiphene is a drug that stimulates the ovary. It is suggested that the clomiphene–like substance is responsible for the higher rate of twins. In West Africa, the rate of twin pregnancy is estimated to be 1:40 deliveries, while in Europe it is

about 1:80. Although it has not been proved, the Yoruba race in Western Nigeria, is said to have the highest rate of twins in the whole world

### 94. What early feelings may suggest that I may be expecting twins?

In twins or multiple pregnancy, most of the normal pregnancy complaints are more serious or exaggerated. They also occur earlier than in single pregnancy. These include the feeling of being nauseated and frequent, severe vomiting episodes called hyperemesis gravidarum. Hyperemesis gravidarum may lead to severe loss of body water and salt causing dehydration. Sometimes with multiple pregnancy, you may not be able to tolerate any food by mouth despite being hungry. Sputum may well up in your mouth and you may spit a lot. Your tummy also enlarges more rapidly.

### 95. What is the average duration of a twin pregnancy?

Averagely, twin pregnancy is about 37 weeks as opposed to 40 weeks in singleton pregnancy. This means that many women with twin pregnancy may run into labor at about 36 – 37 weeks. With higher order multiple pregnancies, e.g. triplets, the duration of pregnancy is much less and labor commonly starts before 30 weeks. Unfortunately, many triplets die after birth, unless they are in hospitals with appropriate facilities to manage premature babies.

### 96. What problems may arise in a woman with multiple pregnancy?

In twin pregnancy, most of the problems encountered in singleton pregnancies are exaggerated or become worse. These include prolonged, excessive vomiting which may lead to dehydration. Pregnancy induced hypertension, anemia, bleeding during pregnancy and childbirth, excessive birth water, abnormal lie, premature delivery and increased risk of delivery by operation. All these make multiple pregnancy more hazardous to the mother and babies.

### 97. What is the most important problem in twin babies?

The most import problem is prematurity. Many twin babies die because they are immature and cannot withstand the rigors of life outside the womb cavity. Premature babies adapt best to life inside the womb cavity until they become more mature at term. Other problems of twin pregnancy include impaired growth in the womb, poor weight gain, low birth weight, stillbirth, difficult labor and poor ability to survive after delivery.

### 98. How can labor be achieved more safely in multiple pregnancy?

Multiple pregnancy is a high risk pregnancy and problems do arise easily during delivery. Things can easily go wrong with the second twin after the

delivery of the first baby. In order to minimize problems during pregnancy and delivery, the following self-help steps are beneficial:
- Book early for antenatal care in a facility with appropriate manpower and equipment
- Attend antenatal appointments regularly and take drugs as prescribed
- Report pregnancy related problems to the doctor, as early as they occur, so that a remedy can be quickly provided
- Consider the doctor's skills as well as those of other delivery personnel, so choose wisely when booking for antenatal care, in case of emergency situations
- Plan to have ultrasound scans in late pregnancy, to foretell placenta location, presentations of the babies and how they are lying in the womb etc.
- Choose to have a Caesarian section, if the doctor decides that an operation is the best way for delivery. Things are less likely to go wrong with an elective CS rather than an emergency operation because they are planned in advance with access to equipment, theatre, and staff. Emergency situations could lead to avoidable and serious complications for mother and child
- Go to hospital as early as possible. Some women invariably delay going to hospital, in the hope that they may deliver without help. This type of attitude may lead to serious problems for you and your baby

## 99. Is it true that malformed babies are more common with multiple pregnancy?

Although there are no clear explanations, there is a slight increase in the occurrence of abnormal babies in twin and other multiple pregnancies, when compared with singleton pregnancy.

## 100. What is a molar pregnancy?

Molar pregnancy is a condition where the womb is pregnant with placenta tissues instead of a baby. There are 2 types of molar pregnancy; complete and incomplete. Both contain placenta tissues and secrete human chorionic gonadotropin, a hormone produced by the placenta, after implantation. In incomplete molar pregnancy, abnormal baby parts are present, while in complete molar pregnancy, there are no abnormal baby parts. The hCG concentration, which is what is used to confirm normal pregnancy in the laboratory, is usually very high and the womb enlarges much faster. Consequently, the womb is bigger than a normal pregnancy of the same gestational age.

### 101. What symptoms possibly indicate that a woman is carrying a molar pregnancy?

Most women with molar pregnancy will have exaggerated symptoms of normal pregnancy like severe nausea and vomiting, very early in pregnancy. Furthermore, molar pregnancy is associated with severe vaginal bleeding which is usually prolonged. So, severe, prolonged bleeding in early pregnancy and rapidly enlarging tummy are important in detecting molar pregnancy. The bleeding will continue unless the abnormal placenta tissues or molar pregnancy is evacuated completely from the womb. Sometimes, some special drugs may be prescribed by the doctor in addition to evacuating the womb.

### 102. How do fibroids affect pregnancy?

Fibroids are very common in the African environment and in many cases, they coexist with pregnancy, without causing problems. However, in some cases, there may be associated problems which may affect the progress of pregnancy. Women should be aware of these problems so that they can access medical treatment as soon as possible. They should look out for:

- Bleeding: Fibroids coexisting with pregnancy may cause sudden, irregular bleeding which may occur on and off and for variable durations. Sometimes, the bleeding may be severe and prolonged. If not treated, it may lead to shortage of blood or anemia
- Pain: There may be associated pain as the womb begins to enlarge. Pain may also be due to changes which occur in fibroids in pregnancy. These changes are called degenerations. They are of various types, but the particular one that may be troublesome in pregnancy is called red degeneration. Pain due to red degeneration may be severe and unbearable. Red degeneration usually requires hospital admission for effective treatment
- Abortion: A fibroid is like a sitting tenant in the womb. Depending on the location, it may cause various problems. When it is located right inside the womb cavity, it makes it difficult for pregnancy to even take place, and if it does, it may cause poor attachment of the pregnancy to the womb. Since the fibroid occupies and contends for space with the baby, abortion may occur
- Abnormal position of the baby: Fibroids can make the baby to lie in an abnormal position, because it may not permit free movement of the baby. If the abnormal lie persists, the woman may have to be delivered through an operation
- Swollen legs: This is because the huge weight of the womb and fibroids reduces venous blood return from the legs
- Others: Other problems include large tummy, as if the woman is carrying multiple pregnancy

### 103. How soon should a woman get pregnant, after having a fibroid operation?

An interval of at least 6-12 months is advisable, to allow the scars of the operation on the uterus to heal and regain proper strength. If the scar is weak, there is increased risk of tear or rupture of the uterus in subsequent pregnancy or during labor. Therefore, after such an operation, it is important for women to use appropriate family planning methods, so that pregnancy occurs only when the scars have healed properly.

### 104. Why are some women predisposed to mental illnesses while pregnant?

This predisposition is due to a number of reasons. Pregnancy is not a disease but it brings so many changes in the body and mind. When a woman is pregnant, her body is like a battle ground for hormones; both old and new. For this reason, common symptoms like incessant nausea, vomiting, excessive salivation, sleepiness and weakness, may worsen pre-existing emotional and psychological conditions. Financial insecurity, unwanted pregnancy, rejection, controversy over ownership of pregnancy, societal reaction, feelings of guilt, uncertainty about care, support and welfare during pregnancy, fear of labor and anxiety after delivery, may all combine to tip a woman over the edge and cause mental illness.

### 105. What changes occur in the breasts during pregnancy?

When women are pregnant, the breasts undergo remarkable changes due to the effects of the old and new hormones. These changes include:

- Enlargement
- Darkening or increased pigmentation of the areola and nipple. The areola is the area at the centre of the breast that immediately surrounds the nipple. The nipple also becomes harder and more pointed
- Small point-like swellings in the areola become more visible. They are called the glands of Montgomery
- It is possible to express thick yellowish breast milk at the tail end of pregnancy. This type of milk is called colostrum

### 106. Is it possible for a woman to carry pregnancy for many years without delivery?

Medically speaking, it is not possible. Normal pregnancy should not go beyond 42 weeks. After 42 weeks, the placenta which supplies the baby with nutrients from the mother, becomes inefficient and can no more meet the baby's requirements. Many things begin to go wrong. For example, the baby's growth slows down and it may eventually die. Many people who claim to carry pregnancy for years without delivery do so in ignorance. Some cases of such 'unduly prolonged pregnancy' have turned out to be fake pregnancies or pseudocyesis. Masses in the womb and pelvis like fibroids and ovarian cysts, may also be confused with pregnancy.

# DEAR DOCTOR:

**107. How do I use an ovulation kit? In practical terms, how do I go about it?**

You can buy an over-the-counter ovulation kit from a drug store. The pack contains test strips and instructions on how to test your early morning urine. You need to test your urine early in the morning, starting 3 days before your estimated ovulation date. Once the test is positive, it means ovulation is imminent or you might just have ovulated. Therefore, you should ensure that you have sexual intercourse with your husband or partner on the same day. However, remember that it may take up to 12 months or more, for perfectly normal couples to achieve pregnancy. So do not be disappointed. Remain calm and keep trying.

**108. Is it true that I can increase my chance of having a boy child by having sexual intercourse around my ovulation time?**

Yes. Some experts believe that the Y sperm is lighter in weight, moves faster but dies off earlier than the X sperm. Conversely, the X sperm is said to be heavier, slower but able to survive for a longer time in the female reproductive tract. Some doctors believe that sexual intercourse very close to the time of ovulation, is likely to result in a boy child, because the Y sperm swims faster and gets to the egg first. In the same vein, sexual intercourse before ovulation will most likely result in a girl child because the X sperm, which survives for a longer time will still be around and alive to fertilize the egg, when ovulation eventually occurs. So the timing of sexual intercourse around the time of ovulation may influence the gender of the baby. This timing method has not been conclusively proven and is not infallible.

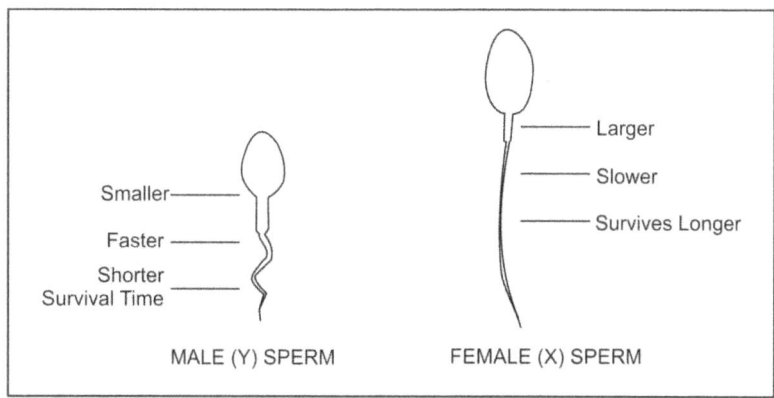

### 109. I have heard that there are several ways of determining the sex of a baby. Is this true?

There are many methods of determining sex which include:

- Sperm sorting - Separation of sperm into X and Y using methods different from DNA analysis. This is partly based on the fact that X sperm cells have bigger heads than Y sperms. This is also done during IVF. Some scientists have claimed that this method may be accurate in up to 70% of cases
- Timing of sexual intercourse - There is a long standing belief that having sexual intercourse at the time or on the day of ovulation, increases the chance of having a baby boy and that having sexual intercourse before the day of ovulation, similarly increases the chance of having a baby girl
- Body salts - Some scientists believe that chemicals in the body called electrolytes can influence the sex of babies. High potassium and sodium salts, low calcium and magnesium salts are said to result in a higher chance of having a baby boy. The opposite is true for a baby girl

There are other suggestions for increasing the chances of the desired sex of a baby but they have not been proven scientifically.

### 110. Can I become pregnant even if my husband withdraws his penis before ejaculating?

Yes, you can. The semen that comes out before ejaculation takes place, contains sperm cells and these can find their way into the fallopian tube and fertilize your egg, especially around your ovulation time. So, the withdrawal method is not a reliable family planning method.

### 111. Is it possible to become pregnant if we practice oral sex?
No, it is not possible to become pregnant, even if you swallow sperm. The sperm cells cannot get to your tubes, so no fertilization can take place.

### 112. I think I am pregnant but how can I be sure?
The first sign is that you would have missed your period. However, there are various other reasons why a woman may miss her period so you should visit your doctor, who will test either your early morning urine or your blood for pregnancy.

### 113. How soon should I have a pregnancy test?
If you miss your menses, you may wait for about 1 week before going for the test. Sometimes, when the test is performed too early, it may be falsely negative. In this case, you may need to wait for another 1 – 2 weeks before a repeat test is done. Blood pregnancy tests are more sensitive than urine pregnancy tests and can be performed earlier. A blood test is likely to be positive at about 1 week after you have missed your period, while urine pregnancy tests are mostly performed two weeks after the period has been missed. If it is positive, then you are likely to be pregnant.

### 114. My pregnancy test is negative despite the fact that I missed my period. What should I do?
It may be that you tested your blood or urine too early. You may need to wait for about 1-2 weeks before having a repeat pregnancy test performed. If you had a urine pregnancy test initially, you may opt for a blood pregnancy test which is more sensitive. Please take note that apart from pregnancy, there are many other reasons why you may fail to menstruate, so it is advisable that you see your doctor.

### 115. Is it true that I may not be carrying a baby, even if my pregnancy test is positive and my tummy is growing, and I have normal signs and symptoms of pregnancy?
It is true. There are some diseases of the placenta that may occur outside normal pregnancy. In such cases, the pregnancy test is positive because the abnormal placenta tissues produce the hCG hormone. The presence of hCG, confirms normal pregnancy in the laboratory. The two main categories of placenta diseases are molar pregnancy and trophoblastic diseases. In these two categories, hCG is produced in high amounts, thus making pregnancy tests persistently positive.

**116. Is it possible for me to be pregnant and still menstruate?**

It is practically impossible. Although you may bleed or spot irregularly, this is not the same as menstruation. There are so many reasons why you may bleed early in pregnancy. Rarely, this may happen when the pregnancy is attaching itself to the womb. Infections, masses like fibroids, orthodox drugs and herbs may cause bleeding. It may also happen if the pregnancy is trying to abort. Bleeding at any time during pregnancy is a bad sign and should be reported to the doctor immediately.

**117. How can you help me to improve my well-being and that of my unborn baby?**

The following tips are beneficial:

- Pregnancy must be planned. It is always better to get pregnant at a planned time and at good interval too. This allows pregnancy to occur when the mother's condition is stable and optimal. This means the mother is in good health, good financial standing and has available family support. The child spacing interval should not be less than 18 months. The maximum number of children should not be more than (3) three
- Ensure that you book for antenatal care in a hospital already familiar with your condition. You should also get booked at a hospital or health center nearest to your home so that you can get there quickly in case of an emergency
- Avoid stress and unaccustomed exercise because they can trigger crisis
- Rest well as much as possible and sleep well too
- Take plenty of fluids (water) at all times and remain well hydrated
- Take your prescribed drugs regularly – do not take drugs not given by your health care providers. Avoid herbal medicine
- Take note of small changes in your health and that of your baby- In particular, always take note and monitor the fetal kicks in the womb. You should count how many times the baby kicks per day and record this in a sheet of paper. If the kicks are no longer felt regularly, you should complain to your doctor immediately
- Memorize your doctor's telephone number and your hospital's help line. Also write them down and keep them where others can easily see them
- Report any case of bleeding to the hospital early
- Make adequate plans and arrangements for labor and delivery well ahead of your delivery date:
    - Assemble items on your delivery list
    - Arrange for finance
    - Arrange for transport

**118. I experienced severe nausea and vomiting in my last pregnancy, now I am afraid to get pregnant again, is it likely to recur?**

You should not be discouraged because of your previous experience. Most times, excessive nausea and vomiting usually subside before 15 weeks of pregnancy. It can recur in subsequent pregnancies but is usually less severe. With the previous experience in your last pregnancy, you should be able to cope better.

**119. What is the role of weight gain in pregnancy?**

It is important that women enjoy good health at the onset and duration of pregnancy. Women who weigh less than 110 lbs at the beginning of pregnancy or those who gain less than 11lbs during pregnancy, run the risk of giving birth to small babies.

**120. What do I do if I start bleeding before my due date?**

As soon as you notice blood, call the attention of a responsible person near you and arrange to get to a hospital as soon as possible. The doctor will find out why you are bleeding and take care of you. Sometimes, you may need to be given blood urgently. This can only be done safely and quickly in a hospital environment. While you are waiting to get to hospital, stay calm. You may apply a clean sanitary towel to the vagina. Keep your legs together and avoid standing. You should lie down on your side. At the hospital, you may also need an infusion to replace your body water, apart from a blood transfusion or an urgent operation, so the earlier the doctor starts treating you, the better for you and your unborn baby.

**121. I am hypertensive. Does this mean I should not get pregnant?**

No, hypertensive women can get pregnant but to avoid adverse effects, the hypertension must be controlled. Doctors now have reasons to believe that mild hypertension may in fact be beneficial to the baby. This is because mild hypertension is associated with better weight gain by the baby. It is therefore advisable for hypertensive women to carefully plan the timing of pregnancy. One way to achieve this is to use a family planning method or device when pregnancy is not desired. It is very important to ensure that the blood pressure is well controlled before and during pregnancy.

**122. I have been told that I will have twins if I have sexual intercourse at certain times. Is this true?**

There is no basis for having sexual intercourse at certain periods or dates in order to achieve twin pregnancy. There are a few factors that increase your chances of twin pregnancy but timing of sexual intercourse is not one of them.

# CHAPTER 13

# Prenatal Care

*Everything grows rounder and wider and weirder and I sit here in the middle of it all and wonder who in the world you will turn out to be."*
– CARRIE FISHER

### 1. What does prenatal care mean?

Pregnancy is a normal physiological event. However, it brings changes to the physical appearance, body chemistry, organs, and systems in the body. Some of the changes can be outwardly recognized as pregnancy advances.

Prenatal care is medical care given to a pregnant woman, which starts very early in pregnancy and continues until she falls into labor or just before delivery. During this period, there are 2 patients being looked after; the pregnant woman and her unborn child. Prenatal care is commonly called antenatal care, so these two terms can be used interchangeably.

### 2. Why is it necessary to have prenatal care (PNC)?

Prenatal care is necessary for the following reasons:
- High risk pregnancy: It helps to identify those women in whom problems may easily develop during pregnancy or delivery. Sometimes, it is possible to identify these women because some of them already suffer from one condition or the other before becoming pregnant. Such diseases include hypertension, diabetes, heart, kidney, and chest diseases. This group falls into the category of women that doctors refer to as high risk pregnancy. It is not always possible to predict those who will develop problems and those who will not, because problems may develop very quickly and unexpectedly; even in those who do not appear sick. This is why pregnant women should be adequately cared for and monitored during pregnancy, delivery, and for about 6 weeks after delivery.
- Existing diseases: In some cases, it is possible to control existing illnesses so that they do not increase in severity during the duration

of pregnancy or delivery. Good examples are diabetes and hypertension which must be controlled adequately so that they do not harm the woman or her unborn baby.
- Well-being and safe delivery: When a woman is pregnant, the doctor looks after 2 patients; the mother and her unborn baby. Both of them should be in good health throughout pregnancy. Prenatal care affords the doctor the opportunity to learn many things about the woman, the baby, and the pregnancy as a whole. This knowledge enables the doctor to plan well ahead of the time of delivery and determine in advance the best way or method to take delivery of the baby. The main objective of PNC is to ensure the safe delivery of a healthy baby that is ready to be nursed by an equally healthy mother

## 3. Is there any evidence that prenatal care affects the outcome of pregnancy?

Yes. There are well documented proofs including those by the World Health Organization (WHO) that have determined that the outcome of pregnancy is much better in women who have prenatal care.

## 4. When should prenatal care normally begin?

Traditionally, prenatal care should start when the pregnancy is about 14 weeks. The first 14 weeks of pregnancy is also called the first trimester. In high risk pregnancy, when problems are expected to develop or get worse, prenatal care should start earlier or as soon as the woman discovers that she is pregnant. In some cases of high risk pregnancy, it is advisable that women suffering from certain diseases attend pre-conception or pre-pregnancy clinics. Despite its importance, pre-conception care is not widely available in developing countries, in contrast to the situation in the developed world.

## 5. What is the importance of pre-conception clinics?

Pre-conception care is good for women who are known to be at higher risk of developing problems or complications during pregnancy. Examples are women who suffer from diabetes, hypertension, those who smoke, and women with genetic disorders.

At the preconception clinic, diseases are treated or controlled, while drugs are changed to those that are known to be safer in pregnancy. Life styles can also be modified to suit pregnancy e.g. reduction of weight in obese women and stoppage or reduction, for smokers. Genetic counseling can also be done for those with disorders. The objective of pre-conception clinics is to enable such women become pregnant, when their health is optimal. This will minimize problems when pregnancy eventually occurs.

6. **How are genetic diseases detected?**

This is an important aspect of care. Ideally, screening for genetic diseases and appropriate counseling should be done for couples, when marriage becomes a strong possibility. This will enable prospective couples to make informed choices before committing to marriage. Screening for genetic diseases is appropriate in some families with affected relatives, in some racial groups or in people from certain parts of the world. Examples are given in the table below:

| DISEASE | TARGET GROUP FOR SCREENING |
|---|---|
| Sickle cell anemia | Africans, African Americans, Caribbean |
| Cystic fibrosis | People with Positive history of affected relatives |
| Tay-Sach disease | Jews, French Canadians |
| B-Thalassemia | People from the Mediterranean, Africans, Indians, Pakistanis |

7. **How often should a pregnant woman attend prenatal clinic?**

Traditionally, the first visit starts at about 14 weeks of pregnancy. Thereafter, the woman is seen once every four weeks until pregnancy is 28 weeks; then once every 2 weeks until pregnancy is 36 weeks. From the 36th week, the woman is seen every week until she goes into labor. However, she may be seen more frequently if there are reasons for the doctor or midwife to get worried about her condition or that of the baby. This type of scheduled visits is called the traditional schedule and is more practiced in developing countries with poor health infrastructures.

8. **What is the disadvantage of the traditional schedule?**

The schedule is cumbersome. The number of hospital visits is too many. Some of these visits are not really necessary in all women. In the developing countries where there is shortage of doctors, too many prenatal visits overstretch the available manpower and reduce efficiency. The schedule is therefore not cost effective.

9. **What is the ideal schedule for prenatal care?**

There is no ideal schedule of visits. Each pregnant woman deserves a plan that is most suitable and cost effective for her. However, the World Health Organization (WHO) recommends that 4 visits are suitable for most pregnant women. The first visit should be when the pregnancy is between 14 - 16 weeks, the second visit at 24 – 28 weeks, and the third visit at 32 weeks of pregnancy. Each of these visits has clearly defined objectives. This schedule seems to be more cost effective.

### 10. What is the main role of Prenatal Care?

Pre-natal care (PNC) has important roles that ensure that the outcome of pregnancy both for the mother and her baby are better and safer. These main roles are:
- PNC helps to prevent diseases during pregnancy.
- PNC helps to establish the basic indices of health and pregnancy parameters for a woman and her baby. These include:
  - Determination of gestational age
  - Monitoring of baby's growth and its well-being

### 11. What are the goals of the first visit?

The first visit is called the booking clinic. This visit is probably the most important of the three recommended visits. In a normal pregnancy, it should take place between 14 – 16 weeks. However, women who already have problems like diabetes, hypertension or recurrent pregnancy losses etc. are encouraged to book earlier. In this visit, the woman is generally assessed to determine her health status and prenatal documentations are made. These include:
- Name and address
- Age and number of pregnancy
- Booking weight, blood pressure
- Urine and blood tests including blood grouping and blood genotype, Rhesus typing or screening, Rubella antibodies status, HIV testing, Hepatitis A, Hepatitis B etc.
- Correct determination of age of pregnancy or gestational age
- Screening through history taking, physical examination and other necessary investigations. Here it is important to find out whether the woman has shortage of blood or anemia. If she does, then urgent actions are taken to correct the situation. Screening also determines whether the woman is high risk pregnancy or not
- Formulation of suitable plan for the individual woman's level of care during pregnancy is done

### 12. What is the goal of the second visit?

The main goal of this visit is to screen for anemia.

Other routine tests are also performed:
- Measurement of the weight to see if the woman is gaining weight normally or not
- Urine tests for sugar and protein
- Physical examination of the womb

- Ultrasound examination of the baby is performed to determine age, number of babies, quantity of birth water, and any abnormality in the baby.

**13.** What happens during the 3rd visit?

This usually takes place at about the 32nd week of pregnancy. During this visit:
- Particular attention is paid to the weight of the woman in order to detect pre-eclampsia, which may manifest as rapid weight gain
- Women are also screened for anemia

**14. What is the importance of the 4th visit?**

This is the last visit before delivery. The focus now is:
- To plan the method of delivery
- To examine for the lie and the presentation of the baby
- To assess the birth canal. Sometimes this may involve an X-ray or CT Imaging of the bones of the birth canal
- The woman is also examined to rule out anemia

**15.** What are the other benefits of PNC?

The indirect benefits of PNC include helpful instructions and health education:
- General hygiene in pregnancy
- Nutrition in pregnancy
- How to identify dangerous events in pregnancy and what to do
- Changing harmful lifestyles like smoking, drinking alcohol, or taking dangerous or illicit drugs
- Getting to know the environment where delivery will take place as well as the personnel that will conduct labor. This particular action fosters friendship and cooperation between the patient and health personnel. More importantly, the doctors and midwives learn how to deal gently and peacefully with the woman during labor

All these important steps have favorable effects on the outcome of pregnancy.

**16. What is the trend in PNC enrollment in the USA?**

There has been tremendous improvement in enrollment for PNC in the USA generally. This represents a shift from the situation in the past. About 4 decades ago, booking for PNC was at a low level especially among the minority groups. However, with concerted efforts from all stake holders, there was a dramatic improvement in enrolment at about the year 1998. Coverage for PNC among pregnant women was over 98%. Fortunately, the largest improvement was in the minority groups especially the African Americans and Hispanics where enrolment was previously lagging.

**17. What are the reasons given by women who do not enroll promptly for PNC?**

There are many reasons why women fail to enroll for PNC on time. In the USA, perhaps the most common is the fact that many women are not aware that they are pregnant. This is mostly due to ignorance of the symptoms and signs of pregnancy. The other reasons include:
- Inability to pay the cost of PNC
- Lack of insurance coverage
- Difficulty in securing appointments for PNC
- Transport difficulties
- Poor appreciation of the need for PNC

Women who have had previous successful PNC and deliveries have the tendency to delay PNC because they are over confident. In the developing countries, the greatest barriers to PNC are:
- Poor public awareness of the importance of PNC
- Lack of reachable clinics
- Poverty
- Taboos and negative beliefs

**18. Why is the gestational age of pregnancy important?**

A normal pregnancy has an average duration of 280 days or 40 weeks. The 40-week duration is divided into 3 semesters with clear goals, both for the milestones of development of the baby, progress of pregnancy and treatment plan, including immunization and delivery. So it is important that an accurate gestational age is determined as early as possible in pregnancy. This is especially because the gestational age is more accurate when determined early in pregnancy.

**19. How do doctors calculate the Estimated Date of Delivery (EDD)?**

EDD is an acronym for estimated dated of delivery. LMP means the date of the last menstrual period. The EDD is calculated by adding 7 days to the date of the first day of the last menstruation and subtracting 3 from the month of the last menses. Lastly, the year in consideration is adjusted if necessary. Here are examples:
- LMP = 10-7-2015

    EDD is calculated as below:

    10 + 7 = 17 = 17th day

    7 − 3 = 4    = April

    Then year is adjusted to 2016.

    So the EDD will be 17 − 4 − 2016 (Please note that the year has been adjusted to 2016 instead of 2015)

- Example 2:
  
  LMP = 15 – 3 – 2015
  
  EDD = 15 + 7 = 22nd day
  
  3 – 3 = 0 (0 means December of same year)

So EDD = 22 – 12 – 2015 (In this example, we do not have to change the year because the woman menstruated early in the year and 40 weeks from that date falls in December of the same year).

EDD calculation is based on the fact that the average length of menstrual cycle in women is 28 days. The method also assumes that ovulation takes place at mid cycle or day 14. "For an accurate estimation of gestational age of a baby and EDD, the menstruation must be regular".

## 20. What routine tests should pregnant women expect to go through when they visit the doctor?

These tests are important. The summary of what the nurses and doctors do during appointments depend on prenatal care plans. The plan depends on whether the patient is a high or low risk pregnancy. Below is an account of the important routine tests:

At each visit, you will be asked some questions:
- Do you have any complaints?
- Have you bled from the vagina?
- Have you drained water or liquor from the vagina?
- Do you feel fetal movements and how often per day?
- Have you experienced abdominal pain?
- Have your eating habits changed?
- Have you been sleeping well?

Some routine tests are also important:
- Your weight will be taken for comparison to ensure that you are gaining weight normally
- Your blood pressure as well as your heartbeats will be measured and also your heart beats
- Your urine will be analyzed for protein, glucose and blood cells
- Your blood will be tested for anemia

Other important examinations include checking the following:
- The size of the womb, most probably with a tape rule to see if the womb is enlarging well
- The movement of the baby
- The presenting part of the baby

A vaginal examination is usually done by the doctor to examine the vagina and neck of the womb to check if:
- The length of the cervix is normal
- The external opening of the cervix is closed
- The feel is normal to touch
- There is bleeding from the womb or leakage of birth water

There are some special laboratory tests that are done on women at risk of diseases like diabetes, Rhesus immunization, neural tube defects etc. So the following blood tests are routinely done at:
- 15th to 20th weeks: alpha fetoprotein for women with risks of Neural Tube Defects (NTDs)
- 24th to 28th weeks: Diabetic screening for women at risks of Diabetes
- 28th week: Estimation of antibodies in Rhesus negative women

In the last 4 weeks of pregnancy, doctors focus attention on the method of delivery. Hence, assessment of the birth canal is carefully done to see if the presenting part of the baby will be able to pass through during labor, to ensure safe and normal delivery.

All these steps are important to ensure that you have good care in pregnancy with the ultimate aim of safe delivery.

**21. Apart from hypertension, what other high risk pregnancy situations exist?**

Some women need special care during pregnancy. Such women include those with preexisting conditions like:
- Diabetes (uncontrolled)
- Heart diseases
- Endocrine disorders like hyperthyroidism
- Kidney diseases
- Sickle cell anemia
- Women who are undernourished
- Women who have anemia even at the beginning of pregnancy
- Women with problems in previous pregnancy which may re-occur such as
  - Preterm labor and delivery
  - Intra uterine growth restriction (IUGR)
  - Bleeding in pregnancy
  - Placenta problems
  - Still birth
- Multiple pregnancy
- Adolescent pregnancy
- Elderly primips

## 22. What are trimesters?

The duration of pregnancy is divided into 3 periods referred to by doctors as 1st, 2nd, and 3rd trimesters. The length of each trimester is as follows:

| | | |
|---|---|---|
| 1st trimester | 1 – 14 complete weeks of pregnancy | 14 weeks |
| 2nd trimester | 15 – 29 weeks pregnancy | 14 weeks |
| 3rd trimester | 30 – 42 weeks of pregnancy | 12 weeks |
| Complete | Total duration of pregnancy | 40 weeks |

Doctors deliberately divided the duration of pregnancy into trimesters for the purpose of monitoring and ease of management of pregnancy. Each trimester represents different milestones of development and different challenges in pregnancy. These can be monitored and managed by the doctor.

## 23. Why is psychosocial screening important?

There is no doubt that psychological and social issues in a woman or her family have remarkable effects on an ongoing pregnancy. These issues must be searched for by asking questions in a manner that is non-judgmental and friendly. The objective is to offer advice or help as early as possible, in order to prevent or limit further adverse effects on pregnancy. Issues that are commonly screened for include:

- Alcohol usage
- Street drugs addiction
- Smoking
- Domestic violence, physical injury etc

These issues can be modified through appropriate counseling. This is an important aspect in curbing habits and ensuring a better outcome for the ongoing pregnancy, especially as they affect the baby in the womb.

## 24. How is the birth canal assessment done?

The objective of assessing the birth canal is to ensure safe vaginal delivery of the baby without harm or injury to the baby or mother. Doctors do this assessment by performing:

- Digital assessment
- X-ray or CT assessment of the birth canal and the presenting part of the baby

### 25. What is a digital assessment?

This is like a preliminary assessment. First, the doctor examines the tummy for the lie and presentation of the baby. Then, he examines the neck of the womb through the vagina to ensure that there are no problems. He then examines the bony parts of the birth canal to see if the birth canal has enough space or capacity to allow safe passage of the baby, during labor and delivery. In this regard, doctors place particular attention to the inlet, canal and outlet of the pelvis. If a woman has had safe vaginal delivery previously, she is more likely to have a repeat safe delivery, especially if the baby is coming head first.

### 26. What about X-ray pelvimetry?

For a woman who is a first timer, if the doctor has any doubt as to whether the capacity of the birth canal is adequate, he may request a further X-ray or CT assessment of the pelvic cavity. These are used to estimate the adequacy of the birth canal. They measure the diameters of the canal at the inlet, midpoint, and outlet. These are called X-ray or CT pelvimetry, depending on whether X-ray or CT is used. CT Pelvimetry is more accurate than X-ray pelvimetry but much more expensive.

### 27. Will radiation during these tests cause harm to my unborn baby?

There is no doubt that prolonged exposure to radiation or massive radiation for a shorter duration can cause damage to babies. However, doctors believe that radiations from investigations like X-ray pelvimetry or CT pelvimetry are not harmful to babies in the womb when properly conducted. Women should not be unduly concerned about these tests.

### 28. What about my baby's presentation?

Over 95% of babies have cephalic (head) presentation at the tail end of pregnancy. This is the most favorable presentation that is appropriate for a safe vaginal delivery. The next common presentation is breach presentation. This means that the baby is born buttocks-first. This happens in about 2-3% of deliveries at term. On rare occasions, babies may present with the shoulder, hand or foot. Presentations except cephalic are regarded as being abnormal and are associated with more problems during delivery. Some of these problems may result in operations or other forms of assistance for safe delivery.

### 29. How does the small womb accommodate the baby?

The womb greatly enlarges throughout pregnancy to accommodate the growing baby, placenta and the birth water. This enlargement is due partly to the actions of the hormones estrogen and progesterone. In the later part of pregnancy, the weight of the baby, placenta and birth water contribute to further enlargement, by stretching the muscle cells and tissues of the womb. Indeed the parameters below illustrate the fact:

| Description | Weight | Volume |
|---|---|---|
| Non pregnant womb | 70g | 10ml |
| Pregnant womb at 40 weeks | 1100g | 5000ml |

This means that the womb at 40 weeks or at the end of pregnancy has enlarged by over 500 times. The weight has increased by over 16 times. No wonder the baby has a big swimming pool of birth water and can jump up and down at will.

## 30. When will the tummy bulge become noticeable?

The womb begins to enlarge once pregnancy has taken place. The enlargement in the upward and downward directions are much more than those at the sides, therefore the uterus appears longer and rises out of the pelvis gradually. At about the 12th to 14th week of pregnancy and beyond, the womb can be seen and touched as a bulge in front and above the waist line. You cannot hide it anymore!

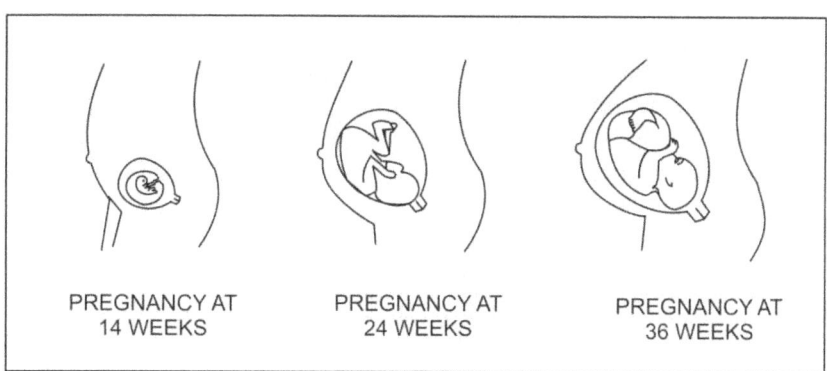

PREGNANCY AT 14 WEEKS    PREGNANCY AT 24 WEEKS    PREGNANCY AT 36 WEEKS

## 31. When do contractions start in pregnancy?

Within the first 13 weeks of pregnancy, a woman may experience some slight contractions which are painless and come at irregular intervals. The number of such occurrences usually increases as pregnancy advances. They are called Braxton Hicks Contractions. Braxton Hicks was the first to talk about this type of contraction. Towards the end of pregnancy, the intensity of Braxton Hicks contractions may increase slightly and the woman may feel them more. At this time, the contractions may cause some discomfort. Some doctors call these contractions 'false labor' because they are different from the womb contractions experienced by women during labor. Braxton Hicks contractions do not make the cervix dilate or shorten in length, as in true labor.

## 32. How is the birth canal able to allow the passage of the baby during labor?

There is a big difference in the vagina of women during and outside pregnancy. Just like the womb, the vagina enlarges. The tissues of the vulva and vagina become soft with a tremendous increase in blood supply. The secretions are also greatly increased. When the vagina and vulva are examined during pregnancy, they appear violet in color because of increased blood supply. This unique appearance is a sign of pregnancy that can be recognized by experienced doctors. It is called Chadwick's Sign. During labor, the vagina and vulva stretches greatly in an elastic fashion to allow the passage of the baby.

## 33. Why do lines appear on the tummy?

Generally, there is increased pigmentation during pregnancy. Doctors believe that the pigmentation may be due to increased stimulation of melanocytes by estrogen and progesterone. Melanocytes are the cells that produce melanin pigment which is responsible for skin color. The effect of increased pigmentation is more visible in outer parts of the body. These include:
- The midline of the tummy where it appears as a blue line; called linea nigra
- Brownish patches on the face and neck, called chloasma or "mask of pregnancy". Chloasma may fade or disappear after delivery

There are individual differences in pigmentation during pregnancy. While many women become generally darker, only few become fairer in complexion during pregnancy.

## 34. Why do women retain water during pregnancy?

In pregnancy, women generally retain more body water. Most women retain a minimum amount of 6500mls of body water and to a large extent, this water retention is due to increased thirst for water by pregnant women and the action of a hormone called vasopressin.

## 35. Is this why my legs are swollen?

Many women experience the occurrence of edema especially in the legs and feet in mid to late pregnancy. This is as a result of the retained water which has reduced osmotic pressure and the fact that the pregnant womb tends to compress on the vessels of the legs. This reduces the amount of blood and water flowing upwards from the legs and feet towards the heart. This stagnation facilitates the accumulation of water in between the tissues of the feet and legs, causing the legs and feet to swell. This is called leg edema in medical parlance.

### 36. Is edema a bad sign in pregnancy?

Edema is common in pregnancy. Ordinarily, it should be regarded as one of the body's normal adjustments to pregnancy. In this case, it should not have any adverse effect on the mother and baby. However, leg edema may be a bad sign if the mother also develops other diseases or conditions in pregnancy. For example:
- Hypertension with protein in the urine
- Heart problems
- Kidney problems

In some of these situations, the edema may be seen in other parts of the body, including the buttocks and the face, causing puffiness.

### 37. What are the problems in adolescent pregnancy?

At both extremes of life, during adolescence and above 35 years, pregnancy is associated with more problems. For adolescents, some of these are:
- Psychosocial
  - Pregnancy ownership problems
  - Street drug use
  - Alcohol use
  - Smoking
  - Domestic violence
  - Poor attendance for prenatal care appointments
  - Poor compliance with doctor's instructions
- Increased desire for abortion
- Premature or preterm birth
- Intra uterine growth retardation
- Low birth weight
- Obstructed labor
- Increased possibility of Caesarian section operation

These reasons and more, make adolescent pregnancy high risk.

### 38. What is the importance of weight gain in pregnancy?

It is important for women to gain weight normally in pregnancy. Appropriate weight gain is dependent on the weight or Body mass index (BMI) before pregnancy. For a woman with a normal weight or BMI, weight gain of 27.5 – 39.6lbs (12.5kg – 18kg) in pregnancy is desirable. 27.5lbs is the average. Of this, 19.8lbs (9kg) is due to the weight of the enlarged womb, growing baby, placenta, birth water, maternal blood, retained fluids and enlarged breasts.

The remaining 7.7lbs (3.5kg) is due to maternal stores of fat. There is a wide range of weight gain that may be regarded as harmless in pregnancy. So there is individual variation. Poor weight gain may suggest problems in pregnancy. The remarkable adverse effect is the delivery of a low birth weight baby i.e. baby weighing less than 5.5lbs (2500g) at birth. Low Birth Weight (LBW) is associated with various complications including early infant death. In the USA, LBW babies are most common among African-Americans.

Accelerated weight gain is abnormal and may herald impending dangers, especially pre-eclampsia. Excessive weight gain may also result in large-for-gestational age babies. This may cause problems during labor and make vaginal delivery unsafe. In such situations, the rate of cesarean operation is increased.

**39. What is the relationship of maternal weight gain to the weight of babies at birth?**

There is medical evidence that supports the fact that maternal weight before pregnancy and the extent of weight gain by the mother during pregnancy, correlates with the weight of the baby. This, to a large extent, is reflected by maternal body water. So, women who gain weight normally in pregnancy, usually give birth to babies with normal weight. Conversely, when a woman's weight gain is less than expected, the baby is more likely to be smaller in weight.

**40. Is it true that some women crave for unusual food in pregnancy?**

Yes, it's true. Some women have been known to demand and strongly crave for unusual foods like the meat of certain animals or meat from certain parts of an animal's body, ice blocks, refrigerator frost, and clay! In some parts of Africa, some types of clay can actually be bought in the market and eaten. The attraction is the sweet nature of the clay. This is more mythical than science. The reason for this type of abnormal demand has remained unexplained. This condition is called pica. Some doctors believe that Pica may be due to iron-deficiency anemia in pregnancy. Of course, malnutrition due to unusual food can easily tip a woman into iron-deficiency in pregnancy. Some cases of pica subside when iron deficiency is treated. In some communities in developing countries, it is not rare for women to crave for new foods during pregnancy. Such women should not be deemed to be taking undue advantage of pregnancy, to force their spouses to provide exotic nutrition. Women are entitled to good nutrition and care in pregnancy, wherever they may be. So this is not pica.

## 41. What are the basic nutritional requirements for pregnant women?

Nutritional requirements in pregnancy vary widely. There are individual differences but the guiding principle is that women should eat well-balanced diets in sufficient quantities. It is difficult to be specific but generally, diets must be able to provide sufficient calories, vitamins, minerals and protein. Diet and delicacies vary from one community to another. The National Research Council in the USA recommends that pregnant women should consume about 2500kcal/day. This should include 60g of protein daily.

Pregnant women should therefore be familiar with the contents and components of the foods available in their communities. However, the general outline should be:

- Vary your diet
- Eat enough foods of animal origin like meat, milk, cheese etc.
- Eat plenty of fruits which will most probably supply many of the vitamins that you need
- Start folic acid supplementation as early as possible in pregnancy; Iron supplementation may be started at the same time. Iron supplementation is more important in the last 20 weeks of pregnancy
- Ensure that your meals are regular and prepared in a hygienic manner
- Before purchasing multivitamins and mineral supplement packs, carefully read the labels, Noting the following:
- Do not use: if the manufacturer says a drug is not approved or is contra-indicated in pregnancy. Be aware that many drugs that cause birth defects do so early in pregnancy
- Take note of the amounts of Vitamins A, B and C and ensure they do not exceed the amounts recommended for pregnant women
- Ensure the salt used to prepare your foods is iodized
- Get a home weighing scale, check and record your weight at regular intervals
- If you notice any problem after eating particular foods, stop eating them and complain to your doctor

## 42. How does iron intake affect pregnancy?

At all times during pregnancy, a woman must have sufficient blood. A normal diet can provide almost all the elements required for making blood, however most diets do not contain enough iron and folate to meet women's requirements in pregnancy. Elemental iron and folic acid are therefore routinely prescribed for women in pregnancy. It is essential for a pregnant woman to have sufficient blood for a number of reasons including:

- The normal physiological anemia of pregnancy: This is because the water component of blood is far in excess of the red blood cells in pregnancy. This is akin to dilution of blood in pregnancy

- Sufficient blood is needed to pass nutrients and other needs to the baby
- Growing babies need to make their own blood by taking the building blocks from their mother's circulation
- It is usual for women to lose blood during labor and delivery, so they must ensure that they do not easily become anemic, should bleeding occur in pregnancy

Elemental iron and folic acid prevent the occurrences of iron and folate deficiency anemia. Folic acid is also given before and during pregnancy as a preventive measure against Neural Tube Defects (NTDs). NTD is a congenital abnormality of the spinal cord and brain in the fetus.

**43. What are the side effects of taking iron tablets?**

Elemental iron, despite its importance in preventing iron deficiency anemia in pregnancy, has its own draw backs, which in the extreme, includes iron-poisoning. This is why it is usually packed in blisters. Iron ingested can also cause diarrhea in some women. Other side effects of iron include:

- Constipation
- Stomach pain and discomfort
- Nausea
- Vomiting

Iron tablets may also stain the teeth for a short while after ingestion and stains the stool, making it black in appearance. This may be worrisome to some women unless they are informed beforehand.

**44. Is it compulsory for all women to take iron and other vitamins?**

It is beneficial for all women to take iron and folic acid as a routine. It is also highly recommended that women carrying multiple pregnancy and other high risk pregnancy take multivitamins as routine supplements. Iron and folic acid are good for women in the following situations:

- Multiple pregnancy
- Epilepsy
- Sickles cell anemia (iron not needed)
- Other hemoglobin diseases
- Substance abuse
- Vegetarians
- Jehovah witness adherents

For these categories of women, multivitamin supplements are deemed compulsory.

**45. Is iodine supplementation necessary?**

Pregnant women are highly advised to use iodized salt in their diet. Iodine is needed by the fetus and there is also increased excretion of this substance during pregnancy. Using iodized salt should be sufficient to prevent iodine deficiency in pregnancy. In parts of the world where iodine deficiency is common, cretinism in children is also endemic. The features of cretinism include:

- Stunted growth or failure to thrive
- Poor appetite
- Poor weight gain
- Chronic constipation
- Jaundice
- Gaping depression at top of the head (open anterior fontanelle)
- Shrill or hoarse voice or cry
- Weak or flaccid limbs
- General lack of activity or poor play

Drugs containing Iodine are not routinely recommended for all women in pregnancy because they can lead to the enlargement of the thyroid gland in the unborn baby (fetal goiter).

### 46. I understand that Vitamin A supplement is not good in pregnancy, please explain.

On the average, 2500 IU of Vitamin A per day is desirable in pregnancy. Doctors believe that high doses of vitamin A, from 10,000 to 50,000 IU daily may cause birth defects in babies. It is therefore important to always read the labels on drugs packaging carefully before procuring them. Excess Vitamin A in the body is toxic and harmful. Most routine diets should provide sufficient vitamin A. The good news is that the type of Vitamin A contained in fruits like carrots and vegetables are not harmful, and does not cause birth defects. So you do not need to worry about eating fruits.

### 47. What about other Vitamins like Vitamin B6, B12 and Vitamin C?

Vitamin B12 is generally reduced in pregnancy. Vitamin B12 is present only in foods of animal origin. Therefore, pregnant women need to take sufficient animal originated foods, especially meat and milk. Vitamin B12 supplements may be more important in vegetarians and multiple pregnancy. These categories of women are at higher risk of B12 deficiency. Similarly, Vitamin B6 supplement may be necessary in women who are likely to be under nourished, including vegetarians and those with multiple pregnancy. Most balanced diets contain sufficient amounts of Vitamin C. Citrus fruits and many other fruits are rich in Vitamin C. Daily supplement of Vitamin C is good, but excess may reduce the level of Vitamin B12 and cause B12 deficiency.

**48. So what is my guide to choice of Vitamins?**

The best approach is to discuss this with the doctor overseeing your pregnancy. However, a good Vitamin supplement package for your daily usage should contain:

- Iron
- Folic acid
- Vitamin A,
- Vitamin C,
- Vitamin D,
- Vitamin E,
- Copper, Calcium and Zinc

**49. Is exercise advisable during pregnancy?**

There is no doubt that exercise is beneficial in pregnancy. The benefits include:

- Improvement in general body functions
- Improvement in the volume of blood and blood flow
- Exercise can lead to shorter duration of labor, and reduction in the risk of fetal distress
- Exercise has been found to reduce the risk of Cesarean section operation. However, unaccustomed or high intensity exercise can lead to spontaneous abortions and babies with low birth weight. Here are some tips on exercise:
    - Exercise is generally good in pregnancy if you are already accustomed to such. Aerobics are recommended. You can continue at about 50% of capacity compared to your pre-pregnant intensity
    - Do not start a totally new exercise method or program in pregnancy
    - If you have been leading a sedentary lifestyle before pregnancy, you can walk but don't jog. In other words, do not be aggressive when exercising
    - If you suffer from diseases such as hypertension, sedentary exercise like walking may be beneficial
    - Do not continue exercise to the point that you become breathless or unduly fatigued. Also, dizziness is a bad sign that you are getting into trouble, so stop immediately
- Caution: be careful and ask for your doctor's advice if you have the following conditions:
    - Severe hypertensive disorder in pregnancy
    - Uncontrolled diabetes
    - Bleeding in pregnancy
    - Heart disease
    - Kidney disease
    - Multiple pregnancy

## 50. What about work?
Working during pregnancy is not bad, especially if you are accustomed to it and can cope safely with the demands of your work. In developing countries, many women need to work during pregnancy in order to meet family, social, and financial obligations. Even in the USA, about 50% of women in their child bearing age are workers. Working while pregnant does not kill but stressful work schedules can have adverse effects. Generally, the guiding principles should be:
- If you engage in a sedentary occupation, stand up from the sitting position at intervals, move around and stretch your legs and rest regularly
- It is not advisable to change your employment to a more demanding work schedule during pregnancy. You may not be able to correctly guess the effect it will have on you
- When existing work or new employment brings fatigue and lack of sleep, you need to be careful. You should discuss with your doctor

## 51. What employment options do pregnant women have?
In most countries, there are laws put in place to ensure that women are not denied opportunities or discriminated against because of pregnancy. Many women in employment automatically qualify for paid maternity leave. This is enjoyed at the tail end of pregnancy and several weeks after delivery, so mothers can rest and nurture their babies. There are usually 2 options available for would-be pregnant or already pregnant women:
- For women who are competitive athletes, fashion models and other jobs that are highly demanding or heavily regimented occupations; the option is to take time off work to get pregnant and nurse their babies, after which they can resume their occupations. This type of leave could be leave of absence without pay, leave of absence with pay, or other kinds of arrangements with employers. Athletes can quit training for a period of time to have their babies and thereafter resume their careers
- If your employment gives you the benefit of paid maternity leave, then this is best for you. Where maternity leave is not paid for, like in the USA and Australia, women tend to work until very late in pregnancy, in order to meet their economic obligations. With this option, the issue of how to cope with the cost of maintaining your pregnancy and nursing your baby still remains a problem

## 52. Can pregnant women travel?
Travelling is not contraindicated in pregnancy. However, if travelling by road, safety and carefulness are watchwords and it is important to use safety belts always. The belts should be made comfortable by passing them under the breasts, below the pregnant tummy and the upper thigh, so that tension is not exerted on the baby. Speed limits must be obeyed and drivers must be

considerate. It is important to move the legs regularly as often as possible. Long journeys could be broken with periods of rest, to allow the legs to be stretched by taking few steps back and forth. Air travel should follow the same principles. Pregnant women should stand up and walk along the aisle at intervals. In the USA, airlines do not object to flying pregnant women, except maybe, during the week of the expected date of delivery or during labor. It is advisable that you ask for your doctor's opinion if you wish to travel at the tail end of your pregnancy.

### 53. What mode of dressing do you advise?

In the past, it was fashionable for pregnant women to wear full length baggy clothing or caftans during pregnancy. Time seems to have changed and the current attitude of an increasing number of pregnant women is to put on body hugs that exhibit their pregnancy. Whichever you may choose to wear, please ensure that it is elastic or loose enough to avoid strapping and tightening up your tummy. Also, bras that support the sagging and enlarged breasts are appropriate in pregnancy.

### 54. Is constipation normal during pregnancy?

Many women experience constipation as pregnancy progresses. This is because the enlarged womb sits on the bowels and compresses them. The compression slows the movement of stool so that more water is absorbed from the stools which become hardened. It is also possible that some hormones like progesterone, slow down bowel movements too. Attempts to force down hard stools during defecation may result in pain and blood stained stool. Apart from hard stools and constipation, the enlarged womb may also compress on the veins in the lower portion of the bowels, anus, and vulva. The compression reduces drainage of blood from the veins in these parts of the body. Consequently, the veins become dilated or swollen. This is called hemorrhoids. Sometimes, hemorrhoids are associated with pain in the anus which can be severe during defecation. Bleeding from the anus may also be noticed after defecation. If you experience some of these symptoms, you should visit your doctor as soon as you can, for advice and treatment.

### 55. What can be done to relieve heartburn?

Some women experience this complaint and it is fairly common in pregnancy. As pregnancy advances, the enlarged womb pushes the stomach and esophagus up, apart from exerting slight compression on them. Also, the muscle or sphincter at the lower end of the esophagus is weakened and is partially open at this part. The muscles of the esophagus and stomach may also be weakened by progesterone. The stomach normally secretes acidic contents. In this situation, the pregnant womb can readily push the acidic content of the stomach into the partially opened esophagus, which is a pipe that connects to the back of the mouth, through which food passes. The

acidified food in the esophagus has a burning effect at the lower chest wall. This is called heart burn. To get some relief, the following tips can help:
- Avoid spicy foods
- Do not lie down soon after eating. You can sit on the bed for a few hours before lying down
- It may be better to take small quantities of food at intervals
- There are drugs that can neutralize the acidic effect on the esophagus. They are called antacids. These include:
  - Magnesium trisilicate
  - Aluminum hydroxide etc.

Please ensure that your antacids drugs do not contain sodium or sodium bicarbonate. These two can be retained and cause aggravation of problems like hypertension and more fluid retention or edema in pregnancy.

## 56. What are the causes of rashes in pregnancy?

There are some skin conditions that may have existed before pregnancy but some women may complain of itchy sensation for the first time, during pregnancy. Some of these important skin problems include:
- Eczema: Eczema is more likely to improve during pregnancy, though most cases of eczema existed before pregnancy.
- Skin eruption: This may occur in pregnancy showing up as itchy urticaria, fever and fast pulse, usually in the last few months of pregnancy. It usually does not have an adverse effect on the outcome of pregnancy.
- Infestations: Conditions like scabies and infestation of bugs may cause rashes but they are not peculiar to pregnancy. Scabies may cause stubborn itching and discomfort but does not adversely affect pregnancy.
- Allergy and drug eruptions: Some women react abnormally
- to both old and new drugs, some of which may show up as itching, urticaria, eczema, breathlessness, and other symptoms. Symptoms like these may constitute an emergency. If this happens, pregnant women must see their doctor without delay. Drugs that are notorious for acute rash and anaphylaxis are penicillin and anti-malarial chloroquine.

## 57. Is sexual intercourse advisable in pregnancy?

Sexual intercourse can be enjoyed in pregnancy, if there are no problems. However, doctors generally advise against coitus in the last 4 weeks. It is true that many women abstain from sexual intercourse in pregnancy but this may be due to lack of desire or unfounded fear of doing harm to their pregnancy. In certain women, it may be better to abstain from sexual intercourse as much as possible, to avoid adverse consequences. Sexual intercourse may not be appropriate in the following situations:

- Women with previous spontaneous abortions
- Women with threatened abortion earlier in pregnancy
- Women with spurious or irregular vaginal bleeding in pregnancy
- Women with serious placenta problems

The position and attitude of the male partner is important in preventing adverse effects. For example, when the male lies on the woman's tummy, there is increased risk of breaking the water prematurely. This may result in infection of the contents of the womb, as well as premature labor and delivery. Always remember that sexual intercourse is better avoided in the last 4 weeks of pregnancy.

## 58. Is alcohol harmful to pregnant women?

Alcohol in any form has not been proved to be safe in pregnancy. In the USA, the surgeon general warns that alcohol use is not advisable for any pregnant woman or in those considering pregnancy. The most documented effect of alcohol is the adverse effect on the fetus. Babies of alcohol users may suffer from fetal alcohol syndrome. This term is used to describe the combination of congenital physical birth deformities and mental problems that occur due to alcohol intake in pregnancy. These features include:

- Growth retardation
- Heart deformities
- Small head
- Flabby tone of muscles
- Deformed face
- Imbecile look or face, etc

It is suggested that women who drink alcohol heavily during pregnancy, also expose the fetus to alcohol ("baby also drinks").

## 59. How does smoking affect pregnant women?

In the advanced countries of the world, notably the USA, about 13% of women still smoke in pregnancy, down from 20% in 1998. Since 1984, the surgeon general has been warning that smoking can cause:

- Fetal injury
- Premature birth
- Low birth weight

Other adverse effects include:

- Placental damage
- Fetal death
- Infant death

Where a woman finds it difficult to quit smoking, psychologists have recommended nicotine medication such as nicotine chewing gum, in place of outright smoking, in those that smoke 11 – 15 cigarettes daily.

**60. What about caffeine?**

Caffeine intake does not cause birth defects in pregnancy but doctors advise that levels should be reduced and specifically, women should not take more than 5 standard cups per day. Where practicable, abstaining is better, especially if caffeine greatly increases your anxiety or makes you unduly nervous.

**61. What can be done about excessive sleepiness and tiredness in pregnancy?**

Many women do experience excessive sleep and fatigue early in pregnancy. This may be due to the effects of the abundant progesterone and other hormones. There are individual variations in the intensities of these complaints and such problems normally subside on their own around the 16th week of pregnancy. No special treatment is needed to be awake and strong again; only patience.

**62. Is it normal for pregnant women to experience an increase in vaginal discharge?**

Many women experience this complaint in pregnancy, so it may be normal in so far as it is not caused by an increased population of harmful germs in the vagina. However, the increased discharge may be due to the effect of plenteous estrogen hormone which causes heavier secretion from the glands of the cervix. This condition is called leucorrhea and it is usually harmless. If you are worried, you may douche with water at intervals. The water should be made mildly acidic by adding vinegar. If this does not work, you should contact your doctor for proper identification of the problem and treatment. Specifically, infections by germs like Trichomonas vaginalis and yeast should be considered if the discharge becomes itchy or offensive in odor.

**63. How can women tell if the discharge is caused by yeast or other infections?**

When the vaginal discharge becomes profuse and offensive, there is high possibility of vaginal infections. Three infections are important. These are Trichomonas infection, yeast infection, and bacterial vaginosis. The information below may help to identify the infections:

| Vaginal Infection and Germs | % of Women Affected in Pregnancy | Features of Vaginal Discharge |
|---|---|---|
| Candidiasis or yeast infection caused by: Candida Albicans | 25% near the end of pregnancy | Copious, irritating discharge that looks like milk curds |
| Trichomonas infection caused by: Trichomonas vaginalis | About 20% | Copious, foamy, yellowish-green, irritating and itchy |
| Bacterial vaginosis caused by:<br>▪ Gardnerellavaginalis<br>▪ Mobilincus species<br>▪ Bacteroides species | 10 – 30% | Copious, extremely foul smelling and irritating |

Once women suspect that the discharge may be due to any of these or other infections, the doctor must be consulted without delay, in order to avoid adverse consequences in pregnancy.

**64. What is your advice on drug use in pregnancy generally?**

There are 3 main categories of drugs that women may have access to during pregnancy:

- The first category is prescribed by your doctor. This category of drugs should pose no danger, if you follow your doctor's instructions
- The second category can be bought are those bought over the counter in pharmacies. These include common pain killers, drugs for cold, vitamins and mineral supplements. However, it is important that you read the manufacturer's labels and instructions on the packages carefully, to be sure that:
  - The drug can be used by pregnant women
  - The amounts of each of the components that make up the drug are not above those allowed in pregnancy
  - The drug has authority approvals like the FDA in the USA. Sometimes, there may be FDA instructions or warnings from other health authorities which are very important

The third category relates to illicit drugs. You should know that most drugs that affect a woman in pregnancy will most likely affect the baby in the womb. This is because many drugs pass through the mother's circulation to the placenta and then to the baby in the womb. There are serious adverse effects of illicit drugs on the woman and her baby during pregnancy. Generally, the side effects of such drugs on the baby are much similar to their adverse

effects on the mother. The difference is the additional effect on the baby's development, both in rate and manner. Some adverse effects of illicit drugs on babies include:
- Congenital abnormalities or birth defects
- Premature delivery
- Growth retardation in the womb
- Low birth weight
- Fetal distress during labor
- Fetal death and early death in infancy
- Withdrawal effects of illicit drugs which manifest after birth; this is because the baby in the womb is a second hand user of illicit drugs. At delivery, the baby's drug supply is cut off and this leads to withdrawal effects

## 65. What are vaccines?

Immunization is carried out by giving vaccines. Vaccines may contain:
- Antibodies from people that have previously had a particular disease or infection
- Particles from the killed organisms or viruses
- Attenuated or partially modified forms of viruses

Solutions which contain killed viruses, live-attenuated, or modified organisms, are given to a person during vaccination. The organism or its particles or products are called antigens. The combination of antigens and antibodies leads to the destruction of the invading viruses and germs. This leads to healing or protection from such infections. At the same time, memory cells are alerted to swing into rapid and further antibody production, when next the same germ invades the body. This means that the vaccinated person is guaranteed freedom from the particular disease caused by the germ. Antibody production can occur at times when they are needed and can last for a life time, even though the levels may fluctuate. Such a person is said to have lifelong immunity. Similarly, antibodies can be injected directly into the body or taken as small drops of vaccine by mouth. In this case, the person does not produce the antibodies. Most immunization in children are of this category. This is because children lack the ability to produce antibodies on their own, because the immunity system in infants is not well developed.

## 66. What are the types of immunity?

There are 2 types: Active and passive immunity. When people produce antibodies by themselves, due to the presence of antigens, the type of immunity that results is called active immunity. This is because the antibodies were actively produced by the person concerned. Antibodies may also be given or transferred to another person. For example, a mother can pass antibodies to her baby, through the placenta. This type of immunity gained by the baby is called passive immunity. This is because the baby did not personally produce the initial antibodies. So immunity can be active or passive in nature.

## 67. What is immunization?

Immunization is a strategy to obtain immunity and protection from a particular infection or disease. This means that the immunized person has freedom from the disease, for as long as the immunization is still effective in the body. Simply put, the body has the ability to produce cells and molecular substances in the blood to combat foreign germs and diseases. These cells are called antibodies and they are 'fighter cells' that fight and destroy invading organisms or germs. Invading germs are regarded as having antigens. The combination of antibodies and antigens lead to destruction of the invading germs. So, antibodies constitute a natural defense mechanism for the body.

## 68. Are there side effects to immunization?

Immunization is a strategic measure to prevent diseases and their attendant adverse effects from occurring in pregnancy. Some women experience side effects after vaccination, but the advantages of immunization far outweigh the side effects of the vaccines. Most side effects are mild and only few women complain that they are discouraged. The side effects of vaccines vary from one individual to the other. Other side effects are infrequent and may depend on the type of vaccine. Common side effects of vaccines include:

- Fever
- Headache
- Chills
- Rashes
- Swelling at the site of injection
- Redness
- Ulcer
- Nausea
- Vomiting

## 69. What are booster doses?

It is usual for the antibody level of a person who has been vaccinated to reduce with time. This means that the vaccination has to be repeated in order to increase antibody levels in the body. The repeat vaccine doses given at predetermined intervals or during times of high risks are called booster doses. They do exactly what their name says – they boost antibody production and immunity.

**70. Does immunization protect against all diseases?**

Unfortunately, protection cannot be guaranteed because we cannot vaccinate against all diseases. For example, there is currently no vaccination against the HIV infection, so the disease cannot be prevented through vaccination. Immunization is specific and one vaccination can only protect against the disease for which the vaccine is made. That is why there are schedules for immunizations against specific diseases in various parts of the world. The particular schedule is largely determined by the diseases prevalent in a particular community or country. For example, immunization schedules during pregnancy and childhood in West Africa are different from the schedules in the United States of America.

# DEAR DOCTOR:

**71. My doctor said that I am a high risk pregnancy because my blood pressure is high. Please what can I since I hope to be pregnant soon.**

Your doctor is right. Hypertension may have adverse effects on pregnancy. Since you are already hypertensive, your pregnancy may fall into the category called essential hypertension, which may not affect pregnancy too adversely, provided it is controlled. Where hypertension is caused by kidney diseases or associated with heart problems, there is a higher possibility of damage to other organs and adverse consequences to you and your baby. You will need more frequent appointments and good care in a hospital with specialist doctors to bring your blood pressure safely under control.

**72. I have big breasts and I am worried that they may enlarge out of proportion if I become pregnant. What is your advice?**

It is true that the breasts will enlarge during pregnancy because of the growth of cells and tissues and the fact that the cells also secrete milk. In terms of change, there is no way to forecast the size of your breasts during. Some women who have small breasts may acquire big breasts during pregnancy, while the breast enlargement in other women with previously big breasts may be much less. My advice is that breast enlargement issues should not discourage you from starting your family, more so since you are not certain if the breast enlargement will be profound. Your attitude should be to get to the bridge first before you think of crossing it. The breasts may not be so much enlarged as to embarrass you after all.

### 73. I went for my first PNC visit today and the doctor put a metal inside me. I was uncomfortable. Does he have to do that?

The test is most probably a speculum examination. This examination is necessary as it allows the doctor to see the vagina, assess the neck of the womb and determine if it looks normal or not. At this time, the doctor may also conduct the following tests:

- Perform smear to exclude cells suspicious for cancer
- Take samples of discharge or fluid from the far end of the vagina to examine for germs like:
  - Chlamydia trachomatis
  - Trichomonas germs
  - Candida or yeast

The three germs mentioned above are definitely associated with adverse effects in pregnancy. Candida infection may cause stubborn irritation and itching which may be distressful to you. Once any of these is detected, treatment can be initiated promptly, in order to prevent adverse consequences.

### 74. Why is a measuring tape used on my tummy during each visit?

This is a common practice in prenatal clinics. After the first trimester of pregnancy, the enlarging womb is visible as a bulge and can be touched above the upper level at the front of the waist. From 18 to 32 weeks of pregnancy, the measurement of the length of the tape in centimeters, corresponds to the gestational age of pregnancy in weeks. That is when the measurement is taken from the surface of the pubic bone in front, to the topmost part of the enlarged womb. This measurement is called Symphisio-Fundal Height (SFH). In other words, a measurement of 20cm by tape, corresponds to a gestational age of 20 weeks. 26cm implies 26 weeks of gestation etc. However, this is only true in singleton pregnancy, with the baby lying vertically in the womb. This is a practical way for your doctor to have a rough estimate of the age of your pregnancy and it is repeated at each visit, up until the 36th – 37th week. After the 36th week, the measurement may be misleading because at this time, the baby may have come down into the brim of the birth canal. Tape measurements are documented as the fundal height in weeks.

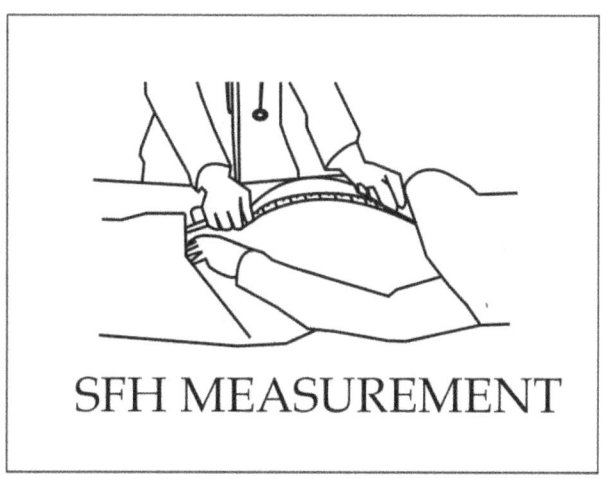

SFH MEASUREMENT

### 75. When should my baby's heart beat be checked?

The doctor must regularly check for fetal heart beats during each visit. Heart beats and fetal movements or kicks, are the 2 simple tests that attest to the fact that your baby is alive. Fetal heart beats can be heard and counted by the doctor or midwife between the 16th and 19th week of pregnancy in many women. At about the 21st week of pregnancy, fetal heart beats can be detected in 95% of women and should be heard in all women at 22 weeks.

### 76. When should I start feeling my baby's kicks?

Babies move about in the womb. They observe periods of rest in between movements. They behave like fish swimming around in the water. The liquor or birth water is their natural swimming pool. The actual time when you begin to feel your baby's kicks or movement depends on your experience. If it is your first pregnancy, you may not notice the first fetal movement (called quickening) until about 25 weeks of pregnancy. For those women who have already experienced pregnancy, the first fetal kicks may be felt as early as 16-18 weeks. Fetal movement is one of the most effective ways to monitor the health of your baby in the womb. Adequate number of daily fetal movements suggest the baby is alive and doing fine. On the average, you should be able to feel 10 movements every 2 hours. As your pregnancy progresses, the movements or jabs become more frequent and stronger. It has been estimated that in the last 12 weeks of pregnancy, fetal jabs movements may be felt 30 times per hour or more.

### 77. When should I be worried about the position of my baby?

How the baby lies in the womb during pregnancy has a great influence on the method of delivery. It may sometimes adversely affect the normal progress of labor. Prior to 33 – 35 weeks of pregnancy, the baby has ample room to swim

about in the birth water, so up to the 34th week, the fetal lie may not be important. After 35 weeks, the majority of babies should have a 'stable lie' which may indicate the way they will come out through the birth canal during delivery. Consequently, in the last 4 weeks of pregnancy, doctors pay special attention to the lie of the baby. The most common fetal lie is longitudinal. This means that the baby is lying vertically inside the womb. With this lie, either the head or the buttock is nearest to the neck of the womb, or to the entrance to the birth canal. Other less common fetal lies are:
- Oblique: when the baby lies in the womb in a slanting manner. The head or buttocks will be to the right or left of the mother's tummy
- Transverse: when the baby lies horizontally in the womb. In other words, the baby lies across the mother's tummy.

So, fetal presentation and lie become important in planning the method of delivery from about the 36th week of pregnancy.

### 78. What test should I do if I am worried about the wellbeing of my baby during pregnancy?

One of the common and important tests you can do is a pregnancy ultrasound scan. Apart from being harmless, it will answer most of the questions that worry expectant mothers. It will tell you the age, the baby's movement, activities of the heart and sometimes breathing movements can be demonstrated. Also, the position of the placenta and adequacy of the birth water can be ascertained. Seeing your baby kicking about in your womb during ultrasound scan strengthens the bond between you and your baby, even at this time. Ultrasound facilities are becoming increasingly available in developing countries and you can repeat the scan as you wish, without any side effects to you or your baby. Where there is more serious concern about the health of the baby, a test called cardiotopogram (CTG) may be ordered by the doctor. This may indicate if the baby is in distress and require urgent attention. In this case immediate delivery may be necessary.

### 79. Now that my breasts are enlarging and I feel some discomfort, what else should I expect?

Early in pregnancy, many women complain of slight tenderness, tension, and tingling sensations in the breast. As pregnancy progresses, the breasts undergo other changes which include:
- Darkening of the skin of the areola, which is the area surrounding the nipple.
- Darkening of the nipple, which becomes more prominent and pointed
- Yellow milk called colostrum can be expressed from the nipples, especially at the tail end of pregnancy. This is necessary towards successful breast feeding.

### 80. Will I be able lose all the weight that I gained when I was pregnant, after delivery?

This is commonly not achievable. Most women lose the highest percentage of weight they gained during pregnancy just after delivery and the next 2 weeks following delivery. Thereafter, weight loss slows down and even when you breastfeed, it is not usually possible to totally return to your pre-pregnancy weight. Most women retain about 3lbs (1.4kg) as an addition to their pre-pregnancy weight and this is more or less permanent.

### 81. Is it ok for me to jog?

Jogging in pregnancy is not suitable for the majority of women. Currently, there is a growing tendency for pregnant women to try out new forms of exercise, including jogging. They even participate in marathons and lawn tennis competitions. These are regarded as extremely demanding exercises and are not advisable. The answer is why jog, when walking is better? So, take a walk.

### 82. My pregnancy is midway but I am finding it difficult to bend down. What is your advice?

You are right. As the tummy grows, it becomes increasingly difficult to bend down and swiftly pick up items or even take a bath. In such a situation, you may gently squat to pick up items and have your bath. If showers are available, you should have your bath while standing. In all situations, please take great care to avoid slips and falls in the bath tub.

### 83. I keep having this nagging headache. What should I do?

Complaints of headache are common in early pregnancy. In the majority of cases, the cause is unknown but sometimes, it may be due to excessive straining to see properly, because of errors in lens refraction in the eyes, brought on by pregnancy. Some are due to infections of the sinuses, which are common in some women. This type of headache may respond to simple pain relievers, vitamins, and antihistamines which should be prescribed by your doctor after examination. It is also important for you to see your doctor because other dangerous causes of headaches like hypertension and migraine, should be ruled out. Where causes cannot be found, the common headaches of pregnancy usually subside in the second half of pregnancy.

# CHAPTER 14
# Labor and Delivery

*"A baby will make love stronger, days shorter, nights longer, bankroll smaller, home happier, clothes shabbier, the past forgotten and the future worth living for."*
– AUTHOR UNKNOWN

### 1. What is labor?
Labor, as the name suggests, is the 'final work' that a pregnant woman has to 'do', in order to deliver her baby. This is the final process that leads to the delivery of her baby from the womb. It normally occurs around the 40th week of pregnancy.

### 2. When is a woman said to be in labor?
Doctors and health workers will regard a pregnant woman to be in labor when she starts having regular uterine contractions. These lead to the shortening and dilatation of the cervix, after 24 complete weeks of gestation. In most developed countries, 24 complete weeks is regarded as the age of viability but in the developing countries, the age of viability is 28 complete weeks. Therefore, the official definition of labor may vary from one country to the other, depending on the gestational age at which the baby can survive outside the womb. As expected, this will depend on the level of neonatal care or support available to newborn babies.

### 3. When does a woman know if she is in labor?
It is interesting to know that the womb contracts throughout pregnancy, but because such contractions are weak and not painful, they are not felt. However, after the 32nd week of pregnancy, the contractions become a little bit stronger, causing some degree of discomfort. These weak contractions are called Braxton Hicks contractions and they occur in an irregular manner. In the next few weeks, when it is time for labor at about the 38th - 40th week,

painful contractions will start. Women are most probably in labor when they start to experience increased, regular, and painful contractions of the womb, which may be preceded by the breaking of the birth water.

### 4. When should expectant mothers report to hospital?

Pregnant women are expected to assemble their baby and delivery items well ahead of their delivery date. This is because they can fall into labor unexpectedly, especially from 4 weeks to the predicted date of delivery. Being prepared for labor in advance will make going to hospital smoother and faster. Women are advised to go to hospital as quickly as possible if:

- The birth water breaks
- They start experiencing painful contractions that come regularly within 10 minutes
- They experience vaginal bleeding: may be with the expulsion of the cervical mucus plug

### 5. What is the meaning of "show"?

Sometimes early in labor, a woman may expel the mucus plug that blocks the cervix during pregnancy. The expulsion of this discharge is usually followed by slight vaginal bleeding. This occurrence is referred to as a "show." A remarkable number of pregnant women notice show just before contractions start. However, if this is not noticed, once women start experiencing regular painful contractions at term, they should pack their things and proceed to hospital.

### 6. What is the best posture of the baby that facilitates normal delivery?

There are generally 2 types of postures that a baby may take in the womb and during delivery. The baby may bend its head forward on the chest by flexing the neck. In this situation, the hand and legs are neatly folded in front of its chest and tummy. Here, the baby is said to be in an attitude of FLEXION. In a well flexed baby, the size of the head is much smaller and more likely to enter or pass through the birth canal safely and faster. The opposite situation occurs when the neck is bent backwards so that the chin of the baby is farther from the front of the chest wall. In this situation, the diameter of the head is increased and it is less likely to pass through the birth canal without difficulty. The baby is said to be in an attitude of EXTENSION. The diagrams below illustrate these situations.

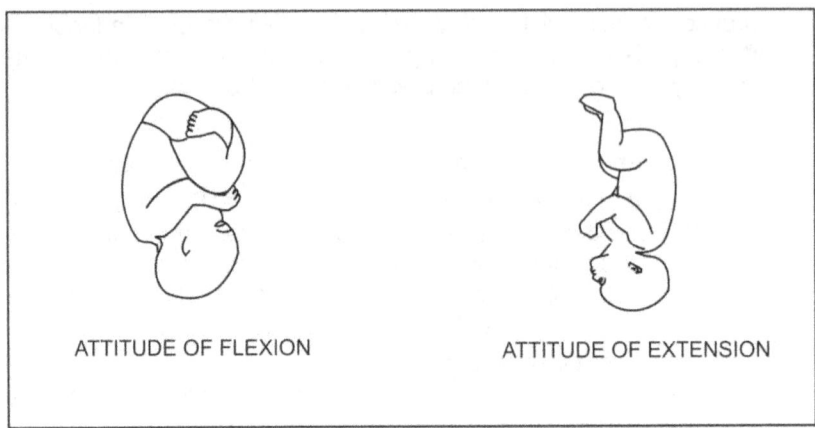

ATTITUDE OF FLEXION          ATTITUDE OF EXTENSION

## 7. When is the baby's head said to be engaged?

The baby's head is said to be engaged when the largest diameter of the head has passed through the inlet of the pelvis. When the woman is examined by doctors, attempts to shake the head from side to side will indicate that the head is fixed. Engagement of the head occurs earlier in first timers from about 38 weeks of pregnancy. In women with previous deliveries, engagement may not occur until labor has started.

## 8. What is molding?

Molding is a term commonly used by doctors and nurses in the labor ward. During labor, the head of the baby undergoes changes in shape and size as it passes through the birth canal. The bones of the head are flat and loosely attached to each other. This enables the shape and size of the head to change easily. During molding, the bones override each other so that the baby's head becomes smaller in size and is able to come down through the birth canal with ease. The shape of the head during this process is determined by its position and the shape of the birth canal at any particular point. Molding is important because it ensures that the "big" head of the baby is made much smaller, making its passage easier and preventing injury to the birth canal. However, because the skull encloses the soft and tender brain of the baby, molding should be moderate and smooth in order to avoid injury.

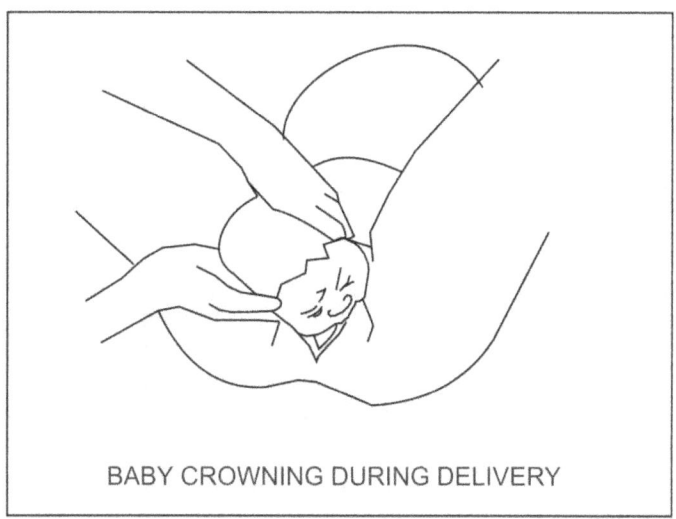

BABY CROWNING DURING DELIVERY

## 9. What is Caput?

As the baby's head passes through the birth canal, it is subjected to forces of contraction from muscles of the womb and other structures in the birth canal. Contractions are needed to push and direct the baby down the birth canal during labor. As the baby's head is squeezed down the canal, the soft tissues of the scalp become swollen. Doctors call this caput succedaneum or Caput for short. This is more commonly seen at the back of the head. Even though the swollen head may worry some young or inexperienced women, Caput is harmless and normally subsides within days after birth.

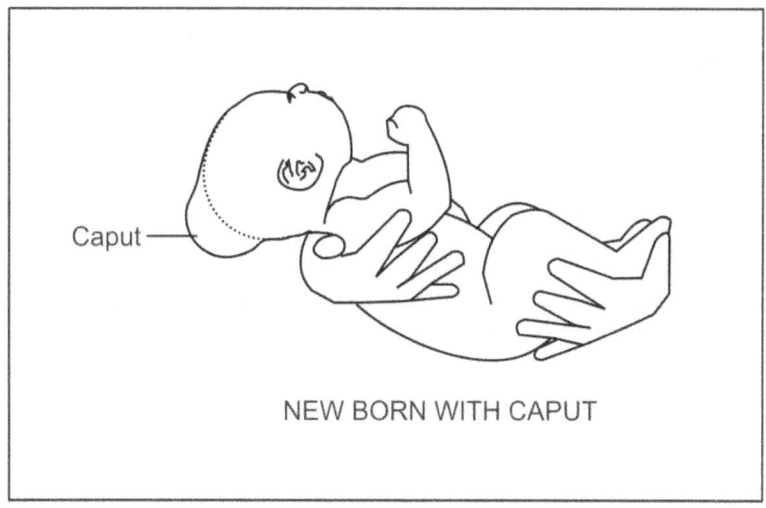

NEW BORN WITH CAPUT

### 10. How is the baby moved through the birth canal during labor?

The main force is provided by the strong contractions of the womb. The powerful contraction is dominant at top of the womb from where it moves downwards. It serves to push the baby in a downward direction in the birth canal. This means pushing the baby from behind. At the same time, contractions dilate the cervix which is also taken up. The barrel shape of the cervix disappears in the process, leaving a circular opening of about 10cm in diameter, when it is fully dilated and baby's head is ready to be delivered. The joints between the bones of the pelvis, soft tissues, cervix, vagina and vulva are all stretched like an elastic band as the contraction pushes the baby downwards from behind. All these work together to expel the baby from the birth canal at the time of delivery. In situations where labor is difficult, bruises and tears can occur along the birth canal, as well as injury to the baby.

### 11. When is a contraction said to be normal?

A normal contraction should be painful, come regularly every 2 – 3 minutes and last for more than 45 seconds. More importantly, in between each contraction, there should be a period of relaxation. At this period of relaxation, the woman can also relax and rest from the pain of contractions. Uterine contractions may be abnormal if they are not effective in dilating the cervix, so that the progress of labor is slow. Sometimes, delivery may happen too quickly. This is because the contractions may be too strong or too aggressive, causing injury to the womb and the fetus.

### 12. What is the normal duration of labor?

The average duration of labor differs and depends on whether a woman is in labor for the first time or has delivered before. For first timers, the average duration of labor is 12 hours. In women with previous experiences of labor, the duration is shorter at 7 hours on the average.

### 13. What is precipitous labor?

When labor is too short or less than 4 hours in duration, it is called precipitous labor. Events in labor happen so fast with excessive force of contraction, causing tear injuries and bleeding to the mother as well as the baby. In this type of situation, safe delivery cannot be guaranteed. In such a situation, both mother and baby run the risk of serious injuries.

### 14. What is prolonged labor?

Prolonged labor means that the duration of labor has far exceeded the average duration. This may be due to the poor contractions, obstruction to the safe passage of the baby through the birth canal and numerous other problems. Both mother and baby become exhausted. In most cases, contractions may be improved upon by using drugs or performing an operation to bring out the baby.

### 15. Of what relevance is the duration of labor to successful delivery?

It is important that labor is conducted in such a way that the mother and baby come out alive and healthy. When labor is prolonged, it usually suggests that there are problems with delivery. The woman may become exhausted and dehydrated. The risk of complications including infection, bleeding, and even death becomes a possibility if help does not come on time. Like the mother, the baby may also become exhausted and distressed, running the risk of death. Therefore, it is important for a woman in labor not to waste precious time at home.

### 16. What are the stages of normal labor?

When labor starts, one of the effects of uterine contractions is that the neck of the womb or cervix, which was closed, begins to open up gradually. The opening up of the cervix is called cervical dilatation. One can regard 0cm as a completely closed cervix. That is when the cervix is not dilated at all. Cervical dilation increases from 0cm and gets to 10cm at the time the baby is ready to be delivered. Therefore, 10cm cervical dilation is also called full cervical dilation.

Cervical dilatation is used to divide labor into 3 stages. These stages are:

> 1st Stage: From the beginning of labor to the time when the cervix is fully dilated. This means that the diameter of the exit point for the baby is 10cm. This stage is further sub-divided into the latent phase and active phase.

> 2nd Stage: This begins from the time of full dilatation to the time when the baby is delivered. Delivery of the baby is expected within 1 hour in first timers and within 30 minutes in women with previous deliveries.

> 3rd Stage: This starts after the delivery of the baby and ends at the expulsion of the placenta. Expulsion of the placenta should take place within 1 hour after the delivery of the baby.

### 17. What is the Latent Phase?

The latent phase begins when contractions starts, up until the cervix is 3cm dilated. During this phase, the timing, duration, and intensity of uterine contractions may vary. So, most women spend more time in this phase.

During this phase and the greater part of the active phase, women in labor may be allowed to walk around the labor ward or drink fluids such as glucose. They are still generally more cooperative, comfortable, and cheerful. In first timers, the average duration of the latent phase is 8 hours. In women who have had previous deliveries, it is about 6 hours.

### 18. What is the Active Phase?

After the passive phase, when the cervix is more that 3cm dilated, labor generally progresses faster. This means increases in the strength and duration of contractions and faster dilatation rate of the cervix. Cervical dilatation happens more rapidly from 3cm to 10cm. At 10cm, the cervix is said to be fully dilated. In the active phase, first timers will achieve 1½ cm of cervical dilatation per hour, while those with previous deliveries will dilate at more than 2cm per hour.

### 19. When is a woman said to be making progress in labor?

Doctors and midwives would normally regard a woman to be making progress in labor if the cervix is dilating at a minimum rate of 1cm per hour, during the active phase of labor.

### 20. What are the general factors that determine the progress of labor?

It is usually not possible for the doctor to predict exactly how labor will progress in any woman. Generally, there are 3 important factors which have been described as the power, passage, and passenger or the 3Ps. These are:
- Power: The efficacy of uterine contractions
- Passage: The adequacy of the birth canal
- Passenger: The parameters of the baby:
  - The size or how big the baby is
  - The lie of the baby
  - Presentation; whether the baby is coming with the head, breech, etc.

These 3Ps summarize the general consideration, for good progress to be made. However, things can suddenly turn out differently from the predicted positions. This is why every woman in labor should be closely monitored.

### 21. How does the shape of a woman's pelvis affect labor?

The shape of the pelvic cavity and diameters of the bones of the birth canal play important parts during labor and delivery. This is because the baby must enter the birth canal through the pelvic inlet, pass through the birth canal into the mid cavity of the pelvis and be delivered from the pelvic outlet. So the inlet, mid cavity and outlet of the pelvis, must be wide enough to allow the passage of the baby safely during labor. There are 4 main types of pelvis. They are:

- Gynecoid pelvis (pronounced: Gy-ne-ko-id): This is the normal female pelvis and is roomy enough to allow the safe passage of the baby. It is present in 50% of women
- Android Pelvis (pronounced An-dro-id): This is the male-type pelvis. It is shaped like a triangle and has a narrow cavity. It occurs in about 20% of women
- Platypelloid Pelvis (pronounced Pla-ti-pe-lo-id): This is also called the flat pelvis. It has a short back to front dimension and longer side diameters, so it appears flat from side to side. The inlet may be too small for the baby to enter the birth canal normally. It is rare and occurs in 5% of women
- Anthropoid pelvis (Monkey Pelvis) (pronounced: An-thro-po-id): In this type, the diameters are longer from back to front and it has a deep pelvic cavity. It occurs in 30% of women

Therefore, the type of a woman's pelvis influences what may happen during labor. Aside from the gynecoid pelvis, other pelvic types more commonly cause obstruction to the safe passage of the baby during labor. They are regarded as abnormal pelvis.

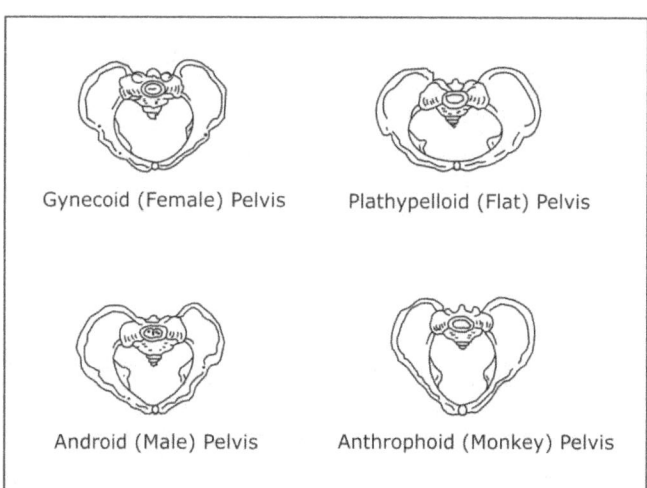

Gynecoid (Female) Pelvis   Plathypelloid (Flat) Pelvis

Android (Male) Pelvis   Anthrophoid (Monkey) Pelvis

## 22.  Can doctors initiate labor?

Yes, they can. It is called induction of labor. There are many reasons why doctors and mid wives may need to induce labor in a pregnant woman. This is more commonly done when a woman has gone past her estimated date of delivery and there are no signs that labor is forthcoming. Doctors may also consider it necessary to initiate labor in the following situations:

- When it is necessary to ensure that labor occurs at a predetermined time. This may be done such that the woman falls into labor when skilled personnel like doctors and nurses are available and facilities in the labor ward are optimal. Labor is planned to take place during the day and on week days, not on weekends. This may be for medical or surgical reasons or due to the fact that the woman is a high risk case. Things are much less likely to go wrong when labor is induced electively
- Sometimes, during the tail end of pregnancy, the life or health of the woman may be in danger because of an ongoing pregnancy. In this case, the baby must be delivered immediately
- Pregnancy may be unduly prolonged or postdated in some women. A postdated pregnancy is one that extends beyond 41 weeks and 6 days. The danger is that the placenta at this time is old and may be inefficient. It may not be able to supply the baby with the nutrition and other requirements that it needs to stay alive and healthy. The baby's health condition may also begin to deteriorate. Another issue is that molding in post-mature babies is poor because the skull is rigid. This makes its passage through the birth canal and delivery difficult. Furthermore, post-mature babies are usually heavy and overweight, resulting in difficult delivery. It is usual for doctors to induce labor as soon as pregnancy is postdated, in order to minimize problems in the mother and baby.

### 23. What are some of the reasons for induction of labor?

There are many reasons why doctors induce labor. Circumstances vary from one woman to another and the attending doctor is in the best position to decide if and when to induce labor. To arrive at such an important decision, doctors take many situations into consideration. In many cases, it is possible to take a decision and plan towards induction well ahead. This guarantees a better outcome. Some of the reasons for induction include:

- Worsening maternal health condition
- Poor kidney function
- Pre-eclampsia
- Increasing severity of Rhesus ISO-Immunization
- Bringing an end to a prolonged pregnancy
- Social reasons may be considered depending on local practice. These include:
  - Specific birthdates or anniversaries
  - Synchronizing with important Holidays and trips

### 24. How is labor induced?

Doctors and midwives use many methods to induce labor. However, the most common method that you may have heard about is using a "drip." A drug called oxytocin is put inside the drip, which helps the pregnant womb begin contractions. The amount of drip that goes into the body is carefully controlled so that contractions are progressive and regulated, resulting in the delivery of the baby. Contractions cause pain which may increase when oxytocin drips are used.

### 25. When is induction of labor appropriate?

Induction is not suitable in all cases of pregnancy even when it may be beneficial. Certain conditions must be met including:
- The baby must be fit with a normal heart rate pattern
- The baby must be lying longitudinally
- There must be no obstruction to delivery through the birth canal e.g.
  - No obstructing fibroid or polyp
  - No major placenta previa
- No cord prolapse
- Women with previous classical cesarean section and other operations on the womb are excluded.

### 26. Generally, what are the complications that may arise from induction?

Doctors take decisions to induce labor for the overall benefit of the mother, the baby, or both. However, on a few occasions, things may go wrong with resulting complications. The major adverse effects of induction of labor include:
- Failed induction: This is usually when there is no cervical dilation up to 3cm, despite sufficient effort and time
- Placenta abruption: This may occur soon after the membranes are ruptured, especially in a situation where there is excess liquor
- Cord prolaspe: The cord may prolapse through the birth canal after the membranes have been ruptured. This creates a surgical emergency
- Fetal distress: The baby may become distressed with manifestation of irregular heartbeats
- Hyper-stimulation: The uterus may be excessively stimulated with very strong uterine contractions that put the baby in distress. This may also cause rupture of the uterus
- Post-partum bleeding: This may occur after prolonged and excessive use of oxytocin or after failed inductions. In these situations, the contraction ability of the uterus may be reduced, thus increasing the risk of bleeding

### 27. Are there any problems linked to the use of oxytocin drips?

An oxytocin drip is no doubt very useful in labor but when it is not used correctly, it can cause other problems. For example, if too much is given, it can lead to a ruptured or torn womb. A ruptured womb is a very serious problem because it is usually followed by serious internal bleeding and the death of the baby. It is more common in women who have had previous operations on the womb and for this reason, such women are usually excluded. Rather, this group of women should always book for antenatal care early in pregnancy and deliver in a well-established hospital, with experienced doctors in attendance. In such situations, there are sophisticated gadgets to monitor the amount of oxytocin given, or it is used with great caution and the strength of womb contractions, heart beats, and other conditions of the baby are usually closely observed. Perhaps the commonest and cheapest way to monitor labor is through the use of the partogram.

### 28. What is a partogram?

When a woman in labor is admitted to the labor ward, it is essential for the events and progress of labor to be monitored very closely and carefully documented. The monitored events include:

> For the mother: The pulse rate, blood pressure, fluid intake, urine output, drugs given, uterine contractions, procedures performed during labor and records of cervical dilatation, effacement and other parameters.

> For the Baby: The heart rate, presentation, descent, engagement and position

These are observed at stipulated times and recorded or plotted on a one-page form with a portion on which a graph can be plotted. Doctors use information on the graph to monitor the progress of labor and determine when further actions are necessary. This record of important events in labor is called a partogram.

### 29. What is cord prolapse?

The fetal membranes wrap the baby, cord, placenta, and birth water inside the womb. When the water breaks, the contents of the womb are exposed to the outside and with the womb opening-up due to cervical dilation, it is possible for the cord to fall through the cervical canal into the vagina. This is dangerous, because during contractions, the cord is usually compressed between the presenting part of the baby, the cervix and pelvic wall. The compression stops the blood supply to the baby which becomes "suffocated." This is called cord prolapse, which means that the umbilical cord has prolapsed through the birth canal. Cord prolapse is one of the common causes of fetal distress. This condition is an emergency which requires the urgent attention of the doctor to prevent fetal death.

## 30. What is the relationship between multiple pregnancy and duration of pregnancy?

A normal pregnancy lasts about 38 weeks on the average, however, the more the number of babies in the womb, the shorter the duration of pregnancy. The approximate rule is to multiply the number of babies in the womb by 2 and subtract the answer from 38 weeks. Examples are given below:

| | | |
|---|---|---|
| Number of babies | 2 (twins): 2x2= 4 AND 38 – 4 | 36 weeks |
| Number of babies | 3 (triplets):3x2=6 AND 38 – 6 | 32 weeks |
| Number of babies | 4 (quadruplets):4x2=8 AND 38 – 8 | 30 weeks |

Therefore, the average duration of a quadruplet pregnancy is roughly 29-30 weeks and the more the number of babies, the shorter the duration of pregnancy. This means that most of the babies will be delivered prematurely with poor chances of survival after delivery.

## 31. What things can women do to help themselves when they are in labor?

There are several little tips that may help. These include:
- Plan ahead – you should put your delivery items together at least one month before your due date. This will include putting a little money aside, at least for transportation, especially if you live far away from the maternity center or hospital. Remember that labor may start suddenly at night
- Be positive – labor is the last piece of work that you will do before holding your baby or bundle of joy. It is important that you think positively, strengthen, and encourage yourself. Labor is painful but necessary. The reward is a bouncing baby. At this time, do not think of terrible events or complications or previous bad incidents. Think about the happy moments that lie ahead. Think positively
- Be focused – think joyfully about the beautiful gift of the baby, which is about to happen. Your health care giver, husband and relatives may keep you company and engage you in positive discussions and actions at this period and in labor. Activities like reading, watching television etc., may take your mind away from the pain
- Abstain from heavy food - at about the time of labor, it is better not to eat heavily. Light food and drinks e.g. tea, oranges, juices are better. If you need energy during labor, you may be given glucose to drink or as an infusion or drip
- Ask questions - during labor, ensure that you tell the health care personnel exactly how you feel, so that you can be properly guided.

Do not do anything on your own unless you are instructed or permitted to do so. When you communicate and cooperate, you are more likely to get help better and faster
- Conserve your energy - during labor, you work. You will need your energy! So, do not waste energy on shouting, quarrelling, or engaging in other aggressive behaviors. If you work-up yourself too much, sweating and swearing, you may become weak and exhausted. You may waste the precious energy that you will definitely need to go through labor, especially when it is time to push
- Help yourself – when the pain of contraction becomes intense, you may be given some painkillers (gas, injections etc.) to help you. Some actions like deep breathing or holding on to somebody (your husband, friend etc.) may improve your ability to cope with the pain. Empathy, comforting words, ancestral praises, and prayers by close relatives, husband, or the attending midwife may strengthen you.

## 32. How can women cope with labor pain?

Pain is a major complaint in labor. There is no doubt that labor pain creates fear and frustration and should be controlled, so that the discomfort of labor is reduced as much as possible. Failure to reduce pain adequately can result in tiredness, exhaustion and dehydration. Some women become disorderly and may refuse to cooperate or obey instructions. Some women may become aggressive and put the doctor under pressure to terminate labor by any means, as quickly as possible, which may result in unnecessary operations. Early in labor, pain may be reduced by giving pain killers like nitrous oxide gas, through a face mask, pethidine or morphine injections and other analgesics. When delivery is imminent, the aggravated pain of contractions may be reduced by giving continued inhalation, injecting a local anesthesia into the birth canal or giving a deliberate cut called an episiotomy. This widens the exit point of the birth canal, to facilitate the baby's delivery.

## 33. When do women feel the urge to push?

As labor progresses and the presenting part of the baby reaches the pelvis after full dilatation, the presenting part distends the vagina and exerts pressure on the rectum. This produces a sensation as if the woman urgently wants to defecate. At the same time, with the wave of contractions of the muscles of her abdomen, she bears down and pushes, thus using her own effort to assist in expelling the baby.

## 34. When should women actually push?

When the presenting part of the baby has descended into the birth canal, it stretches the soft tissues of the fully dilated cervix and vagina and compresses the rectum and anus. At this point, there is an urge to push with each wave of uterine contraction. Some women may begin to "push" prematurely in an effort to help themselves and put an end to the pain. Some do so because of ignorance. It is very important not to push before the cervix is fully dilated and the doctor or midwife says so.

## 35. What is an episiotomy?

An episiotomy is a cut made in the outer genital tract in order to enlarge the outer portion of the vagina, vulva and surrounding muscles. This creates more space and allows the baby to be delivered more easily. It is a neat cut that can be repaired almost immediately after birth. Failure to perform an episiotomy when it is needed, may result in bad tears of the genital tract. This will be more difficult to repair. There is also the increased likelihood of bleeding, infection and ugly scars. So, women should not resist an episiotomy when the nurse or doctor advises it, especially since they are likely to be given injections that make the cut and repair less painful.

## 36. How often is episiotomy performed?

Episiotomy is the second most commonly performed obstetric operation. It is second only to the cutting of the umbilical cord after delivery.

## 37. When is an episiotomy needed?

There are several reasons for giving an episiotomy. These include:
- Widening the lower birth canal, that is, the vagina and vulva
- Preventing tears of the lower birth canal (vulva, vagina and surrounding muscles)
- Preventing the arrest of the presenting baby part (head, breech) at the outer part of the vagina and perineum
- Protecting the head of the baby when delivering small, premature babies
- Delivering large babies with broad shoulders which may prevent safe delivery
- Hastening delivery where such is needed e.g. when the baby is in distress
- Using instruments to assist delivery e.g. when forceps delivery becomes necessary

## 38. What are the advantages of an episiotomy?

The advantages of episiotomy are many and far greater than the discomfort. These advantages include:
- The prevention of ugly tears or injuries of the vagina and the vulva. Ragged tears are more difficult to repair. Sometimes, the tears may extend to involve the anus, which will lead to uncontrolled leakage of stool

- The reduction of complications like severe bleeding. Vaginal bleeding from tears is more difficult to control because the tears are sometimes more extensive, complex and deep
- The reduction of Infections: Infections are more common in genital tears than cuts from episiotomies
- The prevention of surgery: Episiotomies help to avoid surgery in many cases where surgical operations could have been performed when it was difficult for the baby to come out. This may be because the baby was too big or due to a narrow outside opening of the birth canal. In many of such cases, episiotomies may be performed to widen the birth canal and deliver the baby successfully
- Delivery of premature babies: The heads of premature babies are delicate and can easily be injured by excessive pressure, during contractions and pushing. Episiotomies are performed to widen the birth canal so that the heads can pass more freely
- Prevention of deformities of the vagina and vulva: Tears of the vagina and vulva heal with ugly scars. This may result in narrowing of the vaginal opening and lead to future difficulty in penetration of the penis, during sexual intercourse. Also, during subsequent delivery, scars from old vaginal tears are more easily torn than an episiotomy

## 39.  What complications may arise?

Episiotomies are the second most common obstetric operation, second only to cutting the umbilical cord after the birth of the baby. However, it must be performed and repaired correctly. The down side of episiotomy includes:

- Bleeding
- Pain
- Formation of aggregated blood clots called hematoma
- Infection

Later, there may be:

- Ugly scar formation in a few cases
- Pain during sexual intercourse due to a tight vagina or vulva

## 40.  What is the most common position for delivery?

Perhaps the best position is to have the mother in the squatting position. Most people are used to squatting, since it is the position during defecation. This enhances the woman's ability to bear down and is convenient. However, the squatting position makes examination, or manipulation and assistance by the midwife or doctor, clumsy and difficult, during the final exit of the baby from the birth canal. In such a position, it is difficult to protect the baby's head. This can result in serious injury. The popular position is to have the woman, lie on her back on a delivery couch, propped up at an angle, with the limbs folded at the knees and the thighs open in order to facilitate pushing and delivery. Other less common positions include kneeling, sitting supported, standing supported, etc.

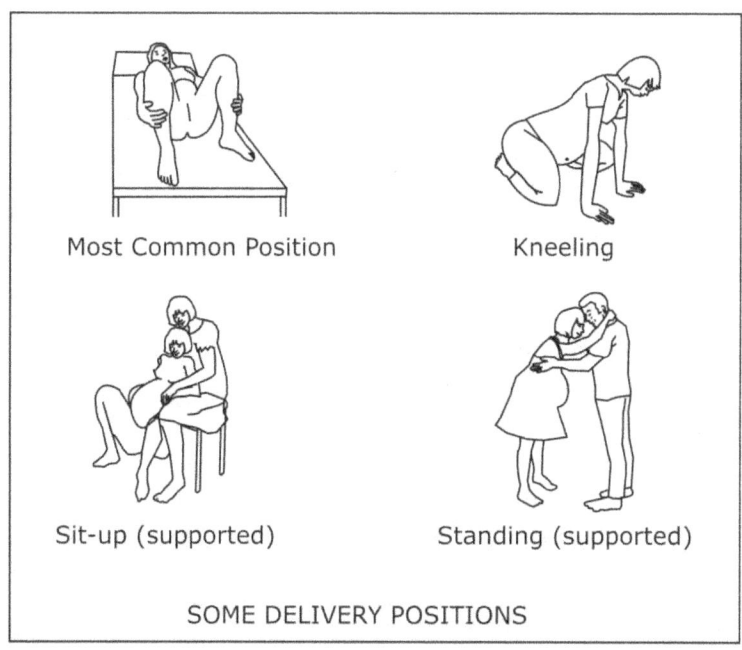

SOME DELIVERY POSITIONS

## 41. What is breech presentation and how common is it?

Breech presentation occurs in 2–3% of women at term. Breech presentation means that the baby will be born buttocks-first, which is a high risk pregnancy, because it is associated with many complications during labor. Such deliveries should occur in a hospital that is well equipped, with specialist obstetricians and experienced midwives.

## 42. What are the dangers of breech delivery?

Labor and delivery in breech are associated with far more problems and complications when compared with situations where the baby comes head first. Such complications include:
- Difficult labor
- Increased probability of surgical operations
- Injury or tear to the mother's birth canal
- Severe vaginal bleeding
- Fetal distress
- Injuries to the baby including:
  - Fracture of the fragile bones
  - Damage to the nerves
  - Damage to the organs of the abdomen
- Fetal death

- Increased probability of infection

### 43. Is it true that deliveries of breech babies must be by operation?

It is not true. An operation is not compulsory. However, delivery of breech babies must be taken in a hospital environment by a senior and experienced doctor. Complications in breech delivery are about 6 times higher than when the baby comes with the head. These complications include injuries to the mother and baby. Sometimes, the baby may die during the process. Once breech is diagnosed near term, it is compulsory that the woman delivers at the hospital, where doctors can take decisions on the best method of delivery.

### 44. What is full term?

A full term pregnancy is one with gestational age of between 37 completed weeks to 41 weeks 6 days.

### 45. What is premature labor?

The term premature labor is used when a woman falls into labor too early before 37 completed weeks of pregnancy. The consequence of premature labor is preterm delivery of babies. According to statistics from the Center for Disease Control and Prevention (CDC), 1 in every 10 births in the USA was preterm for 4 consecutive years up until 2018. This was attributed to pregnancy in teenagers and young mothers.

### 46. What are the causes of Premature Labor?

Labor can occur prematurely for various reasons. These include:
- Genital tract Infections
- Urinary tract infections
- Chorio-amnionitis: this means the infection of the birth water and fetal membranes
- Febrile illnesses
- Bleeding in pregnancy
- Weak or incompetent cervix
- Premature rupture of the membranes
- Injury or trauma in a pregnant woman
- Multiple pregnancy
- Existing systemic diseases in the mother e.g.
  - Uncontrolled hypertension
  - Uncontrolled diabetes

### 47. What is a preterm baby?

A Preterm baby is one that is delivered too early, before 37 completed weeks of pregnancy. In 2017, about 10% of babies were delivered prematurely in the

USA. Among the racial groups, the rate of preterm delivery was higher in African Americans. The major consequences preterm deliveries include low birth weight (LBW). According to the statistics from the Center for disease control and prevention (CDC), in 2016, preterm delivery and LBW were responsible for about 17% of deaths in infants in the USA.

## 48. How does a premature baby look?

Perhaps the first thing that is easily noticed is that most premature babies are small in size, because they are delivered before term. The head is big in comparison to their small, fragile, and slim body. The second is that they are usually inactive, that is, they move their bodies and limbs less often. Other features are:
- Large gaps or fontanelles in the head (depressed area of the head)
- Reddish skin: because of lack of fat under the skin
- Lanugo hairs, which appear whitish, thin and fluffy covering the body
- Swollen feet

These features may be striking to experienced midwives and doctors. Premature babies have premature organs that are poorly adapted to life outside the womb.

## 49. What problems do premature babies have?

Babies are poorly adapted to life outside the womb cavity except at term, when they are fully mature. Even when mature babies are delivered, they must quickly adjust to environmental conditions. This adjustment involves all the organs, especially regarding body temperature control, blood circulation, and breathing. Premature babies have immature organs which are ill equipped to survive outside the womb. The problems include:
- Immature organs: especially the lungs, hence premature babies cannot breathe properly
- Inability to control body temperature: the skin of premature babies cannot conserve or regulate heat. This is because they lack the type and quantity of body fat of mature babies. They have brown fat which cannot hold heat, so they lose body heat rapidly and become cold. This is the reason why they are kept inside incubators, which helps to maintain warm air around them
- Feeding problems: many premature babies cannot swallow properly, which makes feeding problematic
- Low immunity and infection: the immune system is not well developed, so premature babies lack the capacity to cope with the normal adult environment. They succumb to infection more easily
- Poor weight gain: this is mainly because they cannot feed properly
- Holes in the heart: the heart is usually intermediate in form. There are more openings than those of mature babies. Sometimes, the holes may not close except through surgical operation. An example is an

abnormal opening between the immature heart and the lung called Patent ductus arteriosus (PDA) in premature infants. This may result in inefficient circulation. Other complications are:
- Bleeding into the brain
- Cerebral birth injury
- Jaundice
- Kernicterus - toxic effect of jaundice on the brain

## 50. Which organs are more likely to be damaged in premature babies?

Almost all organs are affected by prematurity. These include:

Immature lungs:
- Difficulty in breathing
- Stoppage of breathing at intervals
- Increased infection

Immature liver:
- Jaundice
- Increased damage by drugs

Immature brain:
- Toxic effect of jaundice (kernicterus)
- Bleeding into the brain

Immature kidneys:

Some drugs that are dangerous to the kidney include:
- Streptomycin
- Gentamycin
- Kanamycin
- Cloxacillin

Immature heart:
- Defect such as Patent ductus arteriosus (PDA) and holes in the heart
- Ineffective blood circulation or perfusion of blood to important organs which may cause
  - Heart failure
  - Pulmonary hypertension
  - Bleeding in the brain
  - Severe pain and disease of the immature bowels called necrotizing enterocolitis.

Other problems include:
- Low blood sugar
- Poor feeding and difficulty in swallowing
- Poor temperature control due to low body fat
- Anemia

- Vision impairment due to refractive errors and damage to the retina
- Delayed developmental mile stones and general sub-optimal performance later in life

## 51. What basic support is required for premature babies?

Premature infants need support in order to survive outside the womb. The aim of support is to keep the baby alive up until it is able to adapt and live independently. So, three critical needs are usually addressed:
- Temperature Control: Babies are kept inside the incubator to keep them warm
- Breathing: Oxygen is usually given inside an incubator setting
- Feeding: Feeding is carefully planned to meet the baby's need without causing upset in the newborn's system

## 52. What is a Cesarean Section (CS)?

A cesarean section is a surgical operation performed by doctors to deliver the baby from the womb. It is commonly done by making a flat cut in the lower aspect of the tummy, to enter the abdomen. Thereafter, another flat cut on the lower aspect of the womb, is made being careful to avoid cutting or injuring the baby. The cut that you see on the outside is therefore not the C/S cut. It is not so important medically speaking, even though women worry more about how it looks, for the sake of beauty. On the other hand, the cut on the womb is more important and doctors are careful to ensure that it heals properly, so that the scar is strong enough to withstand the stress of future pregnancies.

## 53. What are the types of cesarean section?

There are 2 main types of cesarean section that you need to know about because these are the usual ones performed by doctors. They are:
- Classical cesarean section: This is done by cutting through the wall of the womb in a vertical manner. Classical CS is done when the doctor needs ample space, to enhance maneuvering during the operation. This may be because the baby is lying abnormally across the mother's womb. The main disadvantage is that vertical cuts predispose to rupture in future pregnancy or labor, compelling future deliveries to be through cesarean operation
- Lower segment CS: In this type, the womb is entered by making a horizontal cut in the lower part. This is by far the most common type of CS operation. The chief advantage is in its safety and the fact that womb rupture is far less common, than in the classical type. However, the doctor must be able to maneuver and deliver the baby with the little space available. Lower segment CS is appropriate in almost all cases where CS is indicated.

## 54. Why do women request for cesarean section?

Cesarean section is one of the most common operations performed by doctors. It is a major operation, which should only be performed for justifiable reasons. Currently and worldwide, more women are requesting for cesarean section. Some of the reasons for this are anxiety, the pain of undergoing normal labor and improvement in safety, thanks to modern techniques, anesthesia and effective antibiotics. Although there are numerous occasions when a CS operation is requested, in all situations, it is only justified, if the doctor in his or her own judgment, thinks that it will guarantee safe delivery. The situations below serve as a useful guide for the performance of C/S operations.

Cesarean sections MUST be performed in the following situations:
- Baby is lying transversely in the womb
- Major placenta previa: which completely obstructs the baby from coming out from the womb
- Masses like fibroids blocking the womb
- Where multiple operations that involved cutting through the womb were done previously, it is safer that subsequent deliveries be through cesarean section
- In developing countries, where classical CS has been performed previously, it is usual for subsequent deliveries to be through CS

Cesarean section MAY be performed in the following situations:
- On the mother's free-will request: this is becoming more widespread
- Where the baby is too big to pass safely through the birth canal
- In some cases of breech presentation
- Where the baby has had growth restriction or sickness in the womb
- Some cases of multiple pregnancy e.g when the first baby lies across the womb
- Cervical cancer, genital warts, etc.

## 55. What happens when the membranes rupture before the expected date of delivery?

The membranes wrap the baby, the placenta, and birth water and serves as a barrier that prevents germs from the vagina from gaining access to the womb and its contents. So when the water breaks, it is usual for contractions to occur within a short time. However, whether contractions start or not, the expectant mother should proceed to hospital as soon as possible because with the barrier formed by the membranes now broken, germs can enter the womb and cause infection to the womb and its contents. These include the baby, membranes, placenta, and remnants of birth water. This type of infection is a serious threat with severe adverse effects on the outcome of pregnancy, unless treatment is started promptly. This type of infection is called chorio-amnionitis. Women in this very dangerous situation must be treated urgently and monitored in a hospital environment.

### 56. Must women be put to sleep during a C/S operation?

Not necessarily. The act of putting somebody to sleep during an operation or giving drugs that will deaden pain is called anesthesia. There are many types of anesthesia and it is the doctor's role to choose the most appropriate one for you. Doctor's will usually discuss the various options available and explain why a particular type has been chosen. This will depend on the type of operation, area of operation, estimated duration of operation, and the patient's physical and medical conditions. Broadly speaking there are 3 main types:

- Local anesthesia: Local anesthesia means local application or infiltration in order to "deaden" the area of operation
- General anesthesia: General anesthesia involves giving injections to put the patient to sleep. Breathing will be taken over by a machine that delivers oxygen to the lungs
- Epidural or spinal anesthesia: In which an injection is given at the back in between the bones of the vertebra column to "deaden" a section of the body including the site of operation. The patient is awake while the operation is being performed and can also talk to the doctor during the operation. This is safe, is increasingly preferred by both doctors and patients and will probably reduce anxiety and fear

### 57. How soon after the operation can the mother go home?

When the mother has recovered from anesthesia after surgery, she is encouraged to move her legs as soon as she can. Early ambulation is an important way to prevent blood clotting disorders especially thrombo-embolism. If there are no complications after a successful CS, she should be gradually up and about on the 3rd day. Most doctors would let her go home between the 4th and 6th day after operation, as long as she is fit but she will of course continue taking antibiotics, pain killers, hematinics and other drugs at home.

### 58. What are the complications of cesarean section to the woman?

Cesarean operations are commonly performed for various reasons which are beneficial to the mother and her baby. However, things may go wrong during or after the cesarean section. These complications are more common if the operation is done as an emergency or in a hospital that is poorly staffed or equipped. The common problems that may arise include:

- Bleeding: Sometimes, a woman may bleed severely due to C/S operation. Bleeding may occur during the operation or after but bleeding during operation is more common. This may be so severe that the woman may require to be transfused with blood, so doctors always ensure that blood is available in the blood bank before starting a C/S operation. The need for blood is an emergency. The common policy in many hospitals is to request the husband or relations of the woman to donate blood or make available 2 or more pints of blood, well in advance, during the antenatal period. This is routine for all pregnancies in developing countries. Unfortunately, in many cases, this voluntary donation of blood is not done, so blood is not available when urgently needed. Bleeding in pregnancy or after childbirth is the most common reason why women die in developing countries

- Infections: Infections may set in before, during, and after CS operations. When this happens, it makes the operation highly risky and likely to bring problems. Unlike the developed countries, environments in many hospitals in most developing countries are poor in quality and loaded with germs. Hence, infections due to operations are common. The germs may come from the immediate environment, the instruments, theatre, doctor, nurses or the woman herself. Infection is the second most common cause of death of pregnant women in most developing countries
- Wounds: This is most commonly due to infections. Wounds breakdown or healing may be problematic and prolong the woman's stay in hospital with the attendant increase in hospital costs
- Unintended injury: Injuries may occur during C/S operations. This is more common in an emergency C/S, because there may not be sufficient time to adequately prepare the woman, the theatre and staff for the operation. The probability that injury may occur also depends on the facilities available in the hospital and the experience of the doctor. Commonly, injuries do occur to the urinary bladder, urine pipes or ureters, blood vessels of the womb and the surrounding structures. Unfortunately, the baby may receive cuts or injuries but these are usually treated effectively
- Blood clot disorders: Generally, increase in blood clot formation is associated with CS operations. The clot is called a thrombus in medical parlance. Such clots may be dislodged from their sites of formation and carried in the blood pipes to other parts of the body like the lungs and brain. At these sites, the clots can block smaller blood vessels and stop blood supply to the organs. This is called thrombo-embolism and is a dangerous situation
- Long term consequences: Most notable are the greater tendency to undergo C/S in future pregnancies and the ever present risk of womb rupture during future pregnancy or labor. Any woman with a previous operation scar on the womb, is at risk of rupturing her womb and must be supervised carefully during pregnancy, labor and delivery
- Other minor complications include:
  - Swollen limbs at the site of injections and drips
  - Pain
  - Inability to move bowels properly after surgery
  - Urinary problems
  - Ugly scars, etc.

- Death: In any major operation, there is always the possibility, however remote, that the woman may die. Death may occur as a result of mistakes by the doctor while performing the operation, due to anesthesia, effects of drugs, excessive bleeding, or other mistakes

## 59. When is the placenta said to be retained after a normal delivery?
In a normal situation, the placenta should be expelled within 1 hour of delivery. If the placenta remains undelivered after this time, it is said to be retained. When the placenta remains un-expelled after the delivery of the baby, it makes it difficult for the womb to contract and effectively close up bleeding blood vessels, especially those in the placenta bed. This results in bleeding which may be severe and endanger the woman's life.

## 60. How long should women stay in the delivery room?
Most women want to leave the delivery suite in a hurry, especially, if delivery has been normal. However, it is usual practice to observe your vital signs like pulse, temperature, blood pressure, and watch out for any bleeding for the next 1 – 2 hours after delivery. Thereafter, they may be allowed into the post-natal ward which is more convenient and where the nurses will monitor and observe to ensure that her health is further stabilized.

## 61. Why do some women urinate unintentionally after delivery?
Voiding of urine after delivery is as a result of mild injuries or bruising and swelling of the bladder, muscles, and other tissues of the pelvis and birth canal. This is called stress incontinence. Leakage of urine may occur unprovoked or while coughing, sneezing, or changing postures. Stress incontinence of urine is more common in the first 24 hours after delivery. These complaints usually resolve with time.

## 62. What is Lochia?
After delivery, women continue to pass blood-like fluid or discharge from the vagina. These are the little remnants of placenta tissue and membranes mixed with blood. The color is initially red for about 10 days. After that, it then becomes light yellow for about 3 weeks or so. Lastly, it turns whitish or normal. This after-birth discharge is called lochia in medical parlance.

## 63. What is Involution?
After the delivery of the baby, the womb becomes empty and contracts. Over the next few weeks, the womb gradually returns to the approximate size that it was before pregnancy. This takes about 6 weeks. This process of reduction in size is called involution. Gradually, the tummy is firmer and becomes flat once more, but it may be difficult to return completely to its previous shape as many women would wish.

## 64. What is Post-Partum Hemorrhage (PPH)

Post-Partum Hemorrhage (PPH) is a medical term that denotes bleeding after childbirth. Technically speaking, it means that the woman has lost 500mls of blood or more. Hemorrhage is the most common cause of death due to pregnancy in the developing world. Both ante-partum and post-partum hemorrhage account for about 23% of maternal deaths in developing countries. Regrettably, PPH can be prevented and so many women need not die because of lack of blood.

## 65. What are the causes of Post- Partum Hemorrhage?

The common causes of bleeding after childbirth are:
- Poor or Non-contraction of the womb: The womb needs to contract after childbirth in order to close the blood pipes and prevent bleeding. Sometimes, the womb fails to do this, resulting in severe bleeding. In medical parlance, when the womb fails to contract, this condition is called uterine atony
- Retained placenta: In this situation, the placenta is not expelled on time after the delivery of the baby. This prevents the womb from contracting. The placenta site is also more likely to bleed as long as the placenta remains inside the womb cavity
- Other masses in the womb: The presence of other masses in the womb may prevent it from contracting. Such masses include fibroids and polyps
- Injury to the birth canal: Women may sustain injuries to the womb, cervix, vagina, or vulva. Depending on the extent of these injuries, women may lose so much blood that their lives are endangered, unless the wound is closed up immediately by the doctor
- Blood clotting disorders: Some women suffer from blood clotting diseases. The blood cannot form clots that will plug the blood pipes and prevent them from bleeding normally. When a normal person sustains injury, the person bleeds for some minutes until a blood clot is formed, plugging the blood pipe and closing up the wound so that bleeding stops. The substances in the blood (called clotting factors), may be lacking or deficient in some women. Also, blood clots may be formed but the clots dissolve immediately, making them ineffective. This condition is dangerous and difficult for doctors to treat. It is called Disseminated Intravascular Coagulopathy (DIC). In this condition, women bleed continuously and even as they are being transfused, the transfused blood also bleeds away continuously

## 66. Which women risk experiencing Post-Partum Hemorrhage (PPH)?

Women at risk include:
- Grand multips: women with 5 or more full term deliveries
- Multiple pregnancy
- Ante-Partum Hemorrhage: those that bled earlier during pregnancy

- Women with Uterine masses such as fibroids
- Older women are more likely to bleed during or after delivery
- Women with history of PPH in previous pregnancy
- Women with bleeding disorders e.g. Clotting problems
- Women with co-existing infections

It is mandatory that women who might possibly have PPH are delivered and supervised in the hospital and blood made readily available.

# DEAR DOCTOR:

### 67. I have heard a lot about oxytocin drips. Why are women so scared of it?

Many pregnant women are afraid of drips because they believe it causes more pain during labor. Fortunately, this increase in pain is what eventually leads to the delivery of the baby - the bundle of joy. If you are considering it, you have to cooperate with the nursing staff or doctor to bear this pain. Many women expend much energy on shouting and agitation, with attendant sweating and weakness, such that they lack the power when it is time to "push".

### 68. My doctor told me that my cervix is not favorable for induction and booked me for a cesarean. What does he mean?

The final decision is taken to induce labor only if the cervix is adjudged to be favorable. The more favorable the cervix, the more likely it is that induction will succeed. To decide whether the cervix is favorable or not, doctors calculate the Bishop's score. If the Bishops score is not favorable, the cervix may be ripened to make it more favorable before induction. Sometimes, as in your own case, depending on local practice, the doctor may opt for surgery, if the chance of successful induction is low.

### 69. Why does my doctor want to induce labor?

The objective is to get your baby out of the womb before labor begins naturally, so by inducing labor and taking delivery, both yours and your baby's health and life are preserved and complications are prevented. Doctors generally contemplate the induction of labor when it is more beneficial for the baby to be delivered, than to allow the pregnancy to continue. By so doing, adverse effects to the mother, the baby or both, are prevented or minimized.

## 70. How should I behave when I am in labor?

When women are in labor, they do many things that are not helpful. Their actions are understandable because when the pain is too much, they can say or do anything. However, some behavior can actually harm you and your baby or jeopardize your chance of progress of labor and safe delivery. These include:

- Quarrelling – do not quarrel with those who are taking care of you. Respect, cooperate, and obey their instructions. If you have difficulties, tell them. Do not harass them so that they can be focused and friendly while helping you during labor. Remember that no matter how hostile you are, you cannot transfer your pain. If you create unnecessary tension or aggression, the doctor and the nurses may be put under pressure to bring the labor to an end as quickly as possible. This may mean performing an operation that is not necessary
- Absconding – do not leave the labor ward or walk about without permission. Tell the nurses if you feel like standing up or walking around the labor ward area
- Eating – do not eat unless you are permitted. Heavy foods are not allowed in labor. This may encourage vomiting or weakness. If the doctor eventually decides that you will have surgery, you are better off when your stomach is empty
- Unauthorized use of drugs – some women hide all kinds of drugs, including native herbal preparations etc., with the intention of taking them during labor. Actions like these may completely jeopardize your labor

## 71. What are the consequences if I push too early?

Judicious use of pain killers and epidural anesthesia are usually deployed by doctors to prevent women from pushing too early but you should be aware of some adverse consequences.

Each time you push, you expend energy, and increase intensity of the force of the normal contraction, so that the birth canal and your baby are put under too much pressure. The excessive force compresses your baby's presenting part and increases the likelihood of tearing apart the soft tissues of the vagina and vulva. There is therefore an increased likelihood of injury to both you and your baby. As a result:

- You get tired faster
- You may sustain tears and injury to your cervix, vagina, vulva and anus
- Tears may lead to serious bleeding
- The joint of your pelvic bones may be stretched and become loose, resulting in pain and difficulty in walking properly after delivery
- Your baby may sustain injuries, especially to the nerves, limbs, head and brain

- Your baby may experience distress
- If your baby is breech, the head may be entrapped in the birth canal

## 72. Doctor, can I demand for a C/S just to avoid pain?

Yes, although there are other effective ways of minimizing pain during labor. You need to discuss this issue further with your doctor to see if you would be happy with other alternatives, apart from an operation. C/S operations are safe and more or less painless, thanks to improved antibiotics, anesthesia and better skills. For various reasons, a growing number of women now demand C/S operations, the important issue is that it must be safe and appropriate for you and your doctor must be convinced that it is the right thing to do. Discuss any of such concerns with your doctor.

## 73. Why did my doctor instruct me not to eat?

After eating, it normally takes about 6 hours for food to leave the stomach during digestion. When food is retained in the stomach, there is always the possibility that partially digested food, mixed with the acid from the stomach, could pass back or be regurgitated into the esophagus. When this happens, there is an increased possibility of acid burns to the esophagus. The reflux of food may also obstruct the breathing pipe and cause breathing difficulties and complications, if an operation is needed. Consequently, to be on the safe side, doctors like to perform operations on an empty stomach.

## 74. Why must I be shaved if I am going to have a C/S operation?

Firstly, shaving will improve access to the site of operation and make cleaning with antiseptic easier. Secondly, hair traps germs in between the strands. This problem can only be resolved by shaving off the hair, so shaving is necessary for proper cleaning in order to make the skin at the site sterile, to make the incision and to ease future wound inspection and dressing. This also promotes a faster wound healing process.

## 75. Will I continue to have a C/S for subsequent deliveries?

Not necessarily. There are perhaps 2 main reasons why women may continue to have repeat cesarean sections. These are:
- If the reason for the initial CS is permanent or recurrent. For example, a woman may have pelvic deformity due to a road traffic accident, which makes it impossible for safe vaginal delivery. This will always warrant an operation for safe delivery. On the other hand, if the reason for the first cesarean section was transverse lie of the baby, the lie in a subsequent pregnancy may be normal, therefore a repeat operation is not needed
- If the patient has previously had a classical cesarean section: All women who have had classical cesarean sections are encouraged to

have repeat C/S operations for subsequent deliveries. So, whether you will have a repeat cesarean may depend largely on the reason for the first operation and whether it was a classical operation or not
- In developing countries, once a woman has had 2 cesarean sections, the practice in most countries is that subsequent deliveries must be through cesarean operation. This is largely a reflection in the challenges of delays in getting to hospital and the limited capacity available for monitoring women in labor. In developed countries, women with multiple C/S may be allowed to attempt normal delivery subject to intensive, meticulous monitoring during labor. This is a practice borne out of the superior health infrastructure in the advanced world

# CHAPTER 15
# Postnatal Care and Breastfeeding

*"Nursing gives you superhuman powers.*
*How else could I be doing all this when I'm usually*
*a sleepaholic?"*
– GWEN STEFFANI

**1. What is the puerperium?**

During pregnancy, almost all organs and systems of the body undergo different changes. Only few of these changes are permanent. Majorities are reversible and they start soon after the placenta has been expelled. Overall, at the end of the $6^{th}$ week after delivery, almost all the organs and systems go back to the state they were before pregnancy. The period from the time the placenta is delivered till the end of the next 6 weeks after delivery, is called the puerperium. The changes include afterbirth illnesses like bleeding after birth, infections, wound healing, depression, etc. Early during this period, the breast may be engorged and painful but this is necessary to pave way for the establishment of breastfeeding. Most importantly, by the end of this 6-week period, women's bodies should have normalized. The womb, for example, should have returned to its regular size before pregnancy. The after birth discharge, called lochia, should also have completely dried up and been replaced by normal vaginal discharge. A good number of women also resume menstruation during this period, especially those who do not breastfeed their babies exclusively.

**2. What is the most essential treatment for bleeding during childbirth?**

Sometimes, it is possible to predict a woman who will bleed during or after childbirth. Those that are at risk of bleeding include women with previous bleeding episode, fibroids, old women in pregnancy, multiple pregnancy, previous surgery, etc. The most essential step is to make blood available in the blood bank, so that the woman can be transfused as early as the need arises. This is the reason why it is important to sustain the campaign for voluntary blood donation. Blood saves life. The other steps are directed towards managing the various causes of bleeding such as tying of bleeding blood vessels by the doctor, or removing a bleeding placenta from the womb.

### 3. How soon can new born babies be held?

If there are no complications, mothers should be allowed to hold their babies as soon as they are able. It is usual for midwives to place babies on their mother's abdomen soon after delivery, even before the cord is cut, so that they start to make contact with their baby soon after delivery and kick start the bonding process.

### 4. How soon can I be up and about after delivery?

It is a good preventive measure for women to move about, after delivery or operation, in order to reduce the occurrence of thrombo-embolism. Therefore, it is beneficial for women to pace around or take a walk as early as they can, after delivery.

During pregnancy, the risk of clot formation is increased generally. This risk extends to the period after delivery. The danger is that it is possible for a blood clot to be dislodged from the blood pipes or veins and be carried in the blood stream to other parts of the body. Where this occurs, the clots may block smaller blood vessels, cutting off the blood supply to the tissue, leading to the death of such tissue or organs. This condition is called thrombo-embolism. It is a killer, in and out of pregnancy. Generally speaking, there are some conditions that encourage thrombo-embolism. These include:
- Pregnancy, delivery and puerperium
- Infection
- Surgical operations such as C/S
- Those with disorders of blood clotting factors
- Women with sedentary lifestyles
- Those who have had previous history of thrombo-embolism.
- Those who have close relatives that have suffered thrombo-embolism are also at increased risk.

### 5. What are the most important needs after delivery?

Most women are tired and dehydrated after laboring to deliver. There are 4 basic things to do that are important for speedy recovery and well-being. These are:
- Adequate rest and sleep: After a most difficult period, sufficient rest and seep are of utmost importance. This may be difficult if mothers

are sick and separated from their babies due to illness, however support from loved ones will be helpful. Women should discuss all these with their doctors.
- Good nutrition: After delivery and the exhausting period of labor, women also need a nutritious diet and supplements to provide the energy to cope with the initial problems of motherhood and promote recovery and repair processes going on in the body. The doctor and the midwives will be happy to provide guidance on this issue.
- Mobility: Women need to be up and about as soon as possible, because over 65% of thrombo-embolism cases in women occur after delivery. One way to prevent this is to move the legs by taking few steps around the ward environment at regular intervals. Any pain in the legs must be reported to the doctor immediately. After an operation like a cesarean section, women may start by shifting the legs about while on the hospital bed, followed later by light walks as soon as possible.
- Communication: Lastly, always talk and discuss unusual events or feelings with the doctor, nurses and even trusted relatives or friends. Things can easily go wrong soon after birth. For example, unexpected bleeding is dangerous but when the doctor is told, the cause will be found quickly and treatment is commenced promptly.

These 4 issues are basic but highly important to good health and good recovery after delivery.

## 6. Why do women complain of abdominal pain after delivery?

Many women experience lower abdominal pain on and off after delivery. Within a 12-hour period after delivery, the contractions of the womb may occur as regular, low intensity pain. Thereafter, the contractions are generally much less and come at irregular intervals. They are called "After pains." Such after pains may be more painful during breastfeeding, because the suckling of the baby increases the intensity of the contractions of the womb.

## 7. How soon after delivery should food be eaten?

Labor is an energy sapping process. There is no doubt that most women are tired and dehydrated after delivery. If labor and delivery have been normal and natural, they can start by drinking small quantities of fluid or beverage soon after the bed sheets and clothing have been changed. This may be as quick as within an hour of delivery. In a situation where deliveries were complicated or a surgical operation was performed, women are most likely to be on a drip. It takes some time for the bowel to accept food without causing problems. This may be up to 48 hours or more, depending on the situation. The drip contains sugar to serve as a source of energy while waiting for the doctor to give the go ahead to start eating. It is only the doctor that can determine when it is appropriate to take food orally, so women must be patient, trusting that the doctor's goal is a speedy recovery.

### 8. What sort of food should be eaten after delivery?

After delivery, when the doctor or midwife has given the go ahead for food, women can go back to eating foods that they are used to. They need to replenish lost energy so they can be fit as soon as possible. It is also important for them to take plenty of fluids to aid breastfeeding. Most doctors prescribe hematinics and vitamin supplements for women routinely after delivery. This is appropriate because of the blood loss during delivery, as well as the need to repair and restore tissues and organs, to their pre-pregnancy state.

### 9. When does my tummy become flat again?

The process that leads to the womb returning to its original size is called involution. After delivery, the womb can be touched or felt at the level of the umbilicus. It gradually shrinks in size, so that within 10 – 14 days after delivery, it has disappeared into the pelvis and cannot be touched anymore. By the end of the $6^{th}$ week after delivery in most women, the womb would have shrunken to the approximate size that it was before pregnancy. The tummy is once more firm and flat. Abdominal exercise to strengthen the muscles of the tummy, improves the flatness and look of the tummy.

### 10. What causes constipation after delivery?

During labor, the bowel may be compressed or even bruised. Coupled with the loss of tone during pregnancy, dehydration during labor and the fact that women in labor might not have eaten for several hours, it is common for women to be constipated for 3 – 4 days after childbirth. Gradually, as women begin to tolerate food orally, their bowels slowly begin to move again so they are usually encouraged to resume eating, starting with light foods. However, for those who have had difficult or complicated deliveries or surgical operations, the doctor should decide when a woman can begin to eat.

### 11. What is puerperal infection?

A woman is said to have puerperal infection or sepsis if she runs a high temperature continuously for 2 days within the first 2 weeks after delivery. The source of this fever is likely to be from infection, related to the birth canal or reproductive tract. This is important because other sources of fever like malaria, typhoid, etc., in developing countries and Africa in particular, must be excluded. Puerperal sepsis accounts for about 17% of such deaths associated with pregnancy in developing countries. It is second only to hemorrhage. In Africa, where some pregnant women still deliver at home, it is important that women with febrile illnesses after delivery report to a hospital as soon as possible, to obtain diagnosis and prompt treatment.

## 12. After delivery, which symptoms may suggest that a woman is infected?

Most infections after birth are due to bacteria. The germs causing the infections may invade the body from the womb, bruises and cuts in the birth canal, or bowels. Germs may also be passed from other patients and even doctors or midwives that attended to patients. So the period immediately following delivery, can easily be complicated by infections. Generally, the signs listed below may indicate infection:

- Fever
- Headache
- Chills
- Body aches or localized pain over the womb
- Excessive tiredness
- Rapid heartbeats and
- Foul smelling Lochia or vaginal discharge.

Sometimes, the patient may feel sick without being able to say exactly what is wrong but with signs listed above, the doctor must be contacted as soon as possible. Fortunately, very effective antibiotics that are capable of killing most of the common germs are now readily available, so infections can be promptly and effectively treated.

## 13. What are the immediate consequences of an infection after birth?

An infection after delivery is an important issue that can add more distress and frustration to a woman's recovery and her ability to care for her new born infant. Whatever may be the cause, it is important to treat infections promptly and effectively, in order to prevent adverse consequences. The immediate consequences of poorly treated infection include:

- Abscess formation: This means an enclosed collection of pus
- Septic shock: This is a serious emergency
- Swollen tummy with absent bowel movements: This is called paralytic ileus
- Blood clot formation: This is called thrombo-embolism. In a few cases, abnormal blood clots are widely formed and dissolved. This condition is called disseminated Intravascular Coagulopathy (DIC). Blood clot disorders are dangerous and may result in death, unless they are recognized quickly and treated effectively.

## 14. What is the most important long term consequence, if the infection is not effectively treated?

There are many consequences of infection. Infection of the lining of the womb is called endometritis. This infection can progress from the womb to involve the fallopian tubes, the ovaries, and the surrounding tissues, thus leading to Pelvic Inflammatory Disease (PID). In many cases, when PID is not treated effectively, it results in tubal blockage which is the leading cause of female infertility in most developing countries. So, it is important to treat all potential infections properly, including surgical wounds, in order to prevent future infertility.

## 15. What are the advantages of breast feeding?

Breastfeeding is manufactured by the mother for the baby. All the ingredients are sourced locally from the mother's body system. The manufacturing process is natural, without adding anything artificial.

Breast feeding the baby has many advantages both for the mother and baby. These are:

- Economical: The mother is the manufacturer and supplier and therefore breast milk comes cheap and plentiful for the baby. As long as the mother is fit, breast milk supply is guaranteed, so it is economical for the family
- Natural: All the ingredients are sourced locally from the mother's body system. The manufacturing process is natural, without adding anything artificial
- Non-infective: breast milk is clean and unlike artificial milk, the mother does not need to be afraid of infectious diseases like diarrhea in the baby.
- Digestible: breast milk is easily digested and tolerated by most babies without problems, unlike cow milk
- Immunity: Breast milk contains immune cells from the mother. This gives the baby passive immunity against many diseases and infections. This is important because newborn babies have poorly developed immunity in this early period of life. Therefore, breast feeding is one way the mother can further protect her precious baby
- Bonding: Breast feeding promotes bonding and love between the mother and baby. Have you ever seen the joy and passion on the face of mothers, when they breast feed their babies? Also, notice the way babies gaze at their mothers during breastfeeding. The bonding is unmistakable
- Good for the womb: the act of sucking on the breast by the baby releases oxytocin hormone in the mother. Oxytocin helps the womb contract. This reduces vaginal bleeding and facilitates the rate at which the womb returns to the size it was before pregnancy (involution)
- Convenient: it is produced seamlessly and automatically, so long as the mother is fit, well-nourished, and well hydrated

## 16. Are there any disadvantages associated with breastfeeding?

There is no doubt that breast milk is one of the greatest gifts that mothers can give to their infants. The advantages outweigh the few disadvantages. However, the drawbacks include:

- Worries, disruption of your sleep, and other activities
- Milk Intolerance: Very rarely seen, some infants do not tolerate lactose, which is a major component of breast milk. This condition is called lactose intolerance
- Breast engorgement: This is usually due to the inability of the secreted milk to be evacuated on time. This condition can happen if the baby is sick and unable to suck, has congenital deformity of the mouth, is born prematurely or separated from the mother. It can also happen in cases of still birth or infant death. The mother may also be unable to feed her baby, if she has had surgery for delivery or due to other illnesses including inverted nipples. Breast engorgement usually occurs 3 – 4 days after delivery. It is very uncomfortable, painful, and may be associated with fever and chills. The milk should be manually expressed at intervals in order to evacuate the breasts and have some respite. Support for the breasts with a firm bra and alleviation with simple analgesics, are also beneficial. The doctor must be informed as soon as possible. In cases of still birth or infant death where there is no baby to suck the breast, doctors usually prescribe drugs such as bromocriptine (parlodel), to suppress breast milk secretion and dry up the breasts
- Breast milk jaundice: In some instances, some babies develop jaundice during breastfeeding. Doctors are not too sure whether this jaundice is due to breast milk or other conditions
- Inability to suck the breast: This may be due to deformity in the mouth of babies. Babies born prematurely may also find it difficult to suck or swallow until weeks after delivery when they become more mature
- Ineffective or inadequate lactation: Sometimes, milk production by the breast may be inadequate for the baby's need. At other times, milk may be present in the breast but the baby may not be able to suck it adequately. The reasons for inadequate lactation are complex. Sometimes, doctors may institute measures like increase fluid intakes and drugs in order to help milk production but this may not work always. If the baby's suckling does not bring milk into his mouth, the mother may express breast milk manually or through the use of breast pump and feed the baby. It is important to let the doctor be aware of these problems as early as possible, so that appropriate solutions can be instituted
- Mastitis or inflammation of the breasts: This happens in about 1% of women who breastfeed and is common in women with cracked nipples or fissures. It is most commonly caused by the staphylococcus bacteria and manifests with breast pain, fever, and

chills. The doctor must be consulted immediately for treatment. Meanwhile, the baby should not be put to suckle in the affected breast
- Inverted nipples: Women who have inverted nipples may find breastfeeding difficult, unpleasant, and cumbersome

Despite these drawbacks, there is perhaps no reason that is good enough for mothers not to breast feed their babies. Where there are difficulties, the doctor's advice should be sought.

### 17. Why should babies be suckled regularly?

Apart from the excellent nutrition that breast milk provides for babies, there are 3 advantages that women also gain when their babies suck the breast:
- First, when babies suck, it encourages more milk to be secreted in the breast. When milk is secreted and the baby does not suckle to evacuate the milk, the breast becomes engorged
- Secondly, each time the baby sucks on the breast, the hormone called oxytocin is released from the pituitary gland in the brain. Oxytocin makes the womb contract after birth, closing down the open blood pipes in the womb, thereby preventing dangerous bleeding
- Also, when the baby sucks, the womb quickly returns to its original pre-pregnant size

### 18. How frequently should babies be breastfed each day?

On the average, the baby should suck actively for 5 – 7 minutes on each breast 3–4 times per day. This should be sufficient for the baby to empty the accumulated milk in each breast. In the extreme, the baby should not be left on the breast for more than 10 minutes, in order to reduce the possibility of sucking air. This may cause abdominal pain. It is important that both breasts are emptied completely during each breastfeeding, to prevent breast engorgement. Remember that unnecessarily prolonged sucking may result in cracked nipples with great discomfort.

### 19. Why do some attempts to breastfeed, end in failure?

The decision to breastfeed should be taken during the pre-natal period and preparation should start at this period. The problems that can be addressed before delivery include fear, anxiety and how to cope with breastfeeding. Breast problems such as retracted nipples and cultivating the habit of taking plenty of oral fluids, should also be discussed. In summary, the major challenges that may lead to failure include:
- General lack of experience
- Anxiety
- Cracked nipples
- Non-conducive environment
- Family and social issues including lack of economic security or welfare

- Poor nutrition and dehydration
- Illness that makes you unfit or too weak to breastfeed

The baby may also have challenges. Inability to suck may be due to:
- Prematurity
- Deformity of the lips or mouth
- Poor ability to swallow
- Infection and other infant disease conditions
- Rarely, some babies cannot tolerate breast milk
- Other conditions that forbids the baby from taking food orally

## 20. Why do the breasts sometimes become engorged?

Milk secretion is accelerated after delivery. The blood level of estradiol hormone falls fairly rapidly after delivery, but the rate of fall may be slowed down in lactating women. With a remarkable fall, prolactin activity is enhanced such that breast engorgement can occur within 3 – 4 days of delivery. Engorgement may become a problem if:
- The infant is not sucking well
- The infant is premature and cannot be breast fed
- The infant is sick or separated from the mother. In this case rooming-in may make breast feeding possible

To prevent engorgement, women are usually encouraged to commence breastfeeding as early as possible after delivery so that the baby can evacuate the milk in both breasts and prevent engorgement. The severity of pain or discomfort experienced due to engorgement depends on how long the breast milk has accumulated. The discomfort can be reduced by using a firm, supportive bra. The breast milk can also be manually expressed from the breasts or through the use of breast devices that facilitate expression of milk.

## 21. For how long should babies be breast fed?

This is a personal decision but women are generally advised to breastfeed actively for 6 – 18 months. If you are a career woman with little or no time, you may consider breastfeeding for about 6 months. Women should understand that the immune systems of babies are not mature and therefore not effective. This means that infants are at risk of getting sick easily and more often but breast milk contains antibodies which give babies passive immunity against diseases. In other words, the longer babies are breastfed, the more they are protected from sickness. The duration of breastfeeding can be extended as far as practicable. In some communities, it is not unusual for nursing mothers to breastfeed for 3 – 4 years. So it's a personal choice.

## 22. Should babies be given added vitamins?

Some doctors may recommend supplements and vitamins for babies. As the baby grows, vitamin D may need to be given daily for strong bones. Some mothers routinely give vitamin B complex syrups for healthy growth. Please ask your doctor for medical advice, before starting any baby on such drugs.

## 23. Since breast milk contains antibodies, do babies still need to be vaccinated?

Breast milk cannot replace the role of vaccines in babies. Immunization schedules are designed to prevent babies from certain illnesses, regardless of whether or not they are breastfed. It is cheaper and more cost effective to take the vaccines, and prevent such diseases which are dangerous and may be fatal.

## 24. Why do some women choose not to breastfeed their babies?

A woman may decide that she does not want to breastfeed for various reasons. This is usually in consultation with her husband. Apart from making a voluntary decision not to breastfeed, women may be advised not to breastfeed in certain situations by the doctor. Such advice is appropriate in some conditions including open tuberculosis, cancer of the breast, HIV infection, etc. Still birth and deaths of infants soon after delivery, also create problems. In these situations, breast engorgements are more likely. Most doctors prescribe drugs such as bromocriptine, in order to suppress milk production. The residual milk can be manually expressed until the breast is dry. The pain of engorgement can be lessened by the use of routine pain killers, while the breast is held firmly with a supporting bra. It is important for women to inform their doctors about their decision not to breastfeed, during the prenatal period.

## 25. How should a nursing mother handle breast engorgement?

Sometimes, after delivery, the mother may be too sick or too weak to breastfeed her baby. This may lead to accumulation of milk in the breasts. This is called breast engorgement - a painful condition which needs the attention of nurses to give medication for pain and express the breast milk. Normally, a woman should be taught how to take care of her breasts and nipples during prenatal care, in order to make breast feeding easy. Many reasons may be responsible for the inability of the mother to breastfeed her baby. These include severe illness or weakness after delivery, unconsciousness, lack of body fluid or dehydration, nipple problems and situations where the baby is not able to suck the breasts. If this happens at home, where medical help is not readily available, adequate rest with good sleep, good intake of fluids, especially water and frequent squeezing of the breasts, may improve the output of breast milk. During this time, the baby may be given artificial feeds and water. The baby should be put on the breasts as soon as possible.

### 26. What is a breast abscess?

A breast abscess normally starts as a breast infection. It then becomes localized and the area begins to accumulate pus. A localized, collection of pus inside the breast is called an abscess.

### 27. What is the difference between a breast abscess and breast engorgement?

Breast engorgement and abscesses may feel similar, especially in the early stage of the abscess. However, apart from breast enlargement, pain, and chills which may be felt in both conditions, when there is an abscess, part of the breast may be seen to be clearly swollen, tender and warm to touch. Initially, the swelling may be felt as a hard mass with a thicker skin. At the later stage, the skin over the swelling becomes softer and reddish, and may peel off as pus accumulates underneath the skin. There will be fever and pain but the pain is throbbing or biting in nature. Most women with abscesses will experience sweating episodes. Seeing a doctor urgently is necessary, because babies should not be breast fed with the affected breast.

### 28. Under what circumstances should a woman not breastfeed?

In certain situations, it is not appropriate for the mother to breastfeed her baby. In many cases, this is to prevent the transmission of diseases to the baby through breastfeeding. Such situations include:

- Tuberculosis - When the mother is sick with untreated or open tuberculosis, breast feeding is forbidden. This is to prevent the baby from getting infected with the tuberculosis germs which are present in breast milk.
- Breast abscess - A breast abscess contains pus and plenty of germs and therefore not appropriate for the baby. If the abscess affects only one breast, the baby may be fed from the other breast. This should be done safely with the permission of the nurse or doctor, because sometimes the other breast may be infected without the mother being aware
- Epilepsy - Mothers with epilepsy should not breastfeed. Apart from the fact that the drugs used by the mother for the treatment of her condition are secreted in breast milk, she may have a seizure unexpectedly and cause injury to her baby
- Mental illness or puerperal psychosis - It is not safe for a mentally ill mother to breast feed as she may easily harm the baby. However, there is no evidence that mental illness is transmitted through breastfeeding

- Drugs - Some drugs taken by the mother may be secreted in breast milk and may harm the baby in various ways. Such drugs include:
  - Chemotherapy or drugs used by the mother to treat cancer
  - Anti-thyroids or drugs used to treat thyroid diseases
  - Anti-epileptics or drugs used to treat epilepsy
  - Antibiotics like tetracycline and chloramphenicol are not safe in pregnancy
- Cancer of the breast - Breast ulcers, open wounds, burns of the breasts are conditions where breast feeding is not advisable

### 29. What is the remedy for inverted nipples?

One of the benefits of good antenatal care is to identify such problems in time and take steps to correct them during pregnancy. During the latter part of pregnancy, doctors usually teach women with inverted nipples to gently apply traction on the nipples and elevate both for a period of time. This should be done several times daily and may go a long way to resolve inverted nipples, if done diligently before delivery.

### 30. How does smoking affect breastfeeding?

Smoking has no health advantage, whether you are breast feeding or not, so as part of the planning towards pregnancy, you should also plan to quit smoking for the sake of your baby. Babies of smokers are also secondary smokers. The lungs of babies are tender and should not be exposed to smoke and the chemicals it contains. If smoking cannot be avoided completely, the following steps may help:
- Reduce the number of sticks and duration to the barest minimum
- Smoke far away from the baby's location
- Avoid smoking in an enclosed space; step outside the house
- Keep the baby under keen observation to detect any breathing issues as early as possible. Call the doctor immediately if there is any breathing problem or skin change from purple to blue
- Remember that babies born prematurely are at higher risks of developing breathing problems. Perhaps this is a special motivation to quit smoking, at least for the sake of the premature and fragile little baby.

### 31. Is it safe to use herbal medicines when breastfeeding?

This is not advisable. Most drugs available at pharmacies should be obtained through prescriptions. The side effects of prescribed drugs are well documented and predictable. On the contrary, most herbal drugs do not have known formulation, doses, or well documented and verified side effects, so it may be dangerous to take such herbs while breastfeeding. The baby may react to such herbs in an unpredictable manner. In many cases, the doctor may not be able to offer much help because of poor knowledge of the content and effect of such drugs.

### 32. How common is depression during pregnancy and after childbirth?

Depression during pregnancy and after childbirth is a common problem and affects women regardless of age, number of previous pregnancies, social status, and race. Depression occurs in about 13% of cases.

### 33. What is maternal blues?

This is a situation where women experience mild to moderate mood changes soon after childbirth. The mood is that of quietness instead of happiness, dullness instead of cheerfulness, and a tendency towards depression. It is common and occurs in up to 70% of women after childbirth, but it does not last longer than 1-2 weeks and women recover completely. These women are usually non-violent but this situation could re-occur in future pregnancies.

### 34. What is post-partum psychosis?

This is a more serious type of mental illness following childbirth. It occurs in 1 in 600 childbirths. It develops suddenly about one week after delivery. The woman suddenly manifests with severe changes in mood and thought content. She has a distorted perception of herself, others, and her environment. It is a psychotic illness and may manifest as:

- Depression
- Elation
- Hallucination
- Aggression
- Violence

Suicidal tendencies are also common in this category. The cause is suspected to be due to sudden changes in hormonal levels following childbirth. This illness may run in the family, however, these women respond quickly and very well to medical treatment.

### 35. What are the predisposing factors to postnatal depression?

In some women, underlying unresolved emotional problems may be a factor. These include:

- Conflict with spouse
- Dispute over ownership of pregnancy
- Insufficient support: financial, social, etc.
- Worries over change of status from being a spinster to a mother
- Change in body form: fear of becoming ugly

- Perception of emptiness and
- Low self-esteem
- Unclear about how to care for baby

The depression usually lasts for a few weeks and wears off gradually. Support from family members, close relatives, and confidants are important for a quick resolution and recovery.

**36. Which groups of women are more likely to become depressed?**

Those in the high-risk group include women in the following situations:
- Previous personal history of mental illness or depression
- Family history of mental illness
- Marriage or spousal problems
- Young age at pregnancy
- Substance abuse and addiction
- Insecurity due to unemployment and finance
- Poor parental support
- Stressful life
- Bereavement and grief

**37. Can babies become mentally ill, if they are breast fed by mothers who have mental health challenges?**

No, not at all. Mental illness is not transmitted through breast milk. However, it is recognized that some mental illnesses may run in a family (familial tendency) or be inherited. Also, some of the drugs used in the treatment of the mother's illness, may be passed on to the baby through breast milk and this may affect the baby. Overall, breast feeding is beneficial to the baby. With support from family members, this should be encouraged. Breast feeding cements mother and child bonding and may assist the mother in recovery.

**38. After childbirth, what behavior shows that a woman may be suffering from mental illness?**

People who knew her before pregnancy and childbirth are in a position to confirm that the woman's behavior has changed significantly.

Generally, she may be sad, moody or cry intermittently, without any good reason. She may feel irritable or restless without cause. She may be unable to sleep or eat, or eat too much. She may lose interest in her environment and her baby and have feelings of guilt. She may also lose her memory, suffer from low self-esteem and become delusional; seeing imaginary objects or persons. Sometimes she could be dull and unmotivated or obsessive about being less attractive. She may hallucinate; hear strange voices or talk to herself. She could also be listless and complain constantly about many problems at the same time, without real evidence. For example: headaches, body aches, suffocation, chest pain, tiredness, fast and shallow breath, palpitation, etc.

These are not exhaustive and it is important for relatives to notice these strange behaviors early enough to call for help from healthcare givers.

## 39. When should the doctor be called in?

It is important to call the doctor:
- If aggression gets severe or worse
- If the woman is not sleeping
- If suicidal tendencies set in
- If she feels like hurting herself
- If she feels like hurting the baby
- If she looks like she might hurt herself or the baby
- If she finds it difficult to perform usual tasks at home or at work
- If she appears to be confused

## 40. How is depression following childbirth different from mental illnesses?

The good news and big difference is that post-partum depression is more easily treatable, with complete recovery, within a short time. Mental illness outside pregnancy and childbirth is more difficult to treat and may not disappear completely.

## 41. What about family planning after delivery?

It is usual practice for the nurse or doctor to advise women on the appropriate method of family planning after delivery. Ideally, this would have been discussed with you during the prenatal period. However, this can be started just before discharge or more conveniently during the first postnatal visit. Please, remember that:

Oral contraceptives or the pills may reduce secretion of breast milk and make breastfeeding difficult. So, pills are not the best if you are breastfeeding:

- Appropriate methods of family planning are:
  - Condom
  - IUCD
  - Spermicides
- Withdrawal method is not effective and is not recommended. Husbands may not be able to keep their promises!
- Sterilization is excellent and permanent but only if couples are certain that they don't want more children. It is meant to be permanent

Always remember that you may become pregnant unexpectedly after delivery if you do not have family planning in place.

### 42. When will the tummy be flat again?

The process that leads to the womb returning to its original size is called involution. After delivery, the womb can be touched or felt at the level of the umbilicus. It gradually shrinks in size, so that within 10 – 14 days after delivery, it has disappeared into the pelvis and cannot be touched anymore. By the end of the 6$^{th}$ week after delivery in most women, the womb would have shrunken to the approximate size that it was before pregnancy. The tummy is once more firm and flat. Abdominal exercise to strengthen the muscles of the tummy improves the flatness and look of the tummy.

### 43. What is the most common genetic abnormality seen at birth?

The most common genetic abnormality in the newborn is called Downsyndrome. It is also called trisomy-21. These children have an extra chromosome of the 21$^{st}$ pair of chromosomes. Down syndrome occurs once in about 600 births. The children may show all or some of the following features:

- Abnormal facial look including:
  - flat poorly developed face
  - short flat nose
  - prominent epicanthic folds
  - small low set ears
- Thickened big tongue with prominent lines. There may be drooling of saliva
- Loose joints of the limbs and waist; thus making walking difficult or clumsy
- Broad hands with short, stumpy, fat fingers
- Growth retardation
- Wide feet
- Mental retardation

## DEAR DOCTOR:

### 44. How soon can I resume sexual intercourse after delivery?

If you have had a normal delivery and have been discharged home by the doctor, you need a period of rest to speed up recovery and make yourself fit to breastfeed and care for your baby. It is good to have a few hours of sleep during the day time. For all these, you need the support of close relatives and your partner. If all things go well at home, the Lochia discharge may stop with 2 – 4 weeks completely. In the absence of lochia, bleeding and pain in the vagina, sexual intercourse can be resumed within the first 3 weeks after delivery. Every caution should be exercised by your partner to be as gentle as he can. Any unusual pain or bleeding after the 'trial' intercourse should be noted and reported to the doctor for his opinion. Another important thing is that before deciding to resume sexual intercourse, it is vital to start an appropriate family planning method. Never assume that it is impossible to get pregnant, even at this time.

### 45. Doctor, I have a watery brownish discharge. I was delivered of a baby girl one week ago. Is this normal?

After delivery, repair processes take place in the placenta site and other parts of the womb. The cells lining the womb, remnants of placenta, blood vessels, and blood cells are discharged during the repair process. This vaginal discharge or fluid is called Lochia. For the first 3 – 4 days after delivery, the Lochia is reddish because it contains altered blood; it is called Lochia rubra. For the next 20 days, the Lochia gradually changes from red to pale yellow or light brownish because it contains much less blood cells, shed tissues of the womb, some bacteria, and inflammatory cells. This discharge is called Lochia serosa. Finally, the discharge gradually becomes thicker, slimy, and much less in quantity. The color turns yellowish white and appears more like the usual vaginal discharge. It is now called Lochia alba or white Lochia. This type of discharge may last till the end of the 6$^{th}$ week after delivery. Lochia normally stops once the healing of the womb is complete.

### 46. I was delivered of a baby girl 3 weeks ago. Since then, I have been experiencing copious reddish vaginal discharge. What do I do?

This type of discharge is called Lochia rubra or red Lochia which appears up to 4 days after delivery. However, the appearance of red Lochia beyond this time may suggest that the womb is not healing properly. This may be due to:
- An injury in the womb during delivery which is not healing
- The presence of small fragments of placenta
- Infection

It is advisable that you visit your doctor to identify the cause and be treated accordingly.

### 47. I noticed bleeding from the vagina 4 days after I was discharged from hospital. What could have gone wrong and what should I do?

Bleeding after delivery is called post-partum hemorrhage. There are many reasons why a woman may experience this problem. They include:
- Presence of small fragments of placenta or membranes in the womb
- Poor involution: usually because of poor contraction, infection or presence of remnants of tissue or masses in the womb
- Wound breakdown: For example, the cut in the womb for a cesarean section operation may break down. Sometimes, wounds of the cervix, vagina, and vulva may break down and bleed

- On very rare occasions, a woman may have chorio-carcinoma, which is a type of cancer of the placenta. Even though the likelihood of this occurring is rare, it is important that your doctor recognizes this so that treatment is started promptly

The important thing is that you should know that abnormal vaginal bleeding is always a dangerous occurrence. There are only two situations in life when bleeding from the vagina is normal; these are during menstruation and delivery, any bleeding outside these two situations are regarded as dangerous. The doctor should be informed immediately.

### 48. My baby's head was so big that I sustained bruises in my vagina and I still have pain. Although it is decreasing, what can I do to lessen the pain?

It is normal for women to experience mild bruises to the cervix, vulva, and entrance to the vagina during delivery. This may cause pain or discomfort in the first few days following delivery. The healing process of the birth canal starts soon after delivery. By the end of the second week, most of the changes in the cervix, vagina, and vulva should have been reversed, so that these parts of the genital tract usually become normal at 2 weeks. Sometimes, there are individual variations and reactions to pain. If there is no associated fever, a simple pain killer may be beneficial. However, if you had had a cut by the doctor which was repaired but is not healing properly, you may need to return to the hospital for a checkup. If infections have set in, you may need a course of antibiotics but this should be prescribed by your doctor after the problem is properly identified.

### 49. Doctor, it has been difficult for me to pass urine since I had my baby yesterday. Is this normal?

Many women experience difficulty in passing urine soon after delivery. It may last for a couple of days and it happens because of mild injuries or bruises to the muscles and lining of the urinary bladder which lead to loss of bladder tone. The good news is that the bladder tone gradually improves with time and the difficulty in urination becomes much less. If there is stagnation of urine, a full bladder and pain, you should let your doctor know this. Unlike the situation above, some women experience frequent urinations for 3 – 4 days after delivery, because the body fluids stored in the body during pregnancy are automatically passed out as urine. So the bladder fills up quickly and there is the urge to urinate more frequently. These 2 conditions are normal and should stop on their own within 1 week of delivery.

### 50. What tips can you give me on how to breastfeed effectively?

Before putting the infant to the breast, you should wash both breasts with mild soap and wipe clean with water. Pay particular attention to the nipple and wash clean with fresh, clean water. Breastfeeding while you are sitting in a comfortable position makes it easy. Once you begin to breastfeed, you will find it easier and derive more pleasure by the day. Breastfeeding can be done when the baby is hungry. This is called demand breastfeeding and may be done every 3 – 4 hours during the day. Below are some more tips that may help you:

- Aim to empty both breasts at the end of the breastfeeding session, by encouraging the baby to spend equal time sucking on both breasts. This may take about 5 minutes on each breast
- Put the nipple of the clean breast into the back of the mouth of the baby
- Ensure that the breast itself does not cover the nostrils of the baby, so that the baby can breathe freely
- Gently squeeze milk into the baby's mouth. The first gush of milk may stimulate the baby to begin sucking
- Be careful to notice when the breast is empty so that the baby does not suck in air instead of breast milk
- Once you are satisfied that one breast is empty, gently open the baby's mouth to tease the nipple out
- Put the baby to suckle the second breast
- At the end of breastfeeding, take a look at your baby to ensure that the baby is comfortable

The initial period may be a learning period but with experience, breast feeding should be a pleasure for you and your baby.

### 51. I have just been delivered of a baby girl. Can I breastfeed with the yellowish breast milk from my breasts?

This type of milk is called colostrum in medical parlance and it is perfect to feed your baby with this yellowish milk. It is secreted in the breast a few days before delivery and up until a few days after delivery. Colostrum as you rightly said, is yellowish and thicker than the usual breast milk but it is tailor-made for the well-being of your baby. It is rich in important proteins, vitamins, and minerals. It contains a good measure of immune substances called immunoglobulin. These are antibodies that help your baby to fight infections and other diseases. This is very important because the immune systems of newborn babies are poorly developed. Poor immunity is one of the reasons why babies are more prone to illnesses.

### 52. If I decide to breastfeed only, will this be sufficient for my baby?

Yes. Breast milk alone is quite sufficient for your baby and it contains all that the baby needs at this time. However, you must ensure that the baby gets enough of it at regular intervals. This means that as the mother supplying the milk, you must eat well, take plenty of fluids and be fit. You may choose to feed your baby "on demand." This means as many times as your baby demands for breast milk but on average, 5 – 7 times per day should be adequate. When a baby is fed sufficiently with breast milk as the main food, this is called exclusive breastfeeding. It is very good and sufficient to supply the nutritional requirements of the baby for at least the first 6 months of life.

### 53. In case of breast engorgement, what should I do?

You can help yourself by taking a common pain killer to reduce your pain. Next is to wash and sterilize a receptacle, clean your nipples and the surrounding area of the breast. Finally, gently squeeze the breast from behind towards the nipple to express breast milk into a container. The expressed milk can be given to the baby if he or she is able to feed, otherwise, it should be discarded. You may repeat this process as many times as it is required. You can also use a breast pump to express the milk. Breast pumps can be purchased over the counter from pharmacies. Always remember to clean and sterilize the pump before use, in order to prevent infection. Also, if you begin to feel hot or have chills or the pain becomes more severe, this could imply that infection is setting in. You therefore need to see your doctor immediately.

### 54. I have cracked nipples. How should I take care of them?

The nipple should be cleaned carefully with water and a towel. Next, it should be smeared with soothing oil or ointment. It is important to rest the breast generally. During this time, you should gently express the breast milk into a clean cup to prevent engorgement. Provided you have observed strict and proper hygiene; the baby could be given the expressed milk.

### 55. I am a working mother, so for how long should I breast feed?

You should breast feed for as long as you can, but most doctors usually recommend that babies should be breastfed for at least 12 months. For the first 6 months of life, exclusive breastfeeding is quite sufficient for the nutritional needs of your baby.

### 56. After 6 months of breastfeeding my baby, what do I need to do?

If you breastfeed exclusively in the first 6 months, this is okay. After this period, you may introduce other baby foods including cereals gradually to satisfy the baby's additional food requirements.

### 57. Can my baby use a pacifier?

Yes. Once your baby has acquired the skill to suckle and breastfeed well, a pacifier is good especially when you put the baby on the bed. The use of pacifiers has also been found to be associated with a reduction in the risk of sudden deaths in infants.

**58. I understand that some of the drugs that I use can be passed on to my baby through breastfeeding. Can you guide me please?**

This is true. The breast milk is part of your body fluid. Generally, it is better to assume that the drugs that you take will be secreted into the breast milk and eventually get to your baby. Fortunately, most of the drugs that you take in normal doses, as prescribed, may not harm your baby or cause any serious side effects. However, illicit drugs like cocaine, heroin, marijuana, etc., are harmful and should not be used.

**59. When I was pregnant, I noticed that my heart was beating faster than usual and my veins shot out. What is the explanation for this?**

During pregnancy, many physiological changes take place in different parts, organs and systems of the body. In the blood supply system, the following remarkable changes take place:

- The blood volume is increased by as much as 40%
- The red blood cells increase by 18%
- The amount of blood pumped out each time the heart beats increases
- The heart rate is increased
- The blood pressure may increase slightly

This is why a pregnant woman experiences faster heart beats and more dilated blood vessels. Some women sweat a lot because more blood is brought to the skin's surface. Many of these changes e.g. blood pressure, reverts to normal soon after delivery and the other parameters revert to normal by the 6$^{th}$ week after delivery. So, the changes that you have noticed are regarded as normal in pregnancy.

**60. Doctor, I suffer from depression. Will my baby contract this mental illness if I breast feed her?**

There is no evidence that psychiatric illness is transmitted or inherited through breast milk. Mental illness is not a disease, like infections that can be transmitted through breast milk. However, when a mother has a mental illness, it is possible for her to injure or harm her baby knowingly or unknowingly. For this reason, it is not advisable for a mentally unstable mother to breastfeed her baby. The baby should be cared for by a responsible relative or nanny. The baby could also benefit from wet nursing or artificial milk.

No. It occurs in women regardless of the number of pregnancies, age and social status. First timers are not at a higher risk of becoming depressed.

# CHAPTER 16

# Cancers of the Cervix and Womb

*"Courage doesn't always roar. Sometimes, courage is the quiet voice at the end of the day saying (I will try again tomorrow)."*
– MARY ANNE RADMACHER

### 1. What is a tumor?
A tumor can be regarded as a swelling or mass. In most cases, the presence of a tumor can be seen or felt, if the tumor is in a location that is accessible. There are two types – benign tumors and malignant tumors.

### 2. What is the difference between benign and malignant tumors?
A benign tumor is not cancerous while the word malignant is used to qualify a mass or tumor that is cancerous. So, a malignant tumor means cancer.

### 3. What is the origin of the word cancer?
Nobody knows for sure. However, it is suggested that the word *carcinos* was coined by Hippocrates, who is widely regarded as "The father of medicine", to describe cells that behave abnormally, like cancer cells. The word carcinos means crab in Greek language. Also, the behavior of cancer cells, share some similarities with crabs. For example, crabs hook onto surfaces tenaciously. Cancer cells also invade normal cells ruthlessly. Furthermore, in horoscopy, the symbol for cancer is a crab.

### 4. How are cancers named?
Cancers are named according to the tissues or organ from which they originated. This is regardless of where they may spread to. So a cancer that

originates from the liver is called liver cancer, while that which originates from the lung is called lung cancer.

## 5. What is the difference between normal and cancer cells?

There are some differences. Normal cells grow in an orderly manner. Normal cells do not destroy other cells and are usually under the control of the various body mechanisms. On the other hand, cancer cells grow in a disorderly fashion. They are not under the control of the usual body mechanisms and they grow and divide many times faster than normal body cells. Cancer cells also destroy other cells, tissues or organs on their path and eat up their host. They possess the ability to disperse all around the body and start new growths or tumors at distant locations.

## 6. What causes cancer?

Doctors and scientists do not fully understand the exact way cancer cells are formed. However, there are both external and internal factors that may promote the formation of cancer cells.

External factors include:
- Chemical agents
- Radiation - sun, radiological and others
- Viruses
- Effects of physical environment - fumes, soot, etc.

Internal factors include:
- Genetic inheritance
- Hormone problems
- Immune problems

These factors may act alone or in combination with one another to initiate or promote cancer formation.

## 7. What are risk factors?

Risk factors are those characteristics of people that make them more likely to develop cancers more than those who do not have such characteristics in the community. These may be natural, artificial, inherited or acquired.

## 8. What are carcinogens?

Carcinogens are substances or things which interact with the body to cause cancers. There are 3 main groups of carcinogens and these are:
- Biological: These are organisms which may be bacteria, viruses and parasites that infect the body
- Chemical: This category includes the king pin of cancer – cigarettes. Others include lead, soot (from chimneys), and alfatoxin which is a contaminant of stored food

- Physical: The most important include ultraviolet rays and ionizing radiation (X-rays)

## 9. How does the severity of cancers compare with their growth rates?

There are different categories and stages of cancers. Most severe and terrible cancers grow at a very rapid rate. So, the rapid rate of growth of a cancer which gives the tumor its huge size is an indication of the severity of the cancer. In other words, huge cancerous masses are likely to be more severe or deadly.

## 10. What is the relationship between cancer and age?

Age is an important factor in the consideration of who gets cancer. Generally, cancer is more common between middle and old age. Even though there are target age groups where some cancers are more common, there is a general increase in cancer between the ages of 55 – 74 years. It is safe to say that after the age of 55 years, the risk of cancer is higher.

## 11. What is the relationship between cancer and the environment?

The environment, both physical and non-physical has been proven to play a crucial role in the risk of developing cancer. The environment includes physical buildings, the air we breathe in, the water we use, the clothes we wear, the conditions at the place of work, the type of work, the food we eat, the beverages we drink and our lifestyle. It is factual to take a position, that all adverse environments increase the risk of developing cancer.

## 12. What is the relationship between cancer and weight?

Generally speaking, people who are overweight by more than 25% have higher death rates from cancer, than people with normal weights or those who are slimmer. So, being overweight increases the general risk of cancer.

## 13. What is the relationship between cancer and alcohol?

Excessive use or abuse of alcohol is associated with the development of various cancers including:
- Liver (due to increased risk of liver cirrhosis)
- Mouth
- Throat
- Esophagus

## 14. What is the relationship between cancer and smoking?

Cigarette smoking is increasing in most parts of the world including the USA, due to the liberalization of social values and more freedom. Cigarettes are the

single most devastating environmental factor causing premature deaths in the USA. Apart from other anti-social effects, smoking accounts for 77% of cancer of the lung in males and 43% in females. Other cancers associated with smoking include cancers of the:
- Mouth
- Throat
- Esophagus
- Urinary bladder
- Pancreas

## 15. What are the most common lifestyles and environmental factors that cause cancer worldwide?

The five most important risk factors for cancer in the world are:
- Tobacco use
- Alcohol
- Obesity/over weight
- Wrong food – lack of fruits and vegetables

Lack of physical exercise / sedentary lifestyle.

These 5 risk factors are responsible for about 33% of cancer. Most importantly, tobacco use is single handedly responsible for 22% of deaths due to cancer. This emphasizes the critical role that stopping of tobacco use, plays in the prevention of cancer and cancer deaths.

## 16. Can cancers be inherited?

Yes. Some cancers may run in some families in the same community. So, existing history of cancers in close relatives like mothers and sisters, may forecast the risk of cancer in other close relatives. This inheritance may be due to mutation or abnormal change in genes e.g. BRCA-1 and BRCA-2 genes which are closely related to the risk of developing breast and ovarian cancers. Some cancers have also been known to occur in some families, in more or less the same way and pattern. Good examples include cancers of the breast, colon and ovary.

## 17. What are screening tests?

Screening tests for cancer are performed to detect changes in the cells or tissues in any part of the body, which may suggest the possibility that such cells or tissues may develop into certain diseases, including cancer, in the future. This is in spite of the fact that the organs or tissues may look grossly normal and function normally, at the time of performing the screening test.

**18. Why are screening tests important with respect to cancer?**

As of now, screening tests appear to be the only way to prevent some types of cancer. For example, a PAP smear is a screening test done for cervical cancer. A PAP smear done at intervals, will detect cells of the cervix that are likely to develop into cancer cells of the cervix, long before they do so, consequently a PAP smear affords the opportunity of surgically removing the cervix, before cancer develops. Women are encouraged to get screened regularly, especially for cancers of the breast and cervix. Screening tests are usually affordable and cost effective. Prevention is always better than cure.

**19. At what age should screening tests for cancer begin?**

It largely depends on the particular cancer being screened for. Screening programs are designed with the nature, characteristics, growth pattern, and epidemiology of a particular cancer in mind. For example, sexual activity or multiple sexual partners, promiscuity, sexually transmitted infections are important factors in the development of cancer of the cervix. Therefore, any woman who is sexually active should do a PAP smear at intervals, regardless of her age.

**20. What are the things that may suggest the possibility of cancer?**

The signs and symptoms of cancer depend on the type. There is an acronym in the word PRECAUTION, which you can use to remember the common complaints that may suggest cancer as stated below.

- P- Pain – constant and increasing
- R- Repeated bouts of diarrhea and constipation
- E- Enlarging mass or growth
- C- Cachexia or severe wasting
- A- Anemia – chronic and unexplained
- U- Ulcer or wound that refuses to heal
- T- Tiredness – without explanation
- I- Incapacitation and impaired functions
- O- Obvious ill health
- N- Notorious cough or hoarseness of voice

The above may point to cancer especially where a precise diagnosis is difficult.

**21. What are the effects of cancer on the body?**

Cancers affect human beings in many ways. People suffering from cancer experience various adverse effects. Cancers affect the physical appearance, the mind, and the emotions. There are some effects that depend on the type of cancer and particular part or organ affected in the body. The severity of the effects also depends on the severity and spread of the particular cancer.

Generally speaking, most people suffering from cancer, experience the following problems:
- Fatigue: chronic weakness and tiredness all the time
- Change in appetite: most people experience poor appetite and difficulty in eating. Few people have increased appetite
- Pain: this may be generalized or related to the organ affected. It is usually a source of worry and may intensify as the cancer spreads
- Weight loss: most cancers cause progressive weight loss with profound changes in appearance. With deterioration in look and appearance, there is low self-esteem. Also, rapid weight loss may indicate failure of treatment, more aggressive disease, or imminent death
- Fear: this is ever present except in a few patients. Fear of death, uncertainty about outcome of treatment, fear about dwindling or lack of support and even life after death create serious anxiety
- Emotional or psychological problems: For many people, the diagnosis of cancer may be seen as a pronouncement of death. Only a matter of time. Sadness, anxiety, depression, anger (why me!) contribute to physical suffering and deterioration in health
- General loss of interest: Loss of interest in the environment and life affairs are common. This may include work, business, loved ones, and relationships, sexual intercourse and previous pastimes. Extreme lack of interest, emotional upset, and physical devastation of the disease may cause rapid deterioration
- Loss of sleep: apart from pain, all other problems mentioned above will result in inability to sleep or lack of it

## 22. What is generally the single most important complaint in women with cancer?

People suffering from cancer may have so many different complaints depending on the type of cancer. However, the complaint of pain appears to be the most common. Pain may come in different ways and people may interpret or express the severity of pain in different ways. Some may complain of serious pain, while for others, the same intensity of pain may be taken as discomfort. Every situation where the reason for pain cannot be easily explained should be worrisome. Pain caused by cancer is usually constant or felt almost all the time. It becomes worse with time. It is also good to look out for other problems that are commonly associated with cancer pain, especially weight loss and the appearance of blood in the stool, urine, or sputum.

## 23. How does cancer generally spread?

Cancer tissues spread in 3 main ways:
- Direct spread: Cancer can spread in a continuous manner to invade nearby structures and surfaces, destroying them as they go. A good

example is the cancer of the ovary, which usually spreads directly to structures surrounding the ovary and the abdominal cavity
- Through blood vessels: Cancer cells can also be carried in blood vessels to various parts of the body. This is called hematogenous spread. Hematogenous spread usually follows the chain of blood vessels and blood supply of the organ involved and its connections. This is the case with cancer of the liver and lungs
- Lymphatic spread: The lymph vessels like blood pipes drain (lymph fluid) from lymph nodes of the various organs of the body, into larger pipes. Some cancer cells are carried into larger lymph vessels to the various lymph nodes and from here, to other parts of the body. The lymph nodes are like soldiers that defend the body during attacks by diseases, including infections, cancer, etc. So in the process of eating up cancer cells, they become enlarged. Enlarged lymph nodes can sometimes be noticed as swellings, in the body of people suffering from cancer

## 24.  What is metastasis?

Metastasis means that a malignant tumor or cancer has implanted at other parts of the body, which is different from the original location of the cancer. For example, a cancer of the ovary may metastasize into the liver. Many deaths due to cancer are as a result of metastasis and destruction of other parts of the body. So, metastasis is an ominous sign in people suffering from cancer.

## 25.  How is the severity of cancer expressed?

Cancer is classified into stages according to severity. Generally, there are four (4) stages with Stage 1 being the least severe and Stage 4 the most severe. Stage 4 means that the cancer is advanced and has spread to involve other parts of the body. The staging system is used to plan treatment and estimate survival prospects.

## 26.  How many will survive cancer globally?

More and more people suffering from cancer live for five (5) years and beyond, with proper management. The number of such people however depends on the type of cancer, the stage or extent of the cancer at the time of diagnosis, the type of treatment and the facilities available. Expertise and experience of those managing the patient are important to the outcome. This is the reason why more people survive in countries with well-developed health infrastructures, like the USA and other Western countries. On the contrary, the diagnosis of cancer in a patient in many developing countries is as good as pronouncing a death sentence on the patient.

### 27. Generally speaking, what are the strategies for survival from cancer?

Many cancers can be "cured" if detected early enough, especially before they manifest at other parts of the body. So, screening to "catch them early" is as important as detecting and treating already established cases. Cancers of the prostate, breast, and cervix are some that can be screened for or detected early to achieve high cure rates.

### 28. What are the major modalities of treatment of cancer?

Generally, cancers are treated through surgical operation, radiotherapy and chemotherapy. In many cases, combinations of these modalities are more effective.

### 29. What is the goal of treatment?

There are two main goals of treatment: the first, of course, is to cure the cancer if possible. This can be achieved if treatment is effectively formulated and started early. Where cure is not foreseeable, the objective is to ensure that the person enjoys a good quality of life which is prolonged as much as possible.

### 30. What is the role of palliative treatment?

On many occasions, it may not be possible to aim for a cure. In such cases, the quality of life of the person is important. Every person so afflicted by cancer, is entitled to enjoy life with decency and dignity, for as long as she lives. Great relief from physical, emotional and social problems and satisfaction can be achieved in patients living with cancer, through palliative care, support, encouragement and empathy by healthcare providers and trusted relatives.

### 31. Why do cancers destroy their hosts?

Cancer cells are destructive in many ways. Cancer cells have terrific ability to divide several times and grow faster than host cells. In doing this, they are autonomous and not under the control of the host's normal body mechanisms. For example, they will absorb as much as they desire of food and blood supply, regardless of the condition of the host. So, whether the host eats or not, cancer cells will feed fat, regardless of whether or not the host already looks lean. Furthermore, there are now indications that some substances in the body including soluble factors such as cytokines are involved in the extreme wasting and weight loss in cancer patients. Cytokines cause massive reduction in the amount of fat and muscles in the body in an abnormal way. This leaves the cancer patient with barely any fat or muscle bulk – only bones!

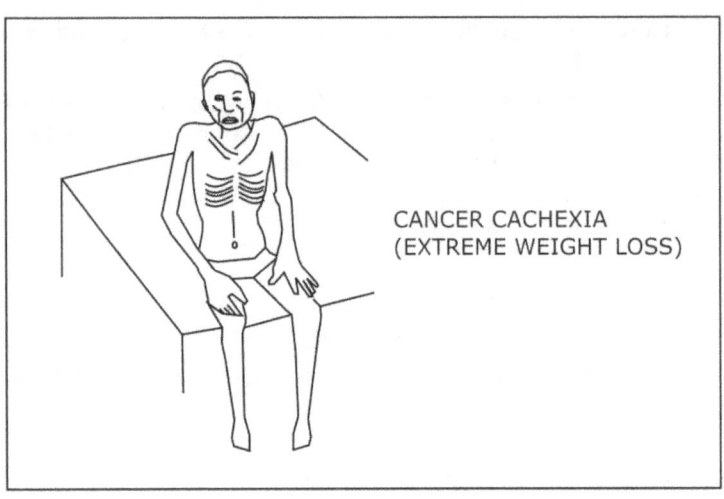

CANCER CACHEXIA
(EXTREME WEIGHT LOSS)

### 32. What are the deadliest cancers globally?

Annually, cancer claims many lives and the death burden is great. According to the World Health Organization (WHO), the breakdown of about 8.8 million deaths due to cancer in 2015 shows the 5 deadliest cancers as stated in the table below:

| POSITION | CANCER | NO OF DEATHS (2015) |
|---|---|---|
| 1st | Lung cancer | 1,690,000 |
| 2nd | Liver cancer | 788,000 |
| 3rd | Colon & rectum cancer | 774,000 |
| 4th | Stomach cancer | 754,000 |
| 5th | Breast cancer | 571,000 |

The greatest fatality is caused by Lung cancer. This is quite unfortunate because cigarette smoking, which is responsible for most of these cases, is a habit forming substance which can be stopped.

### 33. Globally, how many people die of cancer every year?

According to the WHO, cancer is responsible for 1 death out of every 6 deaths and it is the second most common cause of death in the world. In 2018, cancer was responsible for 9.6 million deaths globally. As usual, approximately 70% of these deaths occur in the developing countries, with non-existing or poorly developed health infrastructure.

## 34. How many people die of cancer in the USA every year?

Cancer is the second most common cause of death in the USA, second only to heart disease. According to the national cancer institute (NCI) forecast, about 609,640 people were expected to die of cancer in 2018. Based on the 2011-2015 death statistics, according to the NCI, the death rate due to cancer in both men and women (Cancer mortality) is 163.5 deaths per 100,000 deaths per year. Generally speaking, it is estimated that about 1,600 people die of cancer on a daily basis in the United States.

## 35. What is the trend in the number of deaths due to cancer per year in the USA?

Generally, in the last five decades, the number of deaths due to cancer in men has increased. This is mainly due to deaths from lung cancer in men. On the contrary, the number of deaths from cancer has reduced in women, due to reduction in deaths from cancers of the cervix, womb, liver, and stomach. However, and on a positive note, the NCI has reported a current trend that the overall death rate due to cancer in the USA fell from 1991 to 2015.

## 36. What about deaths due to lung cancer in women in the USA?

Overall, there is an increase in the number of deaths due to cancer of the lung in women because more women now smoke cigarettes.

## 37. What are the 4 most common cancers in women in the USA?

Generally speaking, skin cancer comes first as the most common cancer. However, cancer specialists, by consensus, have excluded skin cancer in the ranking, most probably because a remarkable number are of the non-melanoma type. If skin cancer is excluded, the 4 most common cancers in women in order of occurrences are cancers of the:
- Breast
- Lung
- Colorectal
- Womb

## 38. What is the global economic loss due to cancer?

The devastating effect of cancer wherever it occurs is difficult to quantify in terms of economic and non-economic losses. In the USA, the agency for health research and quality (AHRG) the direct medical costs of cancer in 2015 alone at about $80.2 billion. However, the WHO had previously estimated the global monetary loss of cancer in 2010 at about $1.16 trillion. This amount is more than half the combined annual budgets of all the countries in sub-Saharan Africa. Thus the economic impact of cancer is too huge to contemplate. Furthermore, the disproportionate burden that poor countries bear is worrisome.

### 39. What are the most important risk factors for cancer?

The most important risk factors for cancer hinges on lifestyles and types of diets. These are:
- Tobacco use: this is the most important risk factor
- Obesity or High body mass index (BMI)
- Low intake of fruits and vegetable
- Lack of Physical activity
- Alcohol use

These 5 factors account for about 33% of cases of cancers. Unfortunately, the factors can be changed through modification and adjustment of life styles; thus reducing the scourge of cancer.

### 40. Why is death from cancer so high?

This is partly due to the fact that the exact cause of cancer is still unknown. This makes it difficult to have an effective treatment plan that can achieve a cure for cancer. Other reasons for the high mortality rate from cancer include the followings:
- Ignorance
- Some people with cancer report to hospital late in the disease. Of those who report to hospital, few patients reject or deny diagnosis of cancer and disappear for a remarkably long period of time. Thereafter, they show up in hospital when the cancer has advanced badly
- Wrong diagnosis at the early period mostly due to human error. There may also be some delay in making a final diagnosis
- Lack of facilities or dedicated cancer clinics
- Lack of skilled personnel
- Development of severe complications and multiple organ failure
- Availability of skilled personnel, equipment, and dedicated cancer centers, facilitate diagnosis and best treatment. Such centers are widely available in the developed parts of the world but are grossly lacking in developing countries.

### 41. Globally speaking, is the burden of deaths due to cancer decreasing?

No. It is quite unfortunate that despite efforts by all stakeholders to combat the scourge of cancer, statistics have shown that more people are dying from the disease. Currently, statistics from the WHO have shown that the burden of cancer has risen to 18.1 million new cases and 9.6 million people were expected to die from cancer in 2018.

### 42. Can cancer be prevented?

Since the actual cause of cancer is unknown, it is difficult to institute preventive measures in most cases. However, because some cancers have known risk factors, some of which can be modified or avoided e.g. cancer of the lung and smoking, it is possible to reduce the risk of this cancer by avoiding the risk factors. Regular screening tests like pap smear may ensure early detection and treatment of potential cancers, before they actually become cancerous.

### 43. Are cancers curable?

Practically speaking, cancers can only be cured if all the cancer cells can be removed from the body. It is usually not possible to do so except in rare cases, where the cancer is still confined to one part of the body and can be completely removed. Therefore, doctors talk of a 5-year survival rate which denotes the chance of a patient living for 5 years or more, from the time of medical intervention or treatment of cancer. To do this, doctors classify cancers into stages according to severity.

### 44. Is it possible for a cancer mass to disappear without treatment?

Yes. A cancer mass can slow down its rate of growth or stop growing altogether for unknown reasons. In very rare cases, cancer may actually shrink and disappear completely. This is a rare exception and cannot be predicted. The general norm is that cancers grow and enlarge rapidly. When rarely cancers disappear on their own volition, they equate a "medical miracle".

### 45. How common is cancer of the cervix globally?

Cancer of the cervix is relatively common. It the second most common cancer of the female reproductive tract. The most common is cancer of the ovary. Currently, cervical cancer is being discovered more often in women younger than 40 years.

### 46. How common is cancer of the cervix in the USA?

The American cancer society (ACS) has estimated about 13,170 new cases of cervical cancer for 2019. From this figure, it is further projected that about 4,250 women may die. However, thanks to increased public awareness and the various methods of screening and early detection, cervical cancer is no longer the number one cause of cancer deaths in women in the USA.

### 47. What age is most at risk of cancer of the cervix in the USA?

Cervical cancer is most common between 35- 44 years of age. It is rare in women below the age of 20.

**48. What are the risk factors for cervical cancer?**

There are many risk factors for developing cervical cancer. However, the single most important factor is the infection by the Human papilloma virus (HPV). This virus is responsible in about 91% of cases of cervical cancer. Other risk factors include:

- Other sexually transmitted infections including HIV and Herpes
- Multiple sexual partners
- Smoking
- Exposure to the drug or hormone called diethylstilbesterol (DES)
- Depleted immunity status e.g. AIDS
- Use of oral contraceptives for 5 years or more
- High parity: having given birth several times (3 or more)
- Low socio economic status

**49. What is the trend in the occurrence of cervical cancer in the USA?**

According to the report from the CDC, in the last 40 years, the incidence of cancer of the cervix has reduced significantly. The annual reduction in cancer cases was estimated at about 1.3% per annum. Similarly, the death rate has reduced significantly by about 0.9% annually. This good news is as a result of increased awareness and early screening for cervical cancer.

**50. What is the pattern of occurrence of cervical cancer according to racial groups in the USA?**

According to information from the Centre for Disease Control and Prevention (CDC), the national program of cancer registries (NPCR) data for 2011 - 2015 showed that the Human papilloma virus (HPV) associated cervical cancer is most common in Hispanic women. Black Americans have the second highest rate followed by Caucasian women. However, Black American women have the greatest burden of death from cervical cancer. In other words, more Black women die from cervical cancer than Hispanic or Caucasian women.

**51 How many people die of cervical cancer in the world every year?**

According to the world health organization (WHO), cancer of the cervix accounts for approximately 7.5% of deaths due to cancer in women. The WHO estimated about 311,000 deaths in 2018, with over 85% occurring in developing countries. The cervix due to its location and the nature of its cells is most suitable to different infections and effects of changes in its environment, especially the acidity level. Some of the infections and chemical agents can transform the cells to begin the process of cancer formation.

**50. What is the usual cause of death in cancer of the cervix?**

Surprisingly, most people who succumb to death as a result of cervical cancer do not die as a result of distant metastasis or destruction of distant organs like the liver, lungs, etc. Rather, death is mostly due to the local spread of cancer to surrounding organs, especially the urinary bladder and ureters (urine pipe connecting the kidney to bladder). The extension leads to obstruction of the ureters and cause kidney problems like stagnation of fluid, distension of the kidneys with urine (hydronephrosis) and elevated blood urea which is very harmful.

### 51. How can I reduce my risk of having cervical cancer?

Here are the tips:
- PAP smear- the most important thing is to do regular screening tests, once you are 21. This test is called PAP smear or PAP test.
- HPV test or test for the Human papilloma virus
- Get vaccinated against HPV - this protects against HPV infection. It can be taken as early as 9 years up until 26 years
- Don't Smoke
- Stick to one un infected sexual partner
- Practice safe sex- use condoms
- Avoid unsupervised use of contraceptives; ask your doctor for help
- Limit and plan your family size

### 52. What is a PAP Smear?

A PAP Smear is a screening test performed to see if there is any change or disease that may indicate the risk of developing cancer of the cervix in the future. Normally, it takes a long time or many years for the cells of the cervix to develop into cancer. The change is gradual and progressive. Therefore, if these cells are detected early and removed or destroyed, it is practically possible to prevent cervical cancer from developing.

### 53. How is a PAP smear done?

A PAP smear is done by gently scraping the surface of the cervix with a wooden spatula in order to collect the cells. This process is painless, so you should not be afraid. The cells are then spread on a glass slide, fixed, and sent to a specialist or laboratory, where they are stained and examined for changes that may suggest future development of cancer.

### 54. What is the earliest warning that may suggest cervical cancer?

The cancer may be developing for many years without much to show for it. What is certain is that abnormal cells of the cervix will be shed constantly. So, regular screening for these cells is the key to catch cancer of the cervix as early as possible. However, the most important complaint of cancer of the cervix is abnormal vaginal bleeding in females who are below 40 years.

## 55. What complaints are commonly associated with cancer of the cervix?

Most women suffering from established cancer of the cervix exhibit 4 major complaints:
- Abnormal vaginal bleeding
- Copious watery vaginal discharge (leucorrhoea)
- Bleeding during sexual intercourse
- Painful urination

In most developing countries, many patients report very late to hospital with complaints of severe low abdominal and pelvic pain, accompanied by copious and very offensive vaginal discharge. However, the two most important classical complaints are:
- Prolonged abnormal vaginal bleeding
- Blood stained watery vaginal discharge

## 56. How is the cancer treated?

The type of treatment deployed is usually decided upon by the doctor after a thorough investigation. This will help to determine the type, the severity, and the extent of spread of the cancer. The common modalities of treatment include combinations of surgery, radiotherapy, and drugs depending on the stage and type of the cancer.

## 57. What are the side effects of radiotherapy?

Patients undergoing radiotherapy may experience some adverse effects and complications. Some of the complications are general and almost everybody undergoing such treatments will have them. The important effects include:
- Radiation dermatitis or inflammation: This may appear as sensation of intense heat and "burning"
- Menopause: Women undergoing radiation may stop menstruating due to the effects on the reproductive organs, especially the ovaries and the womb
- Weakness, fatigue and dizziness
- Anemia
- Entero-colitis: Radiation may cause inflammation of the bowels resulting in bouts of diarrhea. This may lead to nutritional deficiency and contribute to weight loss
- Other Skin damages include:
  - Itching
  - Blisters
  - Peeling
  - Cracks
  - Discoloration
- Hair loss: especially around the area being irradiated
- Headache: general aches

- Swelling: due to obstruction of the lymphatic fluid drainage of the area being irradiated, for example, the arm and chest in case of breast cancer
- Radiation pneumonitis: this may manifest as fluid collection in the lungs (congestion) and a troublesome cough

## 58. What are the side effects of chemotherapy?

The effects of chemotherapy depend on the type of drugs involved, the dose, and duration of treatment. These effects are expectedly more severe, if the woman is also receiving radiotherapy. Some effects are more common while others are rare or individualized. The important effects include:

- Nausea and vomiting
- Headache, sometimes the neck may become stiff
- Body pain and aches, muscle pain
- Dizziness
- Exhaustion and weakness
- Burning sensation, especially of the hands and feet
- Tingling sensation and numbness
- Weak skin manifesting as:
  - Skin cracks or easy bruising
  - Mouth ulcers
  - Sore throat
- Stomach upset:
  - Stomach discomfort
  - Diarrhea and dehydration
  - Constipation is less frequent
- Anemia most commonly due to depressed bone marrow formation of new blood cells and destruction of circulating blood cells
- Hair loss – this may happen within 4-6 weeks of starting treatment
- Damage to Brain cells - this is called "Chemo brain" and manifests as cognitive defects such as:
  - Reduced ability to sustain concentration
  - Poor memory and poor thinking ability

Damage to vital organs may occur either during therapy or long after completion. These include:

- Eyes – impairment of vision
- Kidneys- derangement and kidney failure
- Liver- derangement and liver failure
- Heart – heart failure
- Reproductive organs:
  - Damage to the ovaries and destruction of the female eggs
  - Stoppage of menstruation (induced menopause)

### 59. How is HPV contracted?

HPV infection is one of the sexually transmitted infections. So, infection is acquired mainly through normal sexual intercourse with an infected man. However, the infection can be contracted through oral and anal sex, but these are less common. HPV can also be contracted through skin contact with an infected person.

### 60. What other diseases does HPV cause?

The more virulent types of HPV are associated with cancers of other parts of the body. These include:
- Cancer of the penis
- Cancer of the vagina
- Cancer of the mouth and throat
- Cancer of the anus

Even the less virulent types of HPV cause swellings or tumors. These are commonly called papilloma in medical parlance. Examples are anal warts and vulva warts. So, it is very important to prevent HPV infection as much as possible.

### 61. What is cancer of the womb?

Traditionally, the womb has a body and a neck. The body is the big part of the womb that contains the womb cavity, where pregnancy takes place. The neck is the part that joins the body to the vagina. The wall of the womb has 3 layers. These are the outer covering, the middle layer made of muscles of the womb, and inner lining of the womb. The cavity of the inner lining is where pregnancy takes place. It is also called the endometrial cavity. This inner lining is made of endometrial cells, plenty of glands, blood pipes, and nerves. Cancer of the womb usually denotes cancer of the inner lining. It is also called cancer of the endometrium.

### 62. How common is cancer of the womb?

It is fairly common in developing countries, but much less common than cancer of the cervix. Now that women live longer and more women attain the age of menopause and beyond, the expectation is that cancer of the womb will be much more common.

### 63. Which age group is mostly at risk of cancer of the womb?

Cancer of the womb is more common in older women. It is most common in women between the ages of 50 - 65 years, especially those that are also barren.

### 64. Is it possible for young girls to have cancer of the womb also?
Cancer of the womb is most likely to be diagnosed in women who have attained menopause. As mentioned above, majority of cases are between 50-65 years of age. However, cancer of the womb may occur as early as 20 years of age. Doctors are worried when an old woman who has stopped menstruation suddenly begins to bleed from the vagina. A good number of such cases usually turn out to be cancers of the womb.

### 65. How does cancer of the womb spread?
Cancer of the womb usually spreads to involve the neck of the womb in the first instance. With time, the vagina, urinary bladder, and other organs in the neighborhood of the womb, including the lower portion of the large intestines become affected. Therefore, at this stage, the woman may experience problems including waist pain, blood stained, foul smelling, copious vaginal discharge, urine, and stool problems etc.

### 66. Who are those at higher risks of developing cancer of the womb?
Those at increased risks of cancer of the womb include:
- Infertile women that have never given birth
- Obese women
- Diabetic women
- Women who attained menopause late
- Women on oral contraceptive pills
- Women with ovarian tumors
- Women on estrogen hormone treatment
- Women on irradiation treatment

### 67. How do I reduce my risk of cancer of the womb?
- Avoid sedentary lifestyle; engage in regular exercise
- Avoid obesity; maintain a healthy weight at all times
- For a hormone replacement therapy (HRT), discuss your concern with the doctor, combined estrogen and progesterone replacement may be better than estrogen alone
- Use of birth control pills is beneficial
- Progestin secreting intra-uterine contraceptive devices (IUD) are also beneficial
- Green leafy vegetables and fruits are helpful
- Where appropriate and advised by the doctor, removal of the womb will put a permanent stop to the fear of womb cancer

### 68. Does cancer of the womb run in families?
Yes. It is possible to establish positive family history of cancer of the womb in some cases. The risk of cancer of the womb is higher when close family

members or first degree relatives had cancer of the womb. Your first degree relatives are people like your mother and sisters because these people share some genetic characteristics with you.

### 69. What is the most common complaint by women with cancer of the womb?

The most common complaint is that of sudden occurrence of irregular vaginal bleeding, long after a woman has attained menopause. Some women may perceive this bleeding as a re-appearance of their menstruation and this may be a source of confusion. There may also be copious, blood stained, offensive vaginal discharge. Pain may occur in some cases, especially if there is associated infection of the womb.

### 70. What is the treatment for cancer of the womb?

The treatment is to remove the womb through surgical operation. This is called hysterectomy in medical palance. It is usual practice for doctors to also remove the ovaries, tubes and other implicated adjoining tissues at the time of surgery. Radiotherapy and/ or chemotherapy may be added depending on the doctor's findings at surgery.

## DEAR DOCTOR:

### 71. If I am confused as to my choice of treatment, what should I do?

At all times, you must ensure that you understand what the doctor's intentions for your treatment options are. Ask questions if you do not understand or you are confused. Ask for alternatives to the particular option chosen for you. Ask about the benefits and disadvantages. Above all, seek a second opinion from other equally well informed experts. There are centers all around in most countries where you can get information, second opinions and support during and after your treatment.

### 72. Please give me more information about surgery. What are its advantages and disadvantages? The main advantages of surgery are that:

- The mass or tumor is removed and this brings some immediate relief, reassurance, and satisfaction
- Your ovaries can be left behind or preserved. This is important if you are still menstruating or still want children.
- Sexual problems are less
- The disadvantages include:

- Injury may occur to other organs during operation, e.g. urinary bladder, ureters, abnormal leakage, or urine, etc.
- Risk of anesthesia (when the doctor is putting you to sleep)
- Cancer cells can be put into other places unintentionally by the surgeon.

## 73. What about radiotherapy?

It is not an operation, if you are scared of surgery. This is friendlier or acceptable. There is no issue of scar formation that could cause more severe sexual problems including disfigured vagina and pain during sexual intercourse.

## 74. Can I lead a normal life after my womb has been removed?

Yes. The main function of the womb is to carry the baby during pregnancy. Outside pregnancy, it is used for menstruation. So, the main effects are that when your womb is removed, you will not be able to get pregnant or menstruate again. However, you can lead her normal life.

## 75. Can I enjoy sexual intercourse without a womb?

Yes, of course. When the womb is removed, the vagina is normally preserved. The vagina is the most important part of the reproductive tract with respect to sexual intercourse in women. Also, removal of the womb does not affect biological functions, sexual feelings, and enjoyment.

# CHAPTER 17

# Breast and Breast Cancer

*"I think the quality of sexiness comes from within. It is something that is in you or it isn't and it really doesn't have much to do with breasts, or thigh or the pout of your lips"*
– SOPHIA LOREN

**1.   How do women know that their breasts are healthy?**

There are some features that may suggest whether or not your breasts are healthy. These are the skin, nipple, size, and the feel of the breasts.

- The skin of the mature breast is thin, smooth and firm. The area surrounding the nipple is usually slightly darker and may have some spots that look like small pimples. This area is called the areola. You should be quite familiar with the appearance of the skin of your own breasts. Some breasts have dark or light spots, birth marks, and old scars. Most of these spots are harmless and some are as old as you probably can remember. However, it is important to be familiar with the sizes, shapes, numbers, and locations of the spots on the breasts so that any significant changes or alterations may be noticed as early as possible. Remember that during your menstrual cycles, the breast may become fuller and more robust due to congestion. These may also happen if you become pregnant. During pregnancy, breasts become bigger as they begin to secrete breast milk. Existing spots or patches of coloration may become darker or lighter. All these are normal and should not cause any worries, since they are due to changes in hormonal levels and the occurrences of new hormones in pregnancy

- The nipple is normally situated at the center or summit of the breast. It is that elevated, nodule like structure on the breast and is usually darker than the surrounding areas. Most healthy nipples are everted or pointed. Some inverted nipples are normal. However, inverted nipples may pose problems with breastfeeding in the future. When a previously everted nipple gradually becomes inverted or drawn in, it may be necessary to report this to the doctor. The nipple may become inverted or drawn in by masses or diseases, developing in the breast. The most important of such diseases is cancer of the breast, so the doctor's examination and advice are important. As mentioned above, when the nipple discharge appears suddenly thick, yellowish and copious or blood stained, the doctor should be consulted. When the discharge is purulent, it may be difficult to differentiate it from the normal thick yellowish discharge. Pus may suggest an infection or abscess which is usually associated with fever, pain and swelling of the affected breast. If infection or abscess is suspected, the doctor must also be notified without delay.

## 2. How does the normal breast feel?

The breast is chiefly made of fatty tissue, fibrous tissue, and glands. The relative proportions of these components depend on your age and conditions such as menstruation, pregnancy and diseases. Because of its constituents, the breast feels soft in some places and a little harder in other part. Therefore, lumpiness is a relative term. The breast feels naturally lumpy around the time of menstruation, pregnancy, and breastfeeding. Some women may experience increased lumpiness with the use of certain drugs such as family planning pills.

## 3. What self-help activities or tips may help to detect breast problems early?

There are many breast problems which can occur at different times. The key to their early detection is to have a good and detailed knowledge of the shape, size, nipples, skin and textures of both breasts. This is possible through regular observation and inspection of both breasts. Once these are done at regular intervals, changes will be recognized early and reported to your doctor. Observing and feeling the breasts regularly should be part of the lifestyle activities of every female after puberty.

## 4. What is Breast Self-Examination (BSE)?

Breast Self-Examination (BSE) is the practice whereby a woman examines her breasts regularly in a methodical manner, in order to detect if there are problems in her breasts. Focusing on:
- The shape
- General appearance of each breast

- The sizes of the breasts
- The skin
- Feeling the breasts for lumps and pain
- Inspecting and squeezing the nipple for abnormal discharge.

## 5. How is BSE done?

BSE is most appropriately done in privacy. This will ensure that the examination is meticulous and properly done. Where available, BSE is done, standing in front of a large mirror on the wall. The steps are:
- Undress the upper body down to the waist and remove the bra
- Take a general look at the breasts, one at a time, noting:
  - Shape
  - Size
  - Skin
  - Any new appearance.

Note the shape of the nipple and discharge if any.

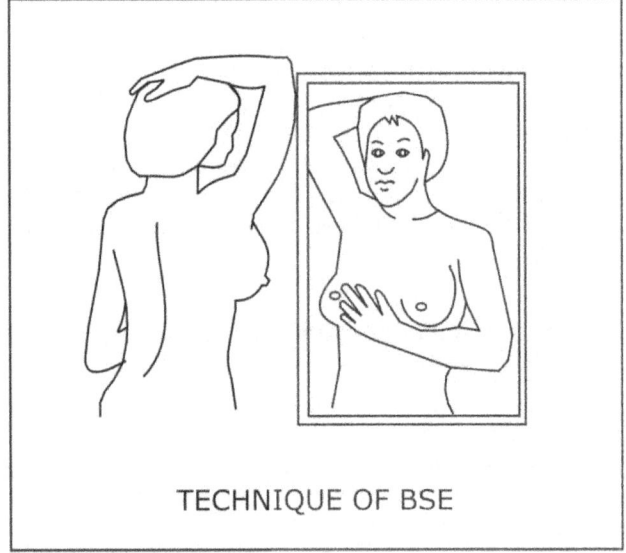

TECHNIQUE OF BSE

- To inspect or feel the right breast, put your right hand at the back of your head. This makes your right breast to hang more freely. In this position, note the appearance of any swelling or bulge
- Chose a point (quadrant) and with the palm feel the texture of the breast in a round-the-clock manner, such that you end at the initial point. Take note of the following:
  - How does the breast generally feel?
    - Normal (no lump or mass)

- Lumpy (many lumps)
- One or two lumps (or mass)
  • If you felt a lump:
    - What is the location?
    - What is the approximate size?
    - Is it hard, soft, or how would you describe it?
    - Is it smooth or regular or not?
    - Is it mobile or not, can you shift it around?
    - Does it disappear sometimes so you have to search for it?
    - Is it painful – how severe?
- Next is to examine the nipple:
  • Note the shape, is it pointed or not?
  • Is there any ulcer or cracking?
  • Gently squeeze it. If the discharge is clear or colored;
    - What is the color?
    - What is the quantity?
- Next lift up the breast and inspect the underneath for any lesion, e.g. rash.
- Finally, inspect and feel the extension of the breast towards the armpit for any mass or lump.
- Record your findings carefully before you forget the details.

Repeat the steps above for the LEFT breast and record your findings. Your findings constitute an important document. You should keep it for future comparison or until your next appointment with your doctor.

## 6. How should women describe the location of a lump or lesion of the breast?

For the purpose of describing problems of the breast during breast examination, the breast is divided into 4 segments called quadrants. These quadrants are obtained by drawing a vertical and a horizontal line across each breast, so that each line passes through the nipple as shown in the diagram below.

The horizontal line divides the breast into upper and lower regions, while the vertical line divides the breast into inner and outer regions. Finally, these divisions result in 4 quadrants which are called:

- Upper Inner quadrant
- Lower Inner quadrant
- Upper Outer quadrant
- Lower Outer quadrant

This division makes it easier to describe the location or site of breast problems. For example, a breast lump which is in the upper part of the breast and close to the midline is correctly described as being located in the upper inner quadrant. If it is at the upper part of the breast and nearer the outside of the chest wall, it is said to be at the upper outer quadrant. Using this method, the location of a lesion or breast mass can be described and understood easily. Take a look at the examples shown in the diagram.

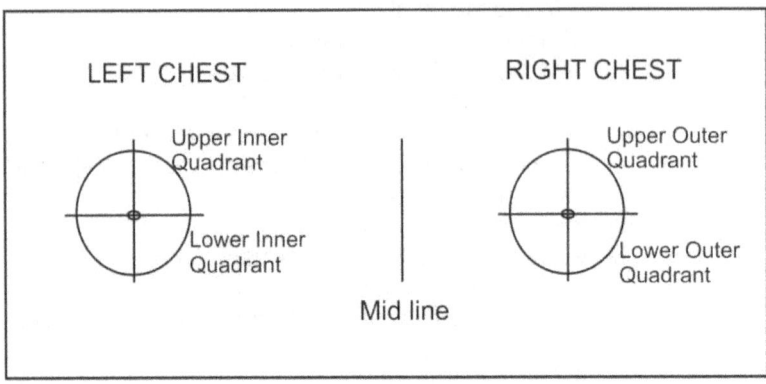

### 7. What is the best way to record my findings?

Findings from BSE are very important and should be documented accurately, in a manner that is simple and easily understood. This documentation can be done through breast mapping. Breast mapping means that you depict your findings during BSE in a pictorial manner on the diagram of each breast, as accurately as possible.

### 8. How is breast mapping done?

Simply put, breast mapping means that you draw your breasts using a free hand, like we do in the biology class. Divide each breast into quadrants and represent your findings in the proper quadrants. The steps are:
- Draw two separate circles about 2 inches in diameter and 1 inch apart. You can make a dot at the center, to represent the nipple area
- Label them as Right (Rt.) and Left (Lt.) breasts

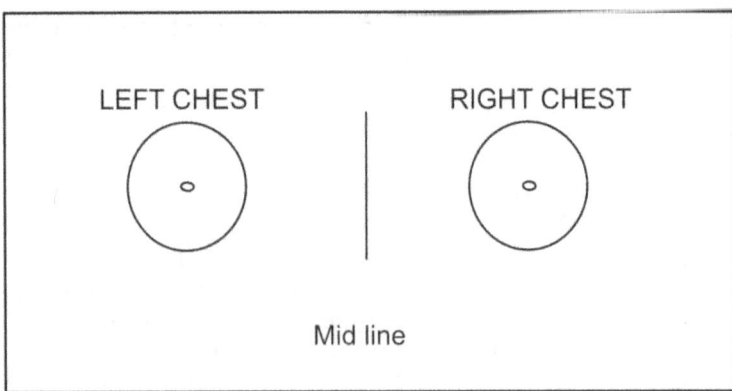

- Divide each circle into 4 quadrants or quarters, by drawing a horizontal line passing through the center and then a vertical line, also passing through the center. The center of the circle where the lines meet represents the nipple

- After examining each breast, draw your findings in the appropriate quadrant of the Rt. or Lt. breast. Your drawings must be free-hand, no shading. For each finding, it is important for you to note the following:
  - Write down the date of the examination. This will enable you to compare changes in the lesion or lump within a time frame
  - In your own words, describe the swelling, lump, lesion on the skin, etc. The important things to note include:
    - Location - which quadrant? Draw the mass or lesion. Draw an arrow to point to the mass. Can you point to it easily?
    - Shape and regularity - what is the shape? Round, spherical, regular wall?
    - Size and texture - a rough estimate or description that will enable you to notice if there is increase or decrease in size in future
    - The feel or how it feels to touch. For example, is it hard, soft, smooth, or coarse when you touch it?
    - Mobility - can your finger move the mass around? Does it disappear at will? Do you have to search for it? Is it fixed?
    - Pain - Do you feel pain with or without touching the mass, lump or lesion? Is this particular place painful?
    - Others - you may add any special thing that you have noticed. This will enable you to give more detailed information to your doctor.

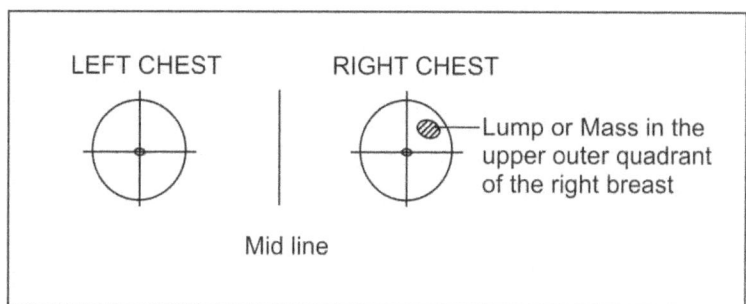

## 9. How often should women examine their breasts?

It is a rewarding habit to take note of any outward change in your breasts as often as you can. Every time you undress to have a shower in a private place, offers excellent opportunities to view and feel your breasts. There is no count that is too frequent. However, it is better to do such self-examinations at regular intervals. This may be once every week or two weeks. Most doctors will advise that you examine your breasts at least once in a month, preferably one week after your menses. Your findings should be carefully noted or recorded in a note book or denoted in your breast map.

## 10. What steps should women take if they have concerns about their breasts?

The first step is to tell the doctor about their concerns. There are 3 main steps that doctors usually take after listening to complaints and asking questions. These are:

- Physical Breast Examination – The doctor will inspect your breasts, touch and feel them to detect problems
- Breast Ultrasound – This may be ordered by the doctor to detect masses in the breast. A breast ultrasound is good at detecting cystic masses of the breast and may also be useful in detecting a few other masses that are remarkable in size. However, many masses and other problems of the breast may be missed. Therefore, ultrasound examination, is not a standard test for breast problems or masses
- Mammogram – This is the X-ray done specifically on the breast. It is the standard test done to detect breast problems. A mammogram test is superior and has more value than SBE and ultrasound examination. Digital mammography, where available, is better in resolution and superior to breast films taken with analog mammogram machines.

## 11. What is a breast lump?

Broadly speaking, a lump may be a small solid tissue or a cyst, which means that it can be felt with the fingers or touched. Some breast lumps are so tiny and free, such that at one moment they can be touched and at other times it is difficult to feel them. That is, they appear and disappear at will. This type of lump is called a "breast mouse." Most breast lumps are harmless. In a few instances, cancer of the breast may begin as a lump, so it is necessary to see a doctor without delay once a breast lump is detected. The doctor will investigate the lump, say what it is and begin early treatment, if necessary.

## 12. What is the difference between lumpiness and a breast lump?

Lumpiness suggests a general feeling of diffuse soft and firm tissues when the breast is examined. On the other hand, most breast lumps are well defined, can be touched, pointed at or held. Some are mobile while a few are not. Breast lumps can be described as soft, firm or hard to touch and it is also possible to describe the shape and estimate the size in many cases. Lumpiness may be natural and harmless but breast lumps must be examined and investigated by the doctor to determine their nature. It is extremely important to determine that a breast lump is not cancerous.

### 13. Why are mammograms important?
Mammograms are used for two main purposes. These are:
- Screening – Sometimes, problems of the breast may not cause complaints at the initial stage. You may not notice any change or have any complaints. Mammograms are used to screen the breast, in order to detect early changes that may transform to a disease in the future. Therefore, mammograms are used to screen the breast for cancer
- Diagnosis – Mammograms are useful in the diagnosis of many diseases of the breast. The common diseases include
  - Breast masses such as:
  - breast lumps
  - cysts of the breast
  - fibro-adenoma
  - Cancer – Breast cancer is the most important reason why doctors order a mammogram test

### 14. Why is it important to do a screening mammogram?
When there is pain or discomfort in your breast, the doctor will most probably ask you to do a mammogram test. However, the most important reason for a mammogram test is to detect cancer of the breast as early as possible. Some breast cancers can grow silently without causing complaints for a longtime. Since you do not feel any pain, the cancer may not be detected on time. So, a regular mammogram examination is useful in spotting such cancers as early as possible. The chances of curing cancer are higher with early detection and treatment.

### 15. How often should I do screening mammograms?
The first thing women should do is to consult a doctor anytime they have concerns or suspect a problem in the breast. The doctor will advise whether or not a mammogram test is needed. However, The American cancer society (ACS) guideline for screening should be followed. The guideline is:
- Women ages 40-44: You have a choice of annual screening mammograms. So you may discuss your choice with your doctor
- Women ages 45 - 54: Do screening mammograms annually. It should be noted that mammograms can be advised by the doctor, if there is need to do so at any time
- Women 55 and older: Do screening mammograms every 2 years or continue annual screening

The ACS has advised that screening should continue so long as you are in good health, and you are expected to live for 10 more years or longer. Some women with high risk of breast cancer (e.g. genetic tendency) should be screened with combined mammogram and MRI. Your doctor should decide this. The benefit of doing screening mammogram before 40 should be discussed with a doctor.

### 16. How painful is it to do a mammogram?

During a mammography examination, the X-ray technician or radiographer needs to compress the breast to make it flatter, before taking the X-ray pictures. This process may cause a little discomfort to some women. However, the advantages of mammogram outweigh the discomfort. Pain should never discourage you.

### 17. What is the most reliable method for detecting breast cancer?

Even though it is good practice to do self-examination of your breasts regularly, it is not usually possible to detect cancers and other breast problems all the time. The best method to detect breast cancer is through a mammogram test, even though in a few instances, mammograms may fail to detect breast cancer. Also, doctors may fail to interpret the X-ray film correctly and the diagnosis of breast cancer may be missed. Currently, digital mammography is becoming more available. Digital mammography is better and may enhance detection of breast cancers.

### 18. What are the draw backs of mammograms?

Mammograms are the best tests to detect breast cancer. Although there are few draw backs, these should not discourage you from having your tests done. These draw backs include:

- Pain – You may feel some pain or discomfort when the X-ray technicians compress your breast to make it flat. Compression is necessary in order to get a good image of the breast
- Little radiation – Radiation from the X-ray during a mammogram test is mild and should not cause any harm. Repeated mammograms at short intervals may be harmful and should be avoided. It is not wise to take a mammogram test without the recommendation of your doctor. If you are concerned about the frequency of taking mammogram tests, you should consult another doctor for a second opinion. In many countries, there are designated societies and institutes that provide help and support for women with breast problems. One of such resource centers is the National Cancer Institute in the USA
- False Interpretation – Sometimes, it is difficult for doctors to interpret mammogram films or pictures and make a correct diagnosis on the basis of the mammogram. It is good practice for radiologists to seek the opinions of other colleagues in such a situation, in order to arrive at the correct diagnosis. This may cause some delay in releasing the

report of your X-ray. It is better for your mammogram result to be delayed than to miss a diagnosis of cancer.

### 19. What are the changes in a mammogram film that may suggest cancer?

The X-ray film may suggest masses. There are two types of masses, benign and cancerous. Benign or non-cancerous masses are likely to be smooth and enclosed with a regular wall. Cancerous masses appear irregular on the mammogram and are sometimes difficult to interpret by specialist doctors. Sometimes, more than one radiologist may need to see the mammogram films and exchange information, before a correct diagnosis is made. The most significant change that may indicate cancer is the appearance of shiny or whitish little specks or spots, called micro-calcifications. These type of spots on your X-ray should not make you panic. There may also be larger shiny areas in the X-ray film. These are called macro-calcifications and are mostly harmless. Only a radiologist should interpret a mammogram.

### 20. If my mammogram shows there is a mass, what should I do?

Benign masses are harmless and should not cause you undue worry, even though they may be associated with breast pain or discomfort. When a mass is suspicious of being cancerous, further tests should be done as soon as possible to confirm the exact nature of the mass. One important test is a biopsy. In this procedure, the doctor takes a sample of the mass or lump for analysis of the cells. This will determine whether the mass is cancerous or not. Sometimes, further imaging may be ordered by doctors, to help determine whether a mass is harmless or cancerous. The imaging includes magnetic resonance imaging (MRI). This test uses magnetic waves to make diagnosis. It is far more expensive than mammograms but sometimes necessary. It is possible to do a biopsy at the same time as the MRI. Also, where there are facilities, a biopsy can be done under ultrasound guidance.

### 21. What is the role of a biopsy?

The biopsy procedure enables the doctor to take a sample of the breast mass and then subject the cells to laboratory tests. This test will reveal whether there are cancer cells or not. Many times, it is also possible to remove the whole breast mass or lumps as a form of treatment. This is called an excision biopsy. That is, the mass is excised so biopsy can serve to detect and to treat breast masses in some cases.

### 22. So what happens after the biopsy procedure is done?

The next step depends on what the mass or lump is. If it is a benign mass, your doctor may decide to leave it alone and watch it over a period of time. He may decide to remove the lump if you are worried or begin to feel pain or discomfort. The majority of doctors will remove a benign mass if they are worried that the mass may transform into cancer in the future, or if the mass is causing serious pain or discomfort. Cancerous breast masses need to be removed and treated with drugs and radiotherapy as early as possible, in order to improve the treatment outcome.

### 23. How common is breast cancer in the USA?
Apart from cancer of the skin, breast cancer is the most common cancer in women in the USA. According to information by the American Cancer Society, the number of new cases of breast cancer in 2016 was estimated at 246,660. A woman has a 1 in 8 chance of developing breast cancer in her lifetime. This is pretty high.

### 24. What are the signs of breast cancer that I may feel or see?
You may feel a lump or a small breast mass; there may be swelling, redness or thickening of the skin of the breast over the mass. This change in the skin of the breast looks like an orange peel. It is called peaud'orange in medical parlance. In addition, you may notice a discrete mass or lymph node enlargement in the armpit. If the mass gets bigger with time, or becomes painful, then it becomes more suspicious. However, a lump may not be painful at all and still turns out to be a cancer. So, any time you notice a lump, you need to see a doctor immediately for further examination. It is important to start treatment of cancer as early as possible, in order to stop the cancer from growing or spreading further.

### 25. How does breast cancer spread?
Breast cancer spreads via lymph nodes and lymphatic vessels. The places that are affected early are the nodes around the breast, usually the armpit and then, other nodes in the chest wall. From here it travels to other parts of the body including the breast on the other side.

### 26. To which organs does breast cancer usually spread?
It is possible for breast cancer to spread to any part of the body. However, the parts most commonly affected are:
- Lungs
- Bones
- Liver
- Brain
- Adrenal glands

### 27. What are the key weapons in the fight against breast cancer?
Cancers are generally regarded as incurable. Therefore, it is best avoided through preventive measures. The following suggestions are helpful:

- Be aware of the various risk factors and avoid them as much as possible. This may entail that you modify your life style to reduce the risk of breast cancer
- Indulge in life styles that will improve your general health. You cannot change your genetic makeup, but by a deliberate decision, you can choose a healthier and safer lifestyle
- Ensure early detection through regular self-breast examinations and doctor's examinations. Ultrasound scan of the breasts and mammogram, when ordered by the doctor, may serve to assure you that all is well with your breasts or not
- Stay active through physical exercise
- Stay off vices, limit alcohol use

## 28. What are the factors that increase the risk of having breast cancer in women?

There are some factors that may increase a woman's risk of having breast cancer. The important factors are:

- Age: Breast cancer is less common in adolescents and young women below the age of 25 years. The rate of breast cancer increases from about the age of 30 years, up until menopause. After menopause, the rate of breast cancer seems to be constant
- Hormonal influence: Long term, inappropriate use or exposures to hormones such as estrogen, are known to increase the risks of cancer in women
- Long duration of child bearing or reproductive life: This is a situation where a woman starts bearing children at a young age and continues childbearing for a long time, up until old age
- Barrenness: For reasons that are not totally clear, barrenness may increase the risk of breast cancer in some women
- Late age at first child: women who have their first baby at a relatively old age, are at higher risks of breast cancer
- Early menarche: Menstruation sometimes starts early in some adolescents, compared to their peers in the community. This generally means that such girls menstruate for a longer duration in life than their contemporaries
- Late age at menopause: just like early menarche, late menopause means more years of menstruation. This increases the risk of breast cancer after 55
- Tumors: Some functional tumors of the ovaries which produce estrogen can predispose to breast cancer
- Obesity: Obese women have increased risk of breast cancer especially after menopause
- Exogenous estrogen e.g. prolonged exposure to estrogen drugs including estrogen hormone replacement therapy is associated with increased risk of breast cancer

- Genetic factors: Some women have genetic predisposition to breast cancer. The risk of developing breast cancer increases in those with:
    - Affected closed relatives e.g. mother and female siblings with BRCA-1 or BRCA-2
    - Multiple affected relatives
    - Situations where breast cancer occurs in relatives at young ages
- Geographical location: The risk of developing breast cancer also depends on geographical location. It is known that Western life style tends to increase breast cancer
- Alcohol: Moderate to heavy alcohol consumption increases the risk of breast cancer
- Environment: Environmental factors or pollutants like fumes and pesticides may increase breast cancer.
- Ionizing radiation: Exposure of the breast to inappropriate ionizing radiation to the chest
- Food: Long term consumption of fatty foods and diets may increase the risk of breast cancer
- Personal history with other breast problems such as lumpy or dense breast
- Sedentary life style: Lack of exercise

## 29. At what age is breast cancer mostly discovered in the USA?

The occurrence of breast cancer increases with age. According to the CDC, most cases of breast cancer in women are diagnosed at about the age of 61 in the USA.

## 30. Is the risk of breast cancer declining in the USA?

According to reports from the CDC, in the last decade, the overall risk of breast cancer has remained unchanged. However, the risk of breast cancer has increased in African American, Asian and Pacific Islander women.

## 31. What symptoms am I likely to notice that indicate that I might have cancer?

Breast cancer may occur without any warning sign. Sometimes, it may be discovered during routine examination by the doctor in a routine visit. However, the following complaints may alert you to possibility of cancer developing:
- Breasts getting bigger rapidly
- Swelling of the breasts or change in size and shape
- Thickening and dimpling of the skin of the breasts like an orange peel
- Appearance of a new breast lump or changes in previous lump whether painful or not
- Breast pain especially if unrelenting

- Drawing in of the nipple from its pointed appearance
- Bloody nipple discharge
- Small nodular or swelling in the armpit

In any situation where you are worried about your breast or suspect an abnormality, you should inform your doctor without delay.

### 32. In specific terms, what is the effect of fertility on breast cancer?

With respect to fertility, the following categories of women are at higher risks of breast cancer:
- Women who have not been pregnant before
- Women who had their first child at 30 years and above
- Women who started childbearing before the age of 12 years

### 33. Doctor, what do you mean by close relatives?

Your close relatives include people like your mother, grandmother, and sisters. These people have close genetic relationship with you. If one or more of this category of relatives have breast cancer, you may be at a higher risk of having breast cancer than other women in your community.

### 34. What should I do if my mother or any of my close relatives have been diagnosed with breast cancer?

If any of your close relatives have been diagnosed with breast cancer, the following may be helpful:
- See the doctor immediately for a thorough breast examination. This is important and should be done as early as possible; not at your convenience
- Be breast self-aware by doing breast self-examination at least once every month
- Do your first time X-ray of the breast or baseline mammogram at least 5 years before the age at which your mother or close relative was diagnosed with breast cancer, or when you attain 35 years of age, whichever is earlier
- Be alert, suspect early, and tell your doctor early if you feel something is wrong with your breasts
- Avoid exposure to factors in your environment that may increase your risk of breast cancer
- Know your BRCA status

### 35. What is the relationship between BRCA and breast cancer?

In some families, two or more members or close relatives might have suffered from breast cancer. In such families, some members or relatives may test positive for the BRCA antigen. Presence of the BRCA antigen strongly suggests the possibility of developing cancer of the breast in such a relative in future. In other words, such a woman has a high risk of breast cancer in the future.

**36. So what do I do?**
If one or more of your close relatives have been tested for BRCA-1 antigen, it is important for you to know your BRCA status. If your test result comes out to be negative and you do not have breast complaints, it suggests that you are free of breast cancer as at the time of testing. However, you will need to do regular BSE and screening mammograms as guided by your doctor. If your BRCA test is positive, it means that the possibility of your developing breast cancer in the future is high. In a situation where close relatives have been diagnosed or died of breast cancer and a living member now tests positive for BRCA, some doctors will advise that both breasts be removed, as a preventive measure of breast cancer.

**37. What are the main methods of treatment of cancer of the breast?**
Currently, breast cancer is treated through surgery and anticancer drugs, depending on the nature and extent of the disease. The aim of surgery is to remove the cancerous breast and some of the surrounding tissues as much as possible. The second treatment is chemotherapy (chemo for short). The doses of chemo drugs are usually carefully calculated and administered as injections/drips at intervals by specialist doctors. Chemotherapy is particularly useful where the cancer has spread from the breasts to other parts of the body.

**38. What is the relationship between breast cancer and oral contraceptives?**
Oral contraceptives may increase the risk of breast cancer in women less than 35 years of age, who have used pills for upwards of 10 years. For this reason, it is very important to seek your doctor's advice on the type of family planning that is suitable for you, and for how long it can be used. Never buy or use pills that are not prescribed for you.

**39. Does smoking increase the risk of breast cancer?**
No. Smoking does not increase the risk of breast cancer. However, you should be aware that smoking is not recommended for good health. Surely, for those who are sick, smoking is more likely to reduce recovery or survival from breast cancer.

**40. What is the relationship between alcohol and breast cancer?**
There is sufficient medical evidence that people who are moderate or heavy consumers of alcohol are at higher risk of developing breast cancer.

Furthermore, as a woman, alcohol has many other bad effects on your health. Light or social drinking may be permissible.

## 41. Doctor, what is the relationship between diet and breast cancer?

Diets high in fat are known to increase the risk of breast cancer. Low fat diets, vegetables, and plenty of fruits routinely taken, reduce the risk of breast cancer.

## 42. Does breast cancer affect only women?

No. Men have breasts and can also be afflicted with breast cancer. If it is not detected early and treated, men also suffer the same fate as women. Even though breast cancer is far less common in men, it is important that men should be breast aware and perform self-breast examination routinely. So, tell your partner or husband.

## 43. Is breast cancer contagious or infectious?

No. Breast cancer cannot be contracted through infection. It is also not transmitted through breast milk. As previously said, you should be aware that the risk of breast cancer is higher if your close relatives have been diagnosed with breast cancer. This does not mean that they infected you.

## 44. In this day and age, should breast cancer be so common?

No. This is because the breasts hang out of the body and can be examined easily by every woman. This makes it possible for breast masses to be detected early, so that cancer can be prevented or treated as early as possible. Unfortunately, most women do not examine their breasts regularly, thereby missing the benefits of early detection.

## 45. How can I reduce my risk of breast cancer?

The risk factors of breast cancer are many. Some of these factors are genetic; you may already have inherited them and cannot do much to effect a change. However, there are many things you can still do to reduce your risk. Here are some of them:

- Do regular breast self-examination (BSE). This is cost effective and convenient
- Do regular Exercise and keep fit
- Maintain a healthy weight
- Avoid or limit alcohol intake
- If you intend to commence birth control pills, seek your doctor's advice. Do not take pills and drugs that have not been prescribed for you.

- If you must be on a hormone replacement therapy(HRT), you must be supervised completely by your doctor
- Breast feeding your baby is beneficial
- Get screened for BRCA early, especially if your close relatives have been diagnosed or died of breast cancer in the past

## 46. What about cosmetic surgery to increase the size of the breasts?

Presently, cosmetic surgical operations are being increasingly performed. This procedure to increase breast size, is especially useful for those who have had parts of their breasts removed for medical reasons. Many women with small breasts have also reported a good degree of satisfaction and restoration of confidence, after this procedure. You should discuss your intention with your doctor for appropriate guidance.

## 47. What if I desire to reduce the size of my breasts?

Some ladies are naturally endowed with big breasts. In some women, the sizes of the breasts may be out of proportion to the body, especially those women with small frames or carriage. This appearance may be perceived as ugly and unacceptable. Again, this type of body build usually comes with flat or masculine bums in many women.

For tall women with good carriage, the psychological and cosmetic problems may be tolerable. For some women with small carriage and big breasts, the craving for breast reduction is ever present. There are two ways to look at the possible remedies. These are:

- Lifestyle - The prominence of the breasts can be reduced by wearing loose dresses combined with firm bras. The dress conceals the size of the breasts while the bra packs them closer and makes them look more compact on the chest
- Surgery - Currently, more women are availing themselves of the services of specialist plastic surgeons for cosmetic reasons. Surgery can be performed by skilled doctors to reduce breast sizes. A breast reduction operation is called reduction mammoplasty. This type of operation is readily available in the developed world. So, for those who are dissatisfied about the looks and sizes of their breasts, mammoplasty is an acceptable solution
- Drugs - Use of drugs such as Danazol can result in the reduction of breast size. However, Danazol is used for other medical reasons on doctor's prescription. It is not recommended to be used for breast reduction.

## 48. Some women experience itching under their breasts. Why is this so and what should be done?

Where the breast folds over the chest wall, it forms a fold of skin between the chest wall and the breast. This is common in fat women, women with big breasts and older women. The skin fold area is commonly warm and wet because of accumulated sweat. Bacteria may breakdown the sweat to form crusts. The crust is an irritant to the skin and may result in itching. Such itching may be prolonged or sustained if the woman sweats frequently or puts on her bra most of the time. Tight fitting bras and hot weather may increase itching. Keeping the underneath of the breast clean and dry is one effective way to reduce it. Weight reduction in obese women may alleviate sweating generally; wearing appropriately sized, slightly loose bras and more frequent cleaning of the underneath of the breasts are beneficial. Sometimes, for the same reason of wetness and warmth, other infections, especially those fungal in origin like eczema and tinea, may occur under the breasts too. These call for appropriate treatment. The underneath of the breast is often omitted or not properly cleaned by some women when bathing, because it is hidden. This attitude may promote itching and infection.

### 49. I experience pain in my breasts at the time of my menses, is this normal? Is there any way I can cure this?

At about the time of menses, it is normal in some women to experience pain, tension or breast discomfort, due to congestion by fluid that happens at this time. This is as a result of hormonal changes leading to menstruation. The breasts and pelvis become congested, leading to breast pain or discomfort and menstrual pain. The pain typically subsides after the menses is over. Pain in the breasts and lower abdomen can also occur with other complaints, in a condition called premenstrual syndrome. There is no cure for this type of pain. However, the severity of premenstrual syndrome reduces with age and childbearing. The pain may be troublesome before menses and is relieved once menses begins. There are treatment regimens that may be beneficial. Analgesics such as Aleve, Advil, and Ibuprofen may be useful. Some women have derived some relief with such unconventional treatments, including the use of evening primrose, exercise, etc.

### 50. Does removing both breasts prevent cancer completely?

No. removal of both breasts does not completely prevent the occurrence of breast cancer. It is not possible for doctors to remove all breast tissue at once, or remove all breast tissue when operating, no matter how hard they may try. So, left over breast tissue could develop into breast cancer but the risk is less than when both breasts have not been removed. Those who have had their breasts removed surgically still need to do screening mammogram at intervals, in order to detect cancer as early as possible.

### 51. If I chose not to do surgery and chemo, what about herbal medicine?

There are various claims and options on the use of herbal care and other nature methods, in the treatment of diseases including cancer. The drugs used include anti-oxidants which come in various forms; green tea, essential oils, combination of various natural herbal preparation, etc. Some testimonies abound on the efficacy of such methods, but they are largely unproven and perhaps it is too early to make a factual statement on their usefulness. However, this remains an alternative if you wish to try them out.

### 52. What is the relationship between the rate of growth of a cancer mass and metastasis?

Most malignant tumors that grow aggressively or are large in sizes are more likely to have metastasized or disseminated. When a tumor has metastasized, hope and the possibility of cure are greatly reduced.

### 53. At what stage do most cancer patients go to doctors for treatment?

Generally, about 30% of patients with cancers present to hospital when the cancers have already metastasized. This is quite unfortunate. This is an indication for public awareness on the need for early diagnosis.

### 54. What part of the breast does cancer mostly start from?

Cancer of the breast can be detected at any part of the breast, but the majority usually arises from the upper outer quadrant. This is the reason why the lymph nodes in the armpit are usually more commonly involved or swollen, in women with breast cancer.

### 55. What is the role of inheritance in cancer?

About 5-10% of all breast cancers are familial or inherited, and about 80% of these familial breast cancers are due to BRCA-1 and BRCA-2 gene mutations. Take a look at the table below:

| BRCA | TYPE OF CANCER |
|---|---|
| BRCA-1 and BRCA-2 | At high risk breast cancer |
| BRCA-1 ONLY | At high risk of ovarian and colonic cancer |
| BRCA-2 ONLY | At high risk of ovary, larynx, and pancreatic cancers |

### 56. What about environmental factors and lifestyles?

The environment plays a big part in the causation of cancers. Many cancers have been traced to environmental exposures to carcinogens and adverse consequences of some lifestyles. The table below gives an insight into the various factors and associated cancers.

| Carcinogens | Source | Cancers |
| --- | --- | --- |
| Carcinogens polycyclic hydrocarbons | Smoke Cigarette / tobacco animal fat – smoked meat, smoked fish | Lung cancer Bladder cancer Sink cancer |
| Aromatic Amines / Azodyes: Some are used to color food | Butter Cherries | Liver Bladder |
| Alfatoxin B1 | Properly stored grains, peanuts groundnuts | Liver |
| Hepatitis B virus Nitrate preservatives (Nitrosamines) | Preserved food | Liver Stomach |
| Asbestors | | Bronchus, GIT cancers and Mesotheliomas |
| Vinyl chloride (Rubber) chromium, nickel (inhaled in industries) | | Lung Skin |
| Insecticides, | | Various cancers |
| Radiation: Sunlight (UV rays) Ionizing and Particulate radiation | | Skin cancer |
| Viruses: HPV Ebstein-Barr virus | Types 16, 18, 31,33, 35, 51 | Found 85% of Cervical Cancer, Burkitt lymphoma B-Cell Lymphoma |

## 57. What is grading?

This is the clinical assessment of a cancer mass that denotes the characteristics of the tumor cells and relates them with the aggressiveness. Cancers are usually graded from I to IV with four being the worst grade.

## 58. What about staging?

This is done using the size of the primary cancer or tumor, the extent of spread to regional lymph nodes and whether metastasis through blood, has occurred or not. Therefore, staging conveys more clinical information than grading and is used by doctors to judge or plan the best form of treatment. It is more important than grading and reported as stage I to IV.

## 59. What are tumor markers?

They are biochemical substances in the blood or body, which when present in abnormal quantities, may suggest the presence or high possibility of a tumor or cancer. Examples are:
- CA-125: which is a tumor marker for ovarian cancer
- CA-19-9: which is a tumor marker for colon and pancreatic cancers
- CA-15-3: which is a tumor marker for breast cancer

## 60. What is the burden of breast cancer in the USA?

Aside from skin cancer, breast cancer is the most common cancer in women in the USA. Breast cancer is more common in Caucasian women that other racial groups. The center for disease control and prevention (CDC) estimates that about 237,000 new cases of breast cancer occur in women every year.

## 61. How many women die of breast cancer in the USA?

The burden of death due to breast cancer in the USA is remarkable. Every year, the CDC estimates that about 41,000 women die of this cancer. Grossly speaking, more Caucasian women suffer from breast cancer. However, African American women are more likely to die of the disease than Caucasians.

## 62. Where can I have my mammogram done?

Mammogram services are available in most clinics, hospitals, and diagnostic centers across the USA. Your doctor should be able to assist you to find one near your location.

## 63. How can I cover the cost of treatment?

In most cases, your insurance policy may take care of the cost from the age of 40 years, depending on the content of your policy. For women with financial issues, who are eligible, the Center for Disease Control and Prevention (CDC) has a program that offers mammograms free or at a much reduced cost. You may tap into this type of program. There are other issues that may bother you about cancer generally or breast cancer in particular. Many organizations,

both government established and NGOs are available to support you in various ways. Some of these are:
- The National Program of Cancer Registries (NPCR)
- Behavioral Risk Factor Surveillance System (BRFSS )
- National Health Interview Survey(NHIS)

# DEAR DOCTOR:

**64. My breasts used to be firm and soft. I am 47 years old and not married yet. I can now feel some little masses when I touch my breasts. Please, help me.**

It is normal for the breasts to feel bumpy or coarse to touch due to changes in the ratio of the fatty and glandular tissues, as a woman gets older. This usually happens at about the age of 45-50 years. The bumps you feel are due to the fat and increased fibrous tissue components of the breast. This change is harmless and natural in women about your age. However, if you are worried or confused, it is advisable to see your doctor for examination. It is a good idea to be sure that what you feel as bumps are not breast lumps or other dangerous breast masses. Most importantly, a cancerous mass or lump must be detected early and removed.

**65. How can I catch a lump early?**

The cheapest and effective way to detect lumps early is to do a self-breast examination at least once a month. Once you feel a lump, however small, you should see the doctor for appropriate investigation and treatment. So, women are encouraged to examine their breasts regularly because it is important to detect breast lumps as early as possible.

**66. If I have already removed my breasts, do I still need to have a mammogram?**

The intention of doctors during surgery for cancer of the breast is to remove all breast tissues. However, it is difficult. Some tissues still remain and may contain cancer cells. Again, most people who have breast removal operations, do so, not as a preventive measure but because the breast is already cancerous. The doctor may recommend follow up mammograms for you, if he thinks they are necessary. There may be a re-occurrence of the cancer, so it is important for you to be examined at intervals in order to determine whether you are still free from cancer or not.

**67. What if I have breast implants?**

As long as breast tissue still remains, cancer is a possibility. Even with the implants in place, a mammogram can still be done very carefully. However, implants usually make interpretations of mammograms more difficult. A digital mammogram is more appropriate.

**68. Doctor, I noticed a small mass beside my right breast. It has been there since I attained puberty and seems to be growing. I also feel some tension and discomfort in this mass during my menses. Please, what could it be?**

Some women have more than one breast on the same side of the chest. Usually, one is fully developed and roughly of the same size as the breast on the other side. The second is usually much smaller and commonly situated beside the one that is well formed, or in front of the armpit of the same side. Less often, it may be located in the right armpit in some women. It is called an accessory breast. This implies that there is a main breast and an accessory breast. One difference is that accessory breasts usually have no nipples. An accessory breast appears like a swelling of fatty tissue. In every other way, accessory breasts have the same texture as normal breasts and undergo the same changes during the menstrual cycle. If an accessory breast is prominent, it may be a source of embarrassment to the woman when she undresses. Otherwise, an accessory breast is harmless. It is advisable to discuss your concerns with your doctor. Some accessory breasts may be removed for purely cosmetic or psychological reasons.

**69. I am 22 years and had my 2nd baby 2 years ago. Now, I notice that my breasts are flat and long like that of a 50- year old woman. Please, is there any drug that can help me to regain the original shape of my breasts?**

I understand your worry. During pregnancy, the breasts enlarge due to hormonal changes in preparation for breast feeding. The skin over the breasts also gets stretched to accommodate the enlargement. The enlargement becomes more pronounced due to breastfeeding, as milk secretion in the breast is established. This means that the principal elements that make up the breast like fatty tissue, breast glands and their secretions increase. As the baby pulls on the breast during sucking, the breasts become elongated. After pregnancy and breast feeding are concluded, the milk gradually dries up and the breast shrinks but it usually does not completely reverse to its original size and firmness before pregnancy. So, losing the lady-like shape and firmness of the breast, the cleavage or groove, are some of the changes that child bearing brings to mothers like you. The breast becomes more elongated and flatter with subsequent pregnancies. The changes may be less dramatic in women who have fewer pregnancies and childbirths. However, even if pregnancy and breastfeeding do not bring flat, elongated breasts, age will

eventually occur and cosmetic damage will follow. The issues that you may need to consider include:
- Right attitude - Shrinking and flattening of the breast is normal. It is physiological. In a positive sense, it is one good price to pay for your baby - "the bundle of joy". Also be aware that change is inevitable after the age of 50. So the best attitude is to see this as natural and do your best to age gracefully. You may also consider bra support for the breasts, to produce an attractive, lady-like appearance
- Surgery - Breast reconstruction and implants may soothe the psychology of some women. The overriding reason is cosmetic. Facilities are becoming more readily available and many doctors will consider performing such surgical reconstructions and implants for cosmetic reasons

## 70. During romance, my husband sucks my breast. I experience lower abdominal discomfort afterwards. What causes this and what can I do?

The act of sucking on the breast or pulling on the nipple causes prolactin hormone to be released from the pituitary gland, in the brain. One of the actions of prolactin hormone is to make breast milk available, when a baby sucks on the breast. However, sucking also causes the release of another hormone called oxytocin. The oxytocin hormone causes the muscles of the womb to contract. It is this contraction that causes pain. So, some women feel pain or discomfort during episodes of romancing the breasts. This type of discomfort also happens when babies suck on their mother's breasts. Although it is perfectly normal, less aggressive romancing with the breasts by your husband, may lessen the amount of oxytocin hormone released and reduce your lower abdominal discomfort. If the pain is significant, use of simple analgesics or pain killers after the act, may be beneficial. I hope this helps and the pain does not discourage you from enjoying romance.

## 71. My right breast is slightly bigger than the left breast, is this normal?

This is a normal finding in most women. Most paired organs or parts of the body like the hands, legs, breasts, etc., are never exactly equal in size. This is natural and should not be a source of worry. However, you may consult your doctor for further assurance, if this is a problem for you.

## 72. If I remove both my breasts, will I still look like a woman?

Most people who have had their breasts removed resort to breast implants in order to look feminine. This type of operation is now widely available. Breast implants maintain the soft texture, shape and contour of the breasts. So, if you are worried about your appearance, a breast implant is a good cosmetic option.

# CHAPTER 18

# Ovary and Ovarian Cancer

*"It will ever be a matter of surprise how so many phenomena of health and symptoms of disease can be determined by two little oval bodies, whose structure does not appear complicated but it is unquestionable that these organs influence the system"*
– EDWARD JOHN TILT

### 1. Where are the ovaries?

The pelvis is the part of the body that extends from the upper part of the thighs and ends at about the waist line. Inside the pelvis are the ovaries, womb, fallopian tubes, vagina, urinary bladder and the lower part of the large intestines.

The ovaries are located deep in the pelvis beside the womb. A woman has one ovary on each side and a normal ovary contains female eggs which are released during ovulation.

### 2. What are the functions of the ovary?

The ovaries are structures that house the female eggs which are necessary for reproduction. Apart from this, the other main function of the ovaries is the production of hormones which are necessary in various situations, e.g.

- Puberty
- Ovulation
- Menstruation
- Growth of the breasts
- Preservation of pregnancy in the first 3 months

3. **What is an ovarian cyst?**

Imagine a balloon that is filled with water. Similarly, a cyst is a collection of fluid which is totally enclosed in a wall. Ovarian cysts are therefore cysts that are located in the ovary.

4. **What is a functional ovarian cyst?**

You may have heard doctors use this term often when they discuss your pelvic ultrasound scan report. Broadly speaking, an ovarian cyst may be benign or cancerous but the majority of cysts are benign. This means that they are not cancers. Many benign cysts are harmless and are caused by the effects of the follicle stimulating hormone. After ovulation, when the egg is released, the shell that is left behind fills with fluid and begins to secret hormones, in preparation for pregnancy. This structure is called corpus luteum in medical parlance. If pregnancy fails to occur, as in many women, the corpus luteum dies off. However, in some cases, instead of dying off, the corpus luteum may grow further to become a corpus luteal cyst. Secondly, at the beginning of each cycle, the ovaries produce 1-2 eggs which are released or made to rupture during ovulation. In some cases, ovulation does not occur and instead of rupturing, the follicles continue to grow to become cysts. They are then called follicular cysts. Corpus luteal cysts and follicular cysts, constitute the majority of benign ovarian cysts in women. They are called functional ovarian cysts. Most functional cysts reduce in size and disappear within 2 to 4 weeks. This is called regression. For this reason, when an ultrasound scan is done and a cyst is discovered, the doctor may tell you to repeat your scan test in about one month, to see if the cyst has regressed or not.

5. **How common are ovarian cysts?**

Ovarian cysts are very common, especially in those women who are still bearing children or ovulating. However, many ovarian cysts do not cause problems or complaints and occur from time to time. More often, cysts grow, regress and then disappear completely. Women may not even notice these occurrences in many cases.

6. **What are the more common types of ovarian cysts?**

There are many types of ovarian cysts. Generally, cysts can be classified into two groups - those that are benign (non-cancerous) and the cancerous cysts. Fortunately, though ovarian cysts are common, the vast majority are harmless. Most times, they are formed from follicles (eggs) after ovulation, during normal menstrual cycles. The two most common benign cysts are corpus luteal and follicular cysts. At the beginning of each menstrual cycle, a woman recruits many follicles from one or both ovaries. Each follicle is a small sac of fluid that contains a female egg called oocyte. The follicles grow gradually and eventually; one becomes the dominant follicle. The dominant follicle then suppresses further growth of the remaining follicles. At about the mid cycle, the dominant follicle ruptures and releases the oocyte. This event is called ovulation. The ruptured follicle grows further to become the corpus luteum as it accumulates fluid. The other follicles gradually shrink in size and disappear, usually before the time of ovulation. It does happen sometimes that the dominant follicle may not rupture. Instead, it accumulates more fluid to form a follicular cyst. Corpus luteal cysts and follicular cysts are the most common functional cysts.

Others less common cysts include:
- Dermoid cyst: They are formed from primitive cells or cells of other parts of the body. It may contain teeth, hair, bone cartilage, glands, etc. It is bilateral in many cases and more common in women
- Endometriomas: These are cysts formed on the ovaries, in women with a condition called endometriosis
- Cystadenomas: These cysts contain clear fluid and may grow so large that the big tummy of the woman may be confused with pregnancy
- The second type of cyst is the cancerous cyst. Fortunately, they are far less common than benign cysts. When a woman attains menopause, the ovaries are less active, since they are no longer engaged in ovulation. Therefore, ovarian cysts are less common in older women and after menopause. When cysts are found in older women, doctors are more worried that the cysts may be cancerous.

### 7. What does the doctor mean by a simple cyst?

Simple ovarian cysts have smooth, regular walls. The walls are not subdivided, so there is only one fluid cavity. The fluid content is most often clear. A good example is a follicular cyst. It is a great relief to both the woman and doctor when a diagnosis of simple cyst is made. This means that the possibility of cancer is remote.

### 8. What about complex cysts?

Complex cysts have thick and irregular walls. The walls are usually subdivided, so that the fluid cavity is partitioned into a number of smaller compartments. The fluids in most complex cysts contain solid tissues debris. Complex cysts may indicate infection or cancer. Sometimes, cysts from infective origins may contain pus or form ovarian abscesses. They may also contain blood if there has been bleeding into the cyst cavity. When complex cysts are seen on ultrasound, doctors may be worried about whether they are cancerous or not.

### 9. What are the common causes of ovarian cysts?

The main causes of ovarian cysts are:

- Hormonal changes: These happen during the menstrual cycles when some follicles do not rupture. Such follicles progress to form follicular cysts. The ruptured dominant or Graaffian follicle, forms corpus luteal cyst. These functional cysts commonly disappear on their own accord without any problems. They may not even be noticed, except through a chance finding during routine ultrasound scan examination
- Infections: Severe infections in the pelvis may occur, for example, during episodes of pelvic inflammatory diseases or sexually transmitted infections. In such conditions, cysts may form in the ovaries. Such cysts are usually painful and may occur on both sides. They may appear as complex cyst on ultrasound scan
- Endometriosis: The cyst that is formed as a result of endometriosis is called an endometrioma. Endometriomas are associated with pelvic pain, especially during menstruation and sexual intercourse.
- Polycystic Ovarian Syndrome (PCOS): This condition is associated with formation of multiple cysts in the ovaries
- Ovarian Stimulation: Currently, ovarian stimulation practice is on the increase. This is a common step in the treatment of infertility, especially now that in vitro fertilization (IVF) is becoming more popular. Stimulation of the ovaries with drugs sometimes leads to multiple cyst formations
- Cancer

## 10. What symptoms are associated with ovarian cysts?

The majority of ovarian cysts are harmless. They do not cause problems and may not be noticed. The cysts just grow up to a size and then regress completely. The few that cause symptoms may do so because of:
- Size
- Site or location
- Twisting
- Rupture
- Bleeding
- Infection of lower abdominal

The main complaints in women with ovarian cysts are:
- Menstrual problems: Most benign ovarian cysts are either follicular cysts or corpus luteum cysts. They are called functional cysts. They secrete hormones according to the nature of their functional cells. Almost all such cysts secrete estrogen hormone. Some secrete progesterone or other hormones. These hormones affect the menstrual period in many women. The menses may become irregular or stop completely. In such situations, the menstrual flow is usually reduced or scanty. When ovarian cysts cause congestion in the pelvis, there may be menstrual discomfort, but this is not common. Endometriomas usually cause painful, irregular and heavy menstrual

bleeding. Under these conditions, it may be difficult for the woman to achieve pregnancy.
- Bloating: As ovarian cysts grow to a large size, the tummy becomes protruded or enlarged. This may cause some discomfort, especially when the urinary bladder is also full of urine or where there are other masses like fibroids
- Pain: Most cysts will not cause pain. However, large cysts may compress on nerves and other organs in the pelvis, causing lower abdominal or back pain. Rarely such pain may be felt down the legs. When pain is severe and of increasing intensity, the doctor should be seen so that the pain can be investigated and treated. Also, with increasing pain, doctors need to ascertain that the cyst is not cancerous. Cysts that form due to infection may also cause severe pain unless the infection is treated on time. Less commonly, ovarian cysts may cause some women to experience discomfort during sexual intercourse
- Pressure and discomfort: Large cysts may cause pressure symptoms and lower abdominal discomfort. Some large cysts may compress or displace abdominal structures like the intestines or the diaphragm. Compression of the intestines may disturb the digestive system and give a sense of bloating. Problems with digestion may also make the woman lose weight. She may appear lean and wasted like somebody suffering from cancer. Doctors call this type of weight loss ovarian cachexia (pronounced ka-ke-xia). Women with ovarian cachexia have a characteristic appearance. The large ovary causes an upward push and displacement of the diaphragm and disturbs its movement during breathing. This leads to breathing difficulty or respiratory embarrassment
- Urinary symptoms: A growing ovarian cyst may incarcerate or compress the urinary bladder. This means that the bladder cannot fill up completely or empty fully in some cases. Such women therefore urinate more frequently. This may be worrisome and distressful.
- Others: Ovarian cysts may have other problems apart from those above. These are however less common and include:
  - Constipation
  - Low back or waist pain
  - Breast tenderness
  - Weight gain
  - Weight loss may be a feature if the cyst is cancerous

## 11. What complications are associated with ovarian cysts?

Complications from benign ovarian cysts are not many. However, most complications will result in severe pain. The common complications include:
- Rupture: Ovarian cysts may break open or rupture suddenly. Ovarian cysts may rupture due to physical injuries such as fall on the tummy. Ruptured ovarian cysts result in sudden, severe sharp abdominal

pain in the lower tummy and waist area. There is a high possibility of internal bleeding during such episodes. When bleeding occurs, the woman progressively feels dizzy and may slump, if medical help does not come quickly. The content of the cyst that is poured into the abdominal and pelvic cavities may cause severe irritation and pain
- Torsion: It is possible for an ovarian cyst to have a stalk or what doctors call a pedicle. This type of cyst is mobile and able to turn and twist on itself. When a cyst is twisted, its blood supply is arrested through the pedicle, causing intense pain on the side where the cyst is located. This is a surgical emergency that needs immediate attention
- Bleeding: In some instances, there may be bleeding or hemorrhage into an ovarian cyst. This usually causes pain on the side where the cyst is located. If the bleeding is heavy, the woman may feel weak and dizzy

All these complications require the urgent attention of the doctor for prompt diagnosis and treatment. Women who have been diagnosed with ovarian cyst and those who have these complaints should see their doctors as soon as they begin to experience worsening symptoms.

## 12. How do doctors diagnose ovarian cysts?

Doctors go through a process in order to arrive at a diagnosis. These include:
- History taking: You will tell the doctor what your complaints are. The doctor will also ask you some questions that may indicate whether you have an ovarian cyst
- Physical examination: This is the next step. The doctor will perform a general examination on you. He will examine your lower abdomen. Sometimes, it may be necessary to examine the pelvis through the vagina in order to see if there is a mass or swelling
- Ultrasound scan: The doctor will most probably order an ultrasound scan examination of the pelvis. This is currently the most popular investigation done to diagnose ovarian cysts. Ultrasound scan is not painful and has no side effects. So, it is acceptable to most women. Ultrasound examination reports are sufficient to make diagnoses of ovarian cysts, in most cases. However, in some cases, the reports may not be sufficient for the doctor to make a reliable diagnosis or decide on the type of treatment. In such situations, other tests such as magnetic resonance imaging (MRI) may be ordered. MRI is expensive and not widely available in many developing countries. Also, blood works such as hormonal estimations, are commonly done before planning a treatment for the ovarian cyst.

### 13. So, what are the types of treatment available?

Most ovarian cysts are harmless. They occur and gradually regress on their own accord, so they don't need to be treated. The doctor may however monitor the size of the cyst for further growth or regression, by asking you to do ultrasound scan at intervals. If treatment is necessary, there are several options:

- Medical/Drug Treatment: Functional cysts may sometimes cause pain and lower abdominal discomfort. The doctor may prescribe pain killers to reduce pain and antibiotics if the cyst was formed due to an infection. Functional cysts occur because the woman ovulates, therefore if a woman does not intend to become pregnant soon, the doctor may decide to suppress ovulation with the use of family planning pills
- Surgery: In cases where medical or interventional treatments are not appropriate, surgical removals of ovarian cysts are done. Samples are taken from the tissue of the cyst for analyses, to find out the type and determine whether it is cancerous or not. However, functional cysts may reoccur after surgery and this is a big drawback
- Intervention: There is a growing practice now, whereby simple functional cysts are drained under direct view using ultrasound scan. This is done through the vagina with an appropriate needle. This may be desirous in women who do not want to undergo surgery and where the cysts are simple and moderate in size. The main advantage of ultrasound cyst drainage is that the procedure does not involve cutting the abdomen and the woman can leave for home after a short rest. Furthermore, with this method, repeated surgeries are avoided when and if ovarian cysts recur

### 14. How can women prevent ovarian cysts?

Most cysts occur because women are still ovulating. Many of these are functional cysts and they form the greatest percentage of benign ovarian cysts. One way for women to prevent such cysts is to prevent ovulation until they wish to become pregnant. Doctors can stop ovulation by prescribing birth control pills, which suppress or prevent ovulation from occurring. This ultimately prevents cyst formation.

### 15. Is it true that some benign cysts can become cancerous?

Yes. Some cysts that have been previously assessed to be benign may transform to cancer at a later time. The reasons for these transformations are not clear. However, when ovarian cysts develop in a woman who had previously attained menopause, there is a high probability that the cyst may be cancerous. This is usually worrisome to doctors.

### 16. When is a surgical operation necessary in the treatment of ovarian cysts?

Your doctor may advise you to have an operation if:
- You have attained menopause when a troublesome cyst is discovered
- The cyst is growing rapidly and causing severe pain or discomfort
- The doctor is worried about it being cancerous
- The cyst is persistent or recurrent (such cysts may also be drained under ultrasound guidance)

### 17. So, are surgical operations needed to remove functional cysts?

When it is certain that an ovarian cyst is simple or functional and not causing unbearable pain, most doctors will do nothing other than ask for a repeat ultrasound scan in about 2-4 weeks. By this time, most functional cysts would have partially regressed or disappeared completely. Sometimes, regression may be slow and the cyst may need more time before it disappears completely. In this case, patience is required for repeat scans to monitor the size of the cyst. If there are complaints like pain and discomfort, or menstruation stops as a result of the cyst, the doctor may decide to remove the cyst through surgical operation.

### 18. Are there no alternatives to surgery?

Nowadays, where ultrasound scan is available, many simple ovarian cysts can be drained, in the hope that the contents will not fill back. The common trend with functional ovarian cysts is re-occurrence after operation or drainage. This may be frustrating for both patients and doctors.

### 19. What is ovarian cancer?

Ovarian cancers are those that originate from the tissues of the ovary. The ovaries are glandular structures on each side of the waist, beside the womb. They contain the female eggs which are released during ovulation. They also produce hormones.

### 20. How common are ovarian tumors?

Tumors of the ovary are common. Fortunately, about 80% are benign, while 20% are cancerous. Generally speaking, cancer of the ovary is far less common in children and young girls. They are more common in older girls and women especially in the age bracket of 40 – 65 years.

### 21. How common is ovarian cancer?

Cancer of the ovary is responsible for 6% of all cancers in women worldwide. In the United States of America, cancer of the ovary ranks as the 5th most common cancer in women. According to the National Cancer Institute, USA, cancer of the ovary accounts for about 3% of all cancers in women. About 20,000 women are diagnosed with the disease every year in the USA.

## 22. What is the death burden of ovarian cancer in the USA?

Of all cancers of the reproductive tracts in women, ovarian cancer is the leading cause of death in the USA. According to the CDC, about 21,000 women die of this disease every year in America. Ovarian cancer ranks as the $5^{th}$ leading cause of death in the USA.

## 23. What age group is most likely to have ovarian cancer?

All women are at risk of ovarian cancer. However, about 90% of ovarian cancer cases occur in women between 45 – 65 years of age. In the USA, statistics from the CDC shows that the highest number of cases of ovarian cancer occurs in women who are 61 or older. The disease is much less common in women below 40. Ovarian cancer is more common in Caucasian women than in Black women.

## 24. What is the most common type of ovarian cancer?

The ovary can be divided into three parts. These are the wall, germ cells, and the inner tissue or stroma. The cells of the wall of the ovary are called epithelial cells. The vast majority of ovarian cancers arise from the cells of the wall. Therefore, they are called epithelial cell cancers. The second type of ovarian cancers which are less common, are formed from the stroma of the ovary and are called non-epithelial cancers. When ovarian cancers are detected in women who are younger than 35 years, they are more likely to be non-epithelial ovarian cancers.

## 25. In terms of treatment outcome, what is the difference between epithelial and non-epithelial ovarian cancers?

Non-epithelial ovarian cancers which occur in younger women, are much easier to treat. The cure rate is also higher, with modern methods of treatment than all epithelial cancers.

## 26. What are the causes of ovarian cancer?

Much like other cancers, doctors do not know the exact cause of ovarian cancer. However, there are some suggestions as to what may be responsible. These suggestions include:

- Chronic or long standing ovulation: There is suspicion that ovarian cancer may occur in women who ovulate for many years. These include women who started menstruation and ovulation very early in life and those who do not stop menstruation until old age

- Induction of ovulation: Doctors may deliberately prescribe drugs to stimulate the ovaries during treatment of infertility. It has been suggested that the use of such ovulation stimulating drugs for several months, may result in ovarian cancer
- Genetic Factors: Cancers of the ovary have been noted to be more common in some families, than the general population. This suggests that genetic factors may play a role in the formation of cancer of the ovary. Women with relatives who have had ovarian cancers are at higher risk of developing the disease. Thus, close relatives of women who have had ovarian cancer should be on the lookout for features of the disease. This may enable the disease to be detected early so that treatment is also started promptly

## 27. Doctor, what genes are you talking about?

The suspected genes that have been linked with ovarian cancer have also been linked with cancers of the breasts and colon. The genes are of two types, namely BRCA 1 and BRCA 2. Both of these normally suppress the development or growth of tumors. In 81% of families where cancers of the breast, colon or ovaries are common, BRCA 1 is found to be defective and unable to suppress tumor growth or cancer. BRCA 2 is defective in 14% of such families.

## 28. So, should I do screening test for BRCA 1 gene?

It is not advisable to do so. Testing for BRCA is available in many places but it is of much less value in screening for ovarian cancer. There is also great difficulty in interpreting the result by doctors. Even when your test is negative, it does not mean that you cannot have ovarian cancer. So, it is difficult for doctors and geneticists to give appropriate advice with confidence, based on BRCA screening test results.

## 29. What about the breast?

BRCA has a stronger association with breast cancer than cancer of the ovary. Despite this strong association, it is difficult to use a BRCA test to foretell women who may or may not have breast cancer. So, BRCA screening test is not universally recommended.

## 30. What are the factors that increase the risk of ovarian cancer?

There are several factors including:
- Age: 90% of cases of ovarian cancer occur in women older than 40.
- Risk is higher if one or more of your close relatives have been diagnosed or died of ovarian cancer
- Risk is higher in women with breast cancer, womb and colorectal cancers

- Women with endometriosis have higher risk of ovarian cancer
- Risk is higher in women with Jewish background

Other risk factors include:
- Early onset of menstruation
- Late onset of menopause
- Infertility or barrenness
- Race (generally more common in Caucasians)

## 31. What are the factors that reduce the risk of ovarian cancer?

The risk is reduced by the following:
- Increased number of pregnancies
- Use of oral contraceptive pills
- Prolonged duration of breast feeding

## 73. Can foods help me?

There are claims that fruits and beverages including coffee, lentils, garlic, tomatoes, grapes and leafy greens can generally lower the risk of cancer but these claims are largely unproven. What is certain is that healthy eating is good.

## 74. Can the use of talcum powder cause ovarian cancer?

Yes. There is a possibility of this happening. This sounds funny but may be true. Some chemicals such as talc powder may increase the risk of ovarian cancer. The skin is like a table tennis net. It is not as water tight as it looks. The skin allows many substances to pass through; even those we apply on it for the sake of beauty or as cosmetics. Some women apply talc or mentholated powder on their skin, in order to keep it dry or beautify it. Somehow, the dusting powder may find its way through the skin, and is eventually deposited in the ovaries. It is not unusual for surgeons to find deposits of dusting powder in the ovaries during surgical operations. Apart from the possibility of causing ovarian cancer, powders have the potential of eroding into the tissues of the ovaries and cause destruction.

## 75. Which screening tests are available to detect cancer of the ovary?

Unfortunately, there are no screening tests that reveal this cancer. This means that women must be alert and report changes in their bodies and other unusual feelings to the doctor as early as possible. The following tips may help:
- Get as much information on cancer of the ovary as possible
- If you have close relatives that have been diagnosed with cancer of the ovary, be alert
- Work closely with your doctor
- Do regular pelvic examinations with your doctor

- Report lower abdominal problems early to your doctor
- Ultrasound scans at intervals may be helpful

Your doctor may order for the estimation of blood CA-125 at intervals, but the test is of doubtful value. CA-125 is also increased in other conditions, including fibroid.

## 76. What is the value of an ultrasound scan?

A Color Doppler ultrasound scan may be combined with a CA-125 blood test. The CA-125 may be done yearly or every 6 months in women with high risk of ovarian cancer. However, doctors are not sure if this is a good screening test. This is because it does not effectively predict the occurrence or non-occurrence of ovarian cancer. Even a negative test does not completely rule out the future occurrence of ovarian cancer. Some doctors believe that combining CA-125 estimation with a Doppler ultrasound may have some value in women who have persistently high levels of CA-125.

## 77. So, what is your advice to women who have high risk tendencies of contracting ovarian cancer?

For such women, some doctors advise removal of the ovaries, for:
- Those that have at least two first degree relatives or more that have been diagnosed with ovarian cancer, breast cancer or colorectal. cancers. First degree relatives are your parents and other female siblings.
- Those that tested positive for defective BRAC 1 and BRAC 2 genes, in whom the risk of ovarian cancer is in the region of 40%.

## 78. Can ovarian cancer be prevented?

Cancer of the ovary is one of the cancers that are difficult to detect or treat. Presently, there is no sure way to prevent cancer of the ovary but the risk of cancer may be reduced:
- In women who have given birth.
- In those who have used oral contraceptives for more than 5 years.
- In women who have breastfed for more than 1 year or more.
- In women who have had their fallopian tubes removed.

## 79. What are the indicative problems or complaints?

The most common complaint is abdominal pain. Other complaints are:
- Lower abdominal swelling, bloating or distension.
- Lower abdominal pain or discomfort.
- Back pain.
- Abnormal vaginal bleeding, especially after menopause.
- Poor appetite, indigestion and feeling full too quickly when eating
- (easy satiety).

- Problem with stooling, usually constipation
- Problems with urination:
  - Frequent urination
  - Painful urination
- Increasing weakness
- Progressive weight loss and wasting
- Cachexia (extreme weight loss)
- Ascites: generalized fluid collection in the abdominal cavity
- Enlarged lymph nodes in the pelvis and other parts

## 80. What are the features that may suggest that an ovarian cyst is malignant?

Unfortunately, most malignant cysts are difficult to recognize and many have spread to other parts of the body by the time they are finally diagnosed. However, the following may suggest the possibility of a malignant ovarian tumor:

- Tumor on both sides (bilateral)
- If the tumor is growing rapidly
- If pain is constant and increasing
- If the cysts appear complex on ultrasound with thick, irregular multi-septate walls and solid tissue materials inside the cyst

## 81. How does ovarian cancer spread?

Cancer of the ovary may be very difficult to recognize. In about 50% of cases, the cancer has spread widely by the time diagnosis is arrived at during surgery. It may spread directly to pelvic organs such as the urinary bladder, fallopian tubes, womb, and large intestines. Further spread will involve the diaphragm, liver and the rest of the intestines. Cancer cells may also be carried in the blood flow to distant organs like:

- Liver
- Lungs
- Neck
- Other parts of the body

## 82. Where does ovarian cancer commonly spread to?

Cancer of the ovary has great potential to spread widely. The common sites of metastasis (spread to other organs) are:

- The abdominal cavity
- Liver
- Lungs
- Bowels and stomach

## 83. How is ovarian cancer diagnosed?

Women suffering from ovarian cancer usually present in hospitals with complaints of ill health that have lasted for some months. The complaints include pain or discomfort in the lower abdomen or deep waist pain. The pain is usually located on one side of the waist and may radiate down the leg on the same side or around the waist and back. Typically, following suspicious complaints by the woman, the doctor interviews her and asks relevant questions that may suggest ovarian cancer. Subsequent steps are physical examination and laboratory investigations. The summary of diagnostic steps may run as stated below:

- Interview or history taking:
  - When the complaint was first noticed?
  - For how long?
  - History of such complaints in closed relatives
  - Major complaints
  - Abdominal pain/discomfort
  - Abdominal swelling, distension, mass
  - Indigestion
  - Weight loss
  - Menstrual upset
- Physical examination
  - Evidence of weight loss
  - Lymph node enlargement
  - Pelvic mass and tenderness
  - Abdomen mass and tenderness
  - Fluid collection or Ascitis in the abdominal cavity
- Laboratory investigations include:
- Blood tests
- Ultrasound of the ovaries and abdomen
- Various types of X-ray examinations of the tummy, kidneys, and pelvis
- Sometimes, Doctors may order for more expensive tests such as CT and MRI in order to clarify diagnosis

However, in some cases of ovarian cancer, diagnosis is only made with certainty, during surgical operations or laparoscopy, when samples of the ovarian tissue are also sent for examination.

## 84. What methods are used to treat ovarian cancer?

Treatment methods depend on the type and extent or severity of the cancer. For early cases of cancer that have not spread beyond the ovaries, surgical operations are performed to remove the ovaries. The womb is also removed if the woman has completed her family. Surgical operations are combined with anti-cancer drugs when the cancer has spread to other organs or parts of the body. The use of drugs to treat cancer is called chemotherapy.

## 85. What are the advantages of surgery?

Perhaps the most important quick win to the patient is the disappearance of the big tummy after surgery. The tummy looks flat after surgery and the patient may derive some satisfaction from this. Other advantages include:
- Reduction in vomiting
- Improved appetite because the bowel is no longer obstructed
- Some weight gain
- The surgeon can cut out parts of the ovarian cancer tissue for further tests, to confirm diagnosis of the exact type of ovarian cancer

## 86. What is the cure rate of ovarian cancer?

By "cure rate" doctors mean how many people will still be alive, 5 years after diagnosis and commencement of treatment. Due to the fact that a great number of cases of cancers of the ovary are diagnosed late, the survival rate is generally low when compared to other cancers of the female genital tract. As indicated previously majority of ovarian cancer are epithelial in origin. According to a review by Ricky Chen in 2017, the 5-year survival rates of epithelial ovarian cancer in the USA are indicated below:

|  |  |
| --- | --- |
| Stage 1 | 90% |
| Stage 2 | 70% |
| Stage 3 | 39% |
| Stage 4 | 17% |

Unfortunately, more than 60% of cases are diagnosed at stages 3 and 4 when the women are already going downhill or very sick with the disease.

## 87. Why is ovarian cancer difficult to treat?

Cancer of the ovary is particularly difficult to treat because the ovaries are hidden, deep in the pelvis. In previous decades, when there was no ultrasound or other effective equipment, to make an early diagnosis of diseases of the ovary, doctors relied largely on their skills and suspicion to make diagnosis. This process usually took a long time, such that by the time diagnoses were made, the cancer would have been more advanced. Currently, ultrasound scan, computed tomography (CT), Magnetic resonance imaging (MRI) is available to make quick and reliable diagnoses. The second reason is that some of the complaints, especially pelvic or waist pain or discomfort, which are present in ovarian diseases, are also experienced by many women around the time of menses. This gives room for procrastination and may lead to delay in going to hospital to see a doctor.

**88. What are the causes of death in this cancer?**

The chief causes of death include:
- Severe infection – due to reduced immunity
- Anemia
- Uremia – This means high level of urea in the body due to renal damage
- Obstruction of the bowels by cancer causing:
  - Vomiting
  - Poor appetite
  - Wasting
- Damage to other organs

**89. Is there any new treatment that may help women?**

Yes. As the knowledge about cancer gets better, so also do new treatments become available. One new treatment for ovarian cancer is immune therapy. A few drugs are now available which may help repair damaged genes like the BRAC genes. These new treatment options should be discussed with your doctor.

# DEAR DOCTOR:

**90. How do I know if I have an ovarian cyst?**

When you have complaints such as pain in the lower abdomen, waist or back, lower abdominal bloating, there is a possibility that you may have an ovarian cyst. The easiest way to find out is to do an ultrasound scan of your pelvis. Ultrasound examinations are good at detecting ovarian cysts and may sometimes enable doctors to know whether the cyst is simple or complex. Anytime you chose to do an ultrasound scan on your own, you need to take the result and probably the picture of the cyst to the doctor, for proper assessment.

**91. Doctor, I am 9 weeks pregnant and have lower abdominal pain. I just had an ultrasound scan which confirmed the presence of an ovarian cyst. What type of cyst could this be?**

Many times, ovarian cysts co-exist with pregnancy without causing any problem. Most of such cysts are corpus luteum cysts. The corpus luteum is needed to produce hormones, especially progesterone, which maintains pregnancy for the first 3 months. Sometimes, ovarian cysts, including corpus luteum cysts, may grow big during pregnancy and displace the womb or compress the urinary bladder. When this happens, the bladder is unable to fill up to full capacity before the woman feels the urge to urinate. The womb grows out of the pelvic cavity after 12 – 14 weeks of pregnancy and leaves the urinary bladder behind. From this time on the bladder can fill-up normally, so that the pain and frequent urination stops.

### 92. So what should I do?

In many cases, the cyst will regress and disappear completely but your doctor must keep watch by ordering ultrasound scan examinations at intervals, to assess the size. Some cysts may grow bigger and co-exist throughout pregnancy. So, it is important that you are closely monitored by your doctor. For the pain and discomfort, simple pain killers may be prescribed for you. For frequency of urination, the doctor may tell you that it is a passing period that will be over in a short while. However, it is important to exclude urinary tract infection as the cause of your pain and frequent urination. Where this is the case, it must be adequately treated. Doctors do not generally perform surgical operation to remove ovarian cysts within the first 3-4 months of pregnancy. This is to avoid removing the corpus luteum, which produces the hormones that are essential for the well-being of the baby at this period. At four months, the placenta usually has taken over the production of hormones from the corpus luteum. So, removing a troublesome ovarian cyst after 4 months of pregnancy may be performed without harm. It is common for doctors to watch the pregnancy very carefully and delay surgical operation till the time of delivery. This is more appropriate because some ovarian cysts may make natural delivery of the baby difficult. In such situations, a caesarian operation will be needed to deliver the baby and the cyst is removed at the same time. Cases that need surgical operation are few. Hopefully, you may not need surgery, but it is important for your doctor to monitor your situation closely.

### 93. Doctor, my ovarian cyst is recurrent and I have had two surgeries for this purpose in the past. So, what do I do next?

It is true that ovarian cysts are common in women in the childbearing age group, but most are harmless. If you have had an operation for removal of a cyst in the past, and the cyst re-occurs quickly, your doctor may not be too eager to perform another surgery, especially if the cyst is not causing problems.

Good alternatives are:
- Removal through a pin-hole incision on the tummy using an instrument called a laparoscope. This is less painful and effective if your doctor is familiar with the technique
- Ovarian cyst drainage with the aid of an ultrasound scan. This is also an effective way of treating simple, small to medium sized ovarian cysts. It is more beneficial if the cyst re-occurs at short intervals with

discomfort or pain. In such situations, it is not practicable to perform surgical operations at short intervals, after each recurrence

**94. My sister who is 38 years old has been diagnosed to have a very large ovarian cyst, and she has lost so much weight. Could this be cancer of the ovary?**

Majority of ovarian cysts that have grown very large are usually benign and not cancerous. You are probably more worried because of the associated weight loss, but this is because such large cysts put pressure on the stomach and intestines. The pressure prevents the woman from eating well and also disturbs digestion. This results in weight loss. Hopefully, this is the case with your sister. Once the cyst is removed, your sister will be able to eat well and her weight will be restored.

**95. My wife had an ovarian cyst which was operated upon. Strangely, the cyst was found to contain a human tooth, hair strands and bones. Is this a spiritual attack rather than a medical problem?**

It is not a spiritual attack. This is a type of benign ovarian mass or cyst found in some women. It is called a dermoid cyst. Dermoid cysts are formed from cells that existed very early, when a baby was just being formed in the womb. At this early stage, such cells have the ability to form any of the organs and tissues found in the normal human being. These include the skin, teeth, hairs, bones, etc. This was the case with your wife. Surely, findings like this may appear strange and disturbing, but they are well documented in medicine and are harmless.

**96. Is it true that ovulation enhancing drugs may cause ovarian cancer?**

Yes. Research findings suggest that incessant ovulation may cause ovarian cancer. This means that when women use drugs that stimulate the ovaries, to produce more eggs, they are at increased risk of ovarian cancer. So, do not indulge in the use of such drugs unless your doctor advises you to do so.

**97. If I am a high risk candidate for ovarian cancer, why can't I remove the ovaries?**

For women with high risk of ovarian cancer like you, surgical removal of both ovaries and fallopian tubes may be helpful. Some doctors advocate this preventive measure. However, if you remove your ovaries prematurely, you may not be able to conceive naturally anymore, unless you store your eggs in an IVF clinical facility. Even the removal of your ovaries does not totally remove the occurrence of cancer. This is because there are some primitive germ cells (cells that occur early in life when the baby is still an embryo) that can transform to ovarian cells. If you are high risk – please talk to your doctor early.

### 98. My doctor advised me to do CA-125 every 6 months, is it really beneficial?

CA-125 is a tumor marker in the blood. Tumor markers can be of value in two ways. The finding of a tumor marker may indicate the presence or high possibility of a cancer. This means that the blood test is positive for the marker. In some cases of cancer, the level of the tumor marker is what is important. In other words, high levels of the tumor marker in the blood, may be a strong indication that cancer is present. CA-125 levels rise in the blood in most cases of ovarian cancer. However, as noted above, increase in the level of CA-125 is not totally reliable and cannot be used to confirm the presence of ovarian cancer, although when the rise is persistent or increasing, doctors are more inclined to suspect ovarian cancer. CA-125 is also used to monitor the progress of treatment of ovarian cancer. A remarkable rise or sustained reduction in the levels of CA-125 may indicate failure or success of treatment respectively. A sudden rise in the level of CA-125 after an initially low level or fall, may indicate reoccurrence of the cancer after treatment.

Furthermore, blood values of CA -125 may be increased in some disease conditions including:

- Fibroids
- Endometriosis
- Pelvic infection

So, your doctor may ask for repeat CA-125 level estimations, if your risk is high or monitor your progress, if you are already undergoing treatment for ovarian cancer.

CHAPTER 19

# Weight Problems and Obesity

*"Most people stop eating not when their stomachs are full but when their plates are empty."*
– MOKOKOMA MOKHONOANA

### 1. When is a woman said to be overweight?
In simple terms, a woman is said to be overweight when her weight is more than what is expected or accepted to be the 'norm' in the society for her age. Sometimes, the use of the term overweight may be subjective. Overweight may be used to mean obesity. In order to assess the degree of obesity objectively, the Body Mass Index (BMI) can be calculated.

### 2. What is BMI?
BMI makes use of the weight of the woman as well as her height. You can calculate your own BMI by dividing your weight in kilograms by the square of your height in meters. The formula is:

$$BMI = \frac{W(kg)}{H(m)^2}$$

By calculating the BMI, some form of standardization is introduced into the assessment of obesity. Remember that some women appear 'fat' because they are shorter while the effect of excess weight may be less noticeable in tall women. So, using the weight and height to calculate BMI, makes it possible to judge obesity better.

### 3. How do doctors use BMI?
The acceptable range of normal BMI is 18 – 24.
Women with BMI below 18 are said to be underweight while those above 25 are overweight. Those above 30 are obese. Furthermore, using the BMI as

the yard stick, the World Health Organization (WHO) classified obesity as below:

| GRADE | TERMINOLOGY | BMI |
|---|---|---|
| Grade 1 | Overweight | 25 – 29.9 |
| Grade 2 | Obesity | 30 – 39.9 |
| Grade 3 | Morbid Obesity | > 40 |

### 4. What is the importance of knowing my BMI?

BMI is an objective way of measuring your weight. It allows you to monitor how rapidly you are gaining weight, because BMI can easily be related to overweight and obesity. Knowing your BMI encourages you to do more to remain healthy. If your BMI value puts you at the overweight or obesity range, then you are motivated to take steps to reduce your weight and normalize your BMI.

### 5. What is morbid obesity?

The word morbid connotes an association with disease. So, when a woman's BMI falls in the range of morbid obesity, she is much more at risk of associated diseases and severe complications such as hypertension and heart diseases. Apart from severe and chronic weight issues and restriction or difficulty in movement, morbid obesity is a closely linked risk of sudden and premature death.

### 6. What is the difference between overweight and obesity?

The difference is in the values of BMI. If your BMI is between 25 –29.9, you are said to be overweight. When your BMI is 30 and above you are obese. Medically speaking, obesity is associated with more medical diseases and conditions and therefore more dangerous than just being overweight.

### 7. When does weight gain become an issue?

It is natural for many women to experience weight gain at middle age, between 40 – 60 years. This is because at this time, there is no more growth, physical activities tend to decline, and the body does not need many calories for its daily activities. However, many women still eat as much as before despite being less active, so being overweight and obesity become troublesome at middle age. Doctors tend to advise that at middle age, women should eat less, exercise more, and be more active.

## 8. What challenges do middle aged women face?

At middle-age between 40 – 65 years, many women begin to experience problems associated generally with advancing age. These problems include:
- Reduced activity and sedentary life
- Weight gain
- Poor bowel movements leading to chronic constipation
- Skin wrinkling
- Breaking hair and appearance of grey hair
- Menstrual problems including menopause
- Poorer memory and forgetfulness
- Emerging diseases:
  - Diabetes
  - Hypertension
  - Joint pains and arthritis
  - Cancer
- Changing body shape:
  - Loss of pretty figure
  - Loss of glamour

Whether a woman will be happy or not, to a large extent, depends on how she handles some of the issues above. If not handled correctly in a positive manner, middle age could be very unpleasant to some women. However, it is inevitable, so it is better to make the best of the situation and take care to be fit physically, emotionally, and psychologically. It is also important for women to be financially healthy at this time.

## 9. How many women in the US have weight challenges?

There are more than 60 million women in this category in the USA, with over 18 million being obese. The trend is such that weight challenges will continue to be an issue for women and a big public health issue for a long time.

## 10. How do people become overweight?

Weight gain can occur in three main ways:
- Familial: In some families, there is a general tendency to be overweight. This is more a case of natural endowment rather than overeating or sickness
- Diseases: There are some conditions or diseases that are associated with weight gain. In many cases, once the condition is over or the diseases are treated, the weight may reduce, even though it may not completely revert to its former state
- Over eating: The food we eat is absorbed and turned into energy. We need energy for our body to function properly and to do our daily work. When we eat just what is needed for our daily functions, there are barely any calories left that can be stored in our body cells. When we eat more than we need, the body only uses what it needs, according

to our activities. The excess is stored in our body mostly as fat and carbohydrate. This results in weight gain. When we eat less than what we need for our daily activities, the balance of our need is taken from our body store, therefore we lose weight. The arithmetic of weight gain is as summarized below:

- Eat exactly what your body needs = No weight gain
- Eat less than what your body needs = weight loss
- Eat more than what your body needs = weight gain

### 11. Is overweight related to wealth?

Yes. Individual as well as national affluence and development have a great influence on the number of overweight and obese persons in a community. With affluence, an average person has the capacity to buy more food items and expand their choices. So more food is eaten and excess calories, accumulated. Secondly, affluence leads to reduced physical activities; we drive cars instead of taking a walk, use the elevator instead of climbing the staircase. Also, in the kitchen there are grinders, dish washers, mixers, etc. You do not need to sweat at all, as long as you have the money to buy whatever you want or need. Countries like the USA and many others in Europe have attained food security. In the USA, food is cheap and comes in bigger portions in more attractive packages. Women enjoy bigger portions of almost everything. So, in summary, the factors responsible for weight gain and increasing obesity rates in the USA include:

- Affluence
- Bigger portions and better packaging
- Food Security - Cheap and available all year round
- Variety – If you do not like this, what about that? "No Obesity in Starvation"

### 12. Does being overweight have any benefit?

There is virtually no documented medical benefit of obesity. However, it is known that so many women may fancy being big for cosmetic and personal reasons.

### 13. How can I lose weight?

It is true that a few people in some African communities are overweight but not because they eat too much. May be they are naturally destined to be overweight or it is inherited. Generally, it is easier to gain weight and far more difficult to lose weight. Once you are overweight or obese, you need to adopt a program of weight reduction in order to lose weight in a healthy manner. This will require discipline and can be very tasking. There could also be various reasons for being overweight such as:

- Eating too much
- Living a sedentary life
- Doing a sedentary job
- Lack of exercise
- Disease conditions: usually you need to ask your doctor why you are overweight
- Uncontrollable appetite
- Snacking
- Unsuitable food, culture

It is important to know the extent of the problem. Check your weight and calculate your BMI. These should form the starting point for a weight reduction program, which may not be as easy as one thinks. You may need the services of a nutritionist, a psychologist, or a doctor in order to map out a program that is attainable, effective, friendly, and healthy. Most weight reduction programs are designed to work in component ways.

## 14. What should the components of a weight reduction program look like?

- Food:
  - Eating less calories
  - Ensuring meals are bulky enough to move the bowels
  - Eating fruits should become a life style. Fruits form bulk, contain a lot of water which the body needs and supply most of the vitamins and trace elements
  - Ensuring a balanced diet that has no nutritional deficiencies
  - Taking nutritional vitamin supplements
  - Combining various edible ways to make different dishes e.g. beans can be made into pastas, cake, or cooked combined with rice, etc. This will stop boredom resulting from eating the same foods all the time
  - Avoiding eating snacks. Many women claim they do not eat much but snack a lot. Eating little portions of food several times a day or snacking with sugary foods, beverages and sweets add up to weight gain. Eating breakfast early in the morning is one of the effective ways of avoiding snacks. It is good to take water in between the standard meals, because this fills the tummy and prevents hunger to a great extent. Women with average build should take about 3 liters or more of water per day
- Exercise:
  Exercise helps to reduce weight in some ways. By exercising, you burn-up calories and store-fat which leads to weight reduction. Other benefits include the fact that exercise tones up all parts of your body and improves your overall level of fitness. One problem of being overweight is clumsiness and lethargy. Lastly, exercise encourages regular bowel movements and prevents constipation
- Life-Long Commitment:

For weight reduction to be effective you need to adopt a healthy lifestyle:
- Exercise must be regular and be part of your lifestyle
- Lifelong commitment to healthy eating habits
- Discipline is required to stop eating between meals
- Measure weight regularly before bathing in the morning

### 15. What are the other benefits of regular exercise?

Apart from helping to reduce weight and prevent abnormal weight gain, exercising regularly either alone or in combination with reduced food intake or healthy eating, has many other benefits. These include lowering the risk of:
- High blood pressure or hypertension
- Bad cholesterol
- Heart diseases
- Chest diseases including breathing problems and cough
- Joint diseases including joint pain
- Cancer: e.g. breast, colon
- Type II diabetes
- Sleep problems: sleep apnea and snoring
- Gall bladder disease

Finally, regular exercise makes you fit and smarter, with less clumsiness and falls.

### 16. What is meant by healthy eating?

There are varieties of food available in different parts of the world, so the choices that are made depend on the type of food available in each community. Some foods and fruits are seasonal in many parts of the world, especially in developing countries. Also, while food is relatively cheap in the USA, Europe, and some parts of Africa and Asia, it is expensive in other parts of the world. Consequently, the cost of food also influences choice. In general, the following are useful tips:
- Eat small breakfasts and drink water regularly to delay hunger
- Eat smaller meal portions - 2/3 to 1/2 sizes. Adjust rations according to the rate of weight loss. For example, start with 2/3 of the usual size, reduce to ½ size and then to something smaller, according to the progress being made
- Dinner should be eaten not later than 7pm and should be about 30 – 40% the usual quantity. It is also desirable to stay active for at least 2 hours after dinner before going to bed. This allows time for digestion and ensures that food eaten at dinner is not just dumped in the stomach
- Avoid saturated fatty food items. Foods like meat and milk contain saturated fatty acids and should be much reduced in the diets, if total exclusion is difficult. Instead, more of unsaturated fatty acid foods like

fish, vegetables and nuts should be taken. Currently, food stuffs with much reduced fat, such as lean milk and lean meat are desirable. One way to reduce fat with meat, is to peel off the fat, burn and remove other obvious fats as much as possible
- Eat more of whole grains. At least 3 ounces of whole grains in the form of oats, cereal, rice, etc., are desirable
- Make it a habit to eat plenty of fruits and vegetables. Oranges, cherry, grapes, mango, garden eggs, and carrots among others are healthy. These can also be mixed or made into a rich coleslaw, salads or smoothies. 'Green' fruits and vegetables such as garden eggs, cucumber, apple, green beans, and broccoli can be made into fruit or vegetable delicacies
- Avoid too much salt. Limit salt intake to not more than 2 – 3g (0.07 - 0.1oz) of salt daily.
- Sometimes, you may need to supplement food elements with calcium and some vitamins but this must be discussed first with a doctor.
- Finally, there are many designer foods and rations that claim to be effective in weight reduction. Be careful about these foods and discuss them with a doctor before making a final choice.

## 17. Why is water so important in weight reduction programmes?

It is generally advisable to increase water intake or cultivate it for an effective reduction program. The benefits include:
- Reduction of hunger – Drinking water early in the morning, fills the stomach and gives a sense of satisfaction. This delays hunger
- Smaller food portions – The usual portions of food can be made smaller and when water intake is increased, it reduces the intense feeling of hunger
- Water reduces dehydration – people who are engaged in weight reduction programs often feel tired and dehydrated due to reduced calorie intake and sweating during routine exercise. So, increased intake of water prevents dehydration, improves tiredness, and promotes a sense of general well-being
- Prevents constipation – Reduced intake of food often leads to constipation. The stool comes out small and harder. Increased intake of water increases the bulk of the stool and makes it soft. The bowel movement improves and constipation is much less
- Reduces hunger pangs – Many weight reduction efforts fail because of the inability to withstand the stress and hunger pangs, resulting from reduced food intake
- Water intake helps to reduce the acidity of the stomach as it fills it up. This leads to reduction in the rate and seriousness of hunger pangs. This may also keep ulcers at bay

### 18. How do I keep my weight down after a successful weight reduction program?

Once you have achieved your desired weight, your next goal is to keep your weight down. To do this, the following may be helpful:

- Entrench your weight loss program into your lifestyle. Those habits you have newly developed must not be abandoned
- Maintain your calorie intake, physical activity and exercise
- Avoid indulgence in unhealthy practices, e.g. excess consumption of alcohol, sweets, etc. Don't eat snacks
- Measure your weight regularly. Learn how to calculate and check your BMI
- Report any suspicious problems to your doctor

Remember always that it is quite easy to gain weight, but it is quite difficult to reverse weight gain. May be you should always keep in mind all the troubles that you went through during your weight reduction program, as a caution not to indulge in weight promoting habits

## DEAR DOCTOR:

### 19. Doctor I am obese, what is my best option to lose weight rapidly?

Do not aim at losing weight rapidly. Rapid weight loss may be dangerous to your health. The best plan is to lose weight steadily, in a way that will not have adverse effects on your health. Most overweight people are anxious to reverse their obesity in the fastest way possible. So, gradual weight loss is your best bet.

### 20. How should I run my weight reduction program?

The details of your weight reduction program are individualized and tailor made for you. However, you can be guided by the following:

- Exercise is universal and can be adapted to suit your work schedules and situation. On the other hand, the type of food eaten varies from one culture to another and from one person to another, according to individual likeness, economic status, and availability. So, your food should be adapted to suit your situation. The amount of weight you intend to lose should determine the amount of calories to be consumed. Choose low calorie foods in the right portions:
- It is desirable to lose 1 – 2 pounds (045 - 0.9kg) every week

- Eat healthy, avoid snacks as much as you can. Inappropriate consumption of sweets, candy, cheese, chocolate, etc., may harm your weight reduction program
- Complement your food program with increased physical activity and exercise
- Measure your weight at the end of every day or more regularly. If you notice reduction, this will encourage you to do more in terms of focus and discipline
- Review your program with your doctor at intervals and let him know of any difficulties you may be having. He will be happy to discuss them with you

## 21. What do you think about the use of weight reduction drugs?

Some obese people resort to the use of drugs to achieve weight reduction. This could be extremely dangerous, especially if the weight loss program is not under the supervision of the doctor. Also, one universal drawback of drugs is the usual rapid weight gain that occurs, when the drugs are stopped. The reduction of calorie intake, increased physical activity, exercise and appropriate lifestyle modifications, are the best ways to lose weight. However, all these require discipline and striving to maintain a normal weight is a lifelong objective.

# CHAPTER 20
# Menopause

*"I wouldn't mind these hot flashes so much...if they would just burn a little fat off my butt and thighs in the process!*
— UNKNOWN AUTHOR

1. **What is Menopause?**

By definition, a woman is said to have attained menopause when she fails to menstruate for 12 consecutive months. Menstruation is a physiological process that results in monthly bleeding in girls and women, starting from puberty up to a time when a woman ages and it finally stops permanently. The word menopause is a medical word that means the final and permanent stoppage of menstruation.

2. **What is the climacteric period?**

The climacteric is a transition period leading up to menopause. During this time, the woman experiences irregular menstrual cycles or skips menses. For example, she may more often miss her periods for weeks or months. Then, she gradually loses her fertility such that on attaining menopause, natural pregnancy becomes practically impossible.

3. **At what time do most women experience the climacteric?**

In most women, the climacteric frequently starts at about the age of 45 years and stops at about 55 years. During this 10-year transition period, many women experience increasing degrees of menopausal symptoms.

4. **At what age does menopause occur?**

Menopause normally occurs in women who are above 50. According to the CDC, menopause often happens in women at about 45-55 years in the USA. In the USA, the average age of most women at menopause is 51 years and is fairly constant. It does not change much from one part of the world to the other, unlike the age of girls at menarche, which generally comes earlier.

### 5. Does menopause happen suddenly?

No. Natural menopause does not happen abruptly. However, artificial menopause may be induced due to the effects of drugs, X- ray treatments, etc. In such cases of artificial menopause, menstruation may stop suddenly. Natural menopause is normally preceded by a transition period, during which menstruation becomes irregular or slows down. During this time, the woman gradually loses her ability to ovulate or ovulates irregularly for a period of time, before it stops finally. She also experiences so many discomforting complaints like hot flushes, night sweats, poor libido, mood changes, etc.

### 6. What are the main types of menopause?

Menopause can be classified into 3 types using the age at which it occurs and whether it is induced or not. Therefore, we have:
- Premature menopause
- Artificial menopause
- Natural menopause

### 7. What is premature menopause?

Most women will experience menopause at about the age of 51 years. However, some women do attain menopause at an earlier age. This may be due to problems of the pituitary gland in the brain, failure or improper function of the ovaries, etc. In some cases, the reasons for the stoppage of menstruation may not be apparent, even after thorough investigations by the doctor. Medically speaking, a woman is said to have premature menopause when she attains menopause naturally before the age of 40.

### 8. What is artificial menopause?

While a woman can naturally or prematurely stop menstruating, menstruation can be stopped or made impossible by the doctor, through the use of some drugs like gonadotropin analogues, drugs used in the treatments of cancers, radiation therapy, or X-ray treatment of cancers, etc. In these situations, where menopause happens due to the effects of drugs, irradiation, or other reasons, the woman is said to have artificial menopause. This means that her menstruation did not stop naturally but by external factors. In some cases of artificial menopause caused by drugs, menstruation may start again after the drug has been discontinued. Artificial menopause caused by irradiation may be more permanent, because the X-rays directly destroy the cells of the ovaries and the lining of the womb. It is also important to know that menstruation automatically stops if the womb is removed, through surgical operation.

## 9. Why is menopause inevitable anyway?

Menstruation is a physiological process. It is controlled by the effects of hormones on the ovaries and the lining of the womb. The Follicle Stimulating Hormone (FSH), secreted by the pituitary gland in the brain, is responsible for stimulating the eggs in the ovaries for the purpose of ovulation during the menstrual cycles. The number of eggs in the ovaries in females is fixed. Unlike males, females do not have the ability to make one single egg on their own. They just recruit eggs from the deposits in the ovaries for ovulation, during their menstrual cycles. The eggs in the ovaries are responsible for the production of estrogen hormone. As women get older, there are fewer eggs left in the ovaries, because many have been recruited and used up during the process of ovulation. Many eggs are recruited at the beginning of each cycle but only one is commonly released at ovulation, the rest simply die off. Therefore, many eggs are wasted at each cycle. Secondly, as women become older, the response of the ovaries to FSH is reduced. Therefore, the amount of estrogen that the few eggs left can produce is much less. As a response to the low estrogen in older women, the pituitary gland increases the supply of Follicle Stimulating Hormone. With time, even with the high level of FSH, the response of the ovaries becomes so poor that ovulation does not take place anymore. For these two reasons, the amount of estrogen in the body becomes insufficient. When compared to pre-menopausal women, estrogen is reduced tenfold in post-menopausal women. This situation of low estrogen is called estrogen deficiency. Most of the complaints by menopausal women are due to this state of estrogen deficiency. So, it is clear that menopause is bound to happen, because estrogen deficiency will surely set in at one time or the other in women at middle age.

## 10. Is it possible to reverse or stop menopause?

When women enter menopause naturally, it should be regarded as irreversible. In some cases of artificial menopause like menopause induced through the use of GnRh, menstruation may return after the drug has been stopped. Women who have attained menopause naturally may be given drugs by their doctors to cause vaginal bleeding. This is not true menstruation. It is called withdrawal bleeding. Doctors are usually worried when a woman begins to bleed after attaining menopause. This type of bleeding may signify problems of the womb, cervix, ovary or vagina. On many occasions, bleeding after menopause may indicate cancer of the womb.

## 11. Why do women become too old to get pregnant, while men can still partake in reproduction even at very old age?

For a woman to conceive naturally, she needs to produce eggs at ovulation. When a baby girl is in the womb, at 20 weeks of pregnancy, she has about 7 million eggs. At birth, this number has reduced to 2 million and typically at puberty, when she becomes physiologically mature to begin her reproductive life, she has only about 400,000 – 500,000 eggs. This represents a great reduction from birth to puberty. From puberty and henceforth, multiple eggs are recruited and used up at each cycle, even though only one is usually released at ovulation. The others are wasted. With time therefore, the remaining eggs are so few such that ovulation becomes difficult and menstruation stops. Without ovulation, there is nothing for the sperm to fertilize, hence pregnancy cannot occur. So, the inability of women to make new eggs to replenish the reserve of eggs in the ovaries like men do, is the reason why their natural ability to conceive at old age is limited.

### 12. Is there any way that a woman who has attained menopause can ever get pregnant?

Yes. Currently, it has become possible, thanks to in –vitro fertilization (IVF) or Artificial reproductive techniques (ART). Stories abound of many women that have achieved conception through IVF, many years after attaining menopause.

### 13. How is reproduction a wasteful process in human beings?

Reproduction in humans is indeed a wasteful process. Imagine the situation where out of about 400,000 eggs available when a girl attains puberty, only about 400 or 1% are utilized for ovulation throughout her reproductive life. The vast majority simply dies off and is wasted with the cyclical menses. Also, a man needs to produce several millions of spermatozoa just to fertilize one female egg. Only one spermatozoon is needed for fertilization but about 15-20 million are needed for normal fertility.

### 14. What is the practical implication of menopause in women?

In practical terms, menopause signifies the end of a woman's reproductive life. This means that the woman may not be able to achieve pregnancy naturally anymore.

### 15. Currently, why is the issue of menopause assuming greater importance in healthcare globally?

Health issues due to menopause are important in the individual lives of women who experience the distress caused by the symptoms. More and more women now live long enough to attain menopause. According to the WHO statistics, 72.0 years was the global life expectancy at birth. Globally, there is a general improvement in longevity across most communities and countries. In the USA, current data from the CDC (2018) put longevity in women at 81.1 years while the overall life expectancy (women and men) is 78.1 years.

| Country | Lifespan |
|---|---|
| United State | 81.3 |
| Britain | 83.0 |
| Germany | 83.4 |
| Canada | 84.1 |
| Australia | 84.8 |
| France | 85.4 |
| Spain | 85.5 |

There are 2 very important implications of the global improvement in longevity. In the first instance, because more women now live above 51 – 52 years, which represents the period when most women attain menopause, more women spend the rest of their lives experiencing the distressful symptoms of menopause. The second issue is that many female cancers are related to old age. These include cancer of the womb. In effect more women may now naturally experience cancer, just because they are predisposed to old age. This improved longevity has a great implication on the global cost of healthcare, since a remarkable percentage has to be allocated to deal with old age problems.

### 16. What are the main complaints about menopause?

At menopause, women do experience many problems but actual complaints vary from one woman to the other. The more common complaints include:

- Hot flashes
- Night sweats
- Frequent tiredness and weakness
- Sleeplessness
- Mood swing
- Anxiety and depression
- Poor libido
- Vaginal dryness
- Frequent urination (day and night)
- Sometimes, urinary incontinence
- Poor concentration ability and lack of attention
- Loss of short term memory and forgetfulness

### 17. What are the early complaints during menopause?

The common complaints of most women at the beginning of menopause are hot flashes. These come with excessive sweating and sleeplessness. This problem typically begins at the time leading up to menopause. The progression may be on for 3-4 years until menopause actually occurs.

### 18. What are the two most common symptoms of menopause?

The two most common complaints in menopausal women are hot flashes and night sweats. These two symptoms are experienced by about 70% of menopausal women. The severity, duration, and frequency of the complaints vary from one woman to another.

### 19. What are the less common complaints?

Apart from the complaints listed above, some women experience other problems even though they are less frequent and sometimes weird. The less frequent complaints include:

- Crying episodes
- Feeling of lightness in the head without any logical explanation
- Lack of interest in most things, including their surroundings
- Difficulty in breathing
- Muscle pain, joint pain

Even though these complaints are less common, they are important. They may also not be readily recognized as symptoms due to menopause. This means prolonged suffering for the woman, because of the delay in seeking for help.

### 20. What are the causes of the symptoms experienced at menopause?

Biologically speaking, doctors certainly know that there is a lack of eggs in the ovaries, as a woman approaches menopause. This leads to the deficiency of the hormone called estrogen. Doctors believe that most of the problems experienced by women at menopause are traceable to estrogen deficiency. The normal level of estrogen in the blood is 50-350 IU/ ml. It is believed that many women will start experiencing the distressful complaints of menopause, when the blood level of estrogen falls below 100 IU/ml.

### 21. What are the medical conditions that may result in menopause?

Apart from the fact that menopause will occur naturally in most women, menopause may occur due to the conditions listed below:

- Premature ovarian failure
- Resistant ovary syndrome
- Removal of the womb - called hysterectomy (obligatory menopause)

- Removal of the ovaries - surgical menopause
- Drugs – e.g.
  - Gonadotropin releasing hormone analogues (GnRh)
  - Chemotherapeutic drugs or drugs used in the treatment of cancer
  - Irradiation therapy

## 22. What is resistant ovary syndrome?

There are some women who attain menopause or early stoppage of menses for reasons that are not clear. In these women, the ovaries appear structurally normal and have abundant follicles. However, despite the apparently normal situation, ovulation and menstruation do not occur.

## 23. Please explain the meaning of hot flashes?

Hot flushes are experienced by many women around the time of menopause. These women feel episodes of body hotness which may last for a few minutes or longer. This feeling of heat in the body is followed by profuse episodes of sweating. Hot flashes may occur many times in a single day or as multiple episodes at nights.

## 24. What is the importance of hot flashes to a woman's health?

Hot flashes are definitely discomforting, inappropriate, and can be most embarrassing. The sweating episodes are associated with severe loss of body water and body salts. This leads to dehydration and severe weakness. When hot flashes happen at night, they interrupt sleep and cause sleeplessness. Depending on how serious the sleep disturbance is, the general health of the woman may be compromised considerably. Continuous inability to sleep is like keeping vigils, which may eventually lead to serious ill health.

## 25. Why do hot flashes and sweating occur?

There are centers in the brain that sense and regulate body temperature. These centers determine how we perceive or feel heat. In menopausal women who experience hot flashes, there is malfunctioning of the regulatory center in the brain, such that the women "feel hot" even at lower temperatures, which other women would normally tolerate. During hot flashes, some women experience or may have panic attacks with each episode of heat. The body readjusts to the heat, by sweating. Sweating helps to lose heat from the skin surface, and because of this, the skin cools down and the woman obtains some relief.

## 26. Why is the issue of poor concentration important?

When a woman is forgetful or cannot sustain proper concentration, she loses track of events and things around her. For instance, she may leave the sitting room to pick something in the bedroom and completely forget this when she gets to the bedroom. Consider a woman who forgets that she had initially turned-on the gas cooker with sticks of lighted matches in her hand. Fire may be the outcome! So, loss of concentration and forgetfulness may endanger a woman's life and the lives of those around her. Secondly, poor concentration and serious forgetfulness means that the woman can be manipulated more easily. She can sign off her fortune by absentmindedly appending her signature on an important document or say yes to an important question when she should have said no. These can be catastrophic!

## 27. What is the effect of menopause on libido?

Libido can be interpreted as the degree of sexual desire or craving. In some women, the change in libido before and after menopause may not be remarkable. However, some women may experience profound changes or totally different degrees of interest in sexual intercourse after attaining menopause. More often, there is reduced desire for sexual intercourse and romantic lifestyles. The reduction in libido may be due to a combination of advancing age and menopause. Certainly, severe symptoms of menopause caused by estrogen deficiency can leave a woman so devastated to the extent of drastically altering her usual and accustomed lifestyle. Health issues like hot flashes, sweating episodes, sleeplessness, vaginal dryness and pain during sexual intercourse, should be carefully discussed with the doctor by the couple. Many of such cases can usually be resolved with the help of the doctor. Hormone replacement treatment may be of value in this situation. Sexual intimacy between couples is an issue that requires mutual understanding and cooperation of the woman and her husband. It should be discussed in such a way that the man understands the situation clearly. The wife needs support and understanding at this time. It is good practice for a couple to visit the gynecologist together, during treatment appointments for a more effective therapy.

## 28. Why do some menopausal women feel pain during sexual intercourse?

One of the effects of estrogen deficiency during menopause is dryness of the vagina. Estrogen deficiency makes the vaginal wall to become wrinkled, and the natural wetness or moisture is remarkably reduced. The dryness creates friction between the penis and the vaginal wall during sexual intercourse. With increased friction as a result of dryness, many menopausal women experience pain during sexual intercourse. Once experienced, pain during sexual intercourse creates fear. This may discourage a woman from further participating in sexual intercourse, just as it will make sexual intercourse non-pleasurable for the husband. So, both the woman and her husband are no longer looking forward to sexual intercourse for different reasons.

### 29. How can women reduce the pain of sexual intercourse associated with menopause?

Many menopausal women are affected by this but they can take some steps to reduce the attendant worries and restore family harmony.

- Dialogue: The first step is to recognize and discuss with your partner the reasons why you are boycotting sexual intercourse. For women, it is because of pain but for husbands, it is because they no longer derive the usual sexual pleasure, especially knowing that it causes pain. Sometimes men may also erroneously think that women are uncooperative or uninterested, especially if they pretend or hide their agony. It is therefore important that women share their problems to enable productive discussions and joint decisions. The next logical step is for the couple to visit their doctor, preferably a gynecologist. Sometimes, the advice of a psychologist is needed
- Adequate foreplay: A longer duration of foreplay and romance before sexual intercourse may increase or facilitate vaginal wetness. It should be noted that generally, vaginal wetness may be more difficult to achieve in menopausal women, hence patience is essential. Achievement of vaginal wetness before penetration will reduce friction and greatly reduce pain during sexual intercourse
- Vaginal lubricants: Sometimes, lubrication of the vaginal wall may not be sufficiently achieved with a longer duration of foreplay. There are proprietary vaginal lubricating creams, many of which contain estrogen. They come in form of creams, gels, etc. They are usually smeared on the vaginal wall during or after foreplay before penetration. Your husband can also apply these creams to the penis before penetration
- The gentleman's attitude: It is very important for your husband to be gentle during sexual intercourse in this situation. Aggressive or 'violent' sex may leave you with vaginal bruises and even lacerations

### 30. Why are old women more prone to bone fracture?

Old women have increased risks of bone fracture due to estrogen deficiency. In about 20% of bones in the body, estrogen plays an important part in maintaining their structure and strength. Lack of estrogen leads to greater bone destruction and reduced formation of new bone tissues. This leads to reduction in bone density and bone strength. So, bones of the vertebra column at the back, the radius in the forearm and the femur in the thigh, become more prone to fracture in old women or after menopause.

### 31. What is the reason why some women stoop at old age?

At old age and after menopause, there is gradual loss of bone material due to estrogen deficiency. Therefore, there is a reduction in bone density and strength. The vertebrae are the bones which, in conjunction with the muscles of the back, keep the back straight in the erect position. Due to the estrogen deficiency, the vertebral bones become smaller in size or shrink and the joints between them also become stiff and less mobile. In some instances, the gel lubricating the joints may dry up, allowing the joints to collapse. For these reasons, the curve of the vertebral column at the back becomes pronounced and more prominent at old age. So, old women appear shorter with bent backs and waist. This is the typical stooping of old age:

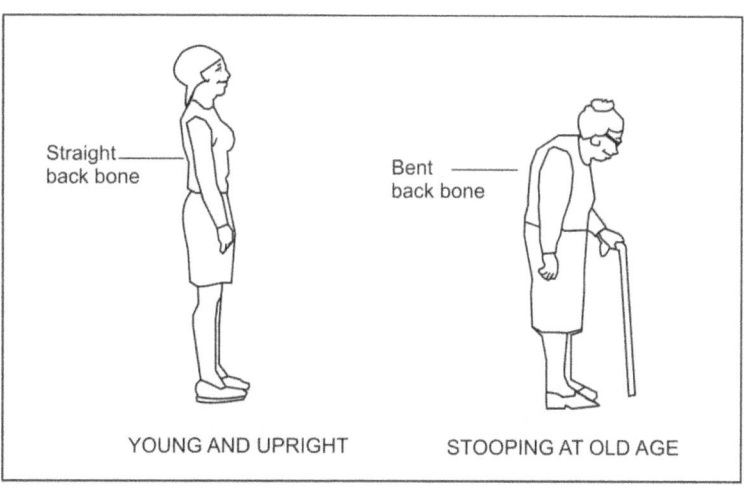

## 32. Does estrogen affect the blood circulation?
Yes. Doctors believe that estrogen deficiency is associated with an increase in total cholesterol and low density lipoprotein (LDL). These are the bad cholesterols. Bad cholesterols accelerate the formation of plagues, which narrow the lumen of blood vessels in the body, including the vessels of the heart. This may result in total blockage. Blockage of the vessels of the heart results in heart attacks. So, estrogen deficiency is one of the reasons why menopausal women are more prone to heart attacks.

## 33. Can the problems of menopause result in psychiatric illness?
No. There is no medical evidence to support this. However, the severity of the problems of menopause may be increased in women who have background histories of anxiety and other neurotic complaints. Similarly, anxiety and depression may become worse in the presence of severe menopausal symptoms.

## 34. Do I need family planning even after menopause?
You are not expected to get pregnant since you are no longer menstruating but you are not 100% safe from unwanted pregnancy within the period just a

few months before and after menopause. Doctors advise that women should use family planning up until 1 year after the final stoppage of their menstruation. The reason is that it is possible for menstruation to come on and off, in the last 3-5 years before menopause and 1-2 years after. If, in any of such cycles, ovulation also takes place, then pregnancy is a possibility. This situation is not common but it happens. So use family planning until one year after menopause, so that pregnancy does not spring a surprise.

### 35. Will all women experience the complaints of menopause?

Most women will experience the effects of estrogen deficiency when they attain the age of menopause. The type, duration, and severity of these complaints vary from one woman to another. Doctors also believe that there are individual differences in the pattern and severity of symptoms according to culture and race. For example, Black women tend to experience hot flashes more than White women. About 80% of Dutch women experience hot flashes at menopause, while hot flashes are rare in women of the Mayan tribe in Mexico.

### 36. What should the appropriate attitude of women be, when menopause finally happens?

Age is sure to catch up with every woman, no matter how hard she tries to prevent it. Obviously, people like to look as young and fresh as ever, but aging is inevitable. The right attitude of women should be to accept menopause as a natural occurrence and manage the effects as wisely as possible. Denial of menopause is of no use. It is better to adopt the right lifestyles that will make you to age gracefully and be in good health. Hormone therapy, when prescribed by the doctor, may reduce the severity of many of the problems experienced by many women at menopause.

### 37. How should women prepare for menopause?

Information is important, so they should be informed in advance. If they are well informed, they will be better prepared and should fare better when they attain menopause. They need to read widely and become familiar with the key problems and the remedies available. Important challenges like hot flashes, excessive sweating, sleeplessness, poor concentration and forgetfulness. Reduced sexuality is also associated with menopause.

### 38. Should doctors treat all menopausal complaints?

No. The decision whether to treat or not usually depends on the severity of the specific complaints. The main treatment for menopausal problems is hormonal replacement. Hormonal replacement therapy (HRT) has many side-effects. Therefore, it is not suitable for all women. Before embarking on HRT, doctors normally conduct tests to identify those women that are suitable and exclude those that are not.

### 39. When do I need to call the doctor in?

Menopause is a natural occurrence. In some women, it may be less troublesome and tolerable. However, for many women, menopause may be such an unpleasant experience. You will need the help of your doctor when the symptoms of menopause begin to affect the quality of your domestic life, disturb your work, or cause distress in your marital harmony. It becomes even more important to seek help because some of the symptoms of menopause like loss of memory may endanger your life or those of others.

### 40. Is it possible for all menopausal women to benefit from HRT?

No. There are some women who should not be given HRT. These include women who have cancers of the womb or breast, hypertension, liver disease and those prone to blood clot or thrombus formation (thrombo-embolism). All caution should also be exercised in women with uterine fibroids, breast lumps, and migraine. For this category of women, HRT should only be given by specialist doctors after thorough investigations and appraisals.

### 41. To what extent may treatment with estrogen help me?

Estrogen replacement therapy is good but it is not suitable for use by all women, and of course, it cannot solve all the problems associated with menopause. At the age when a woman is past menopause, it is possible that some of the problems mentioned above are not due to estrogen deficiency alone. Some other issues of old age may be responsible, at least in part. For example, at the age of 60 years, a woman, may be depressed because she lost her husband, or because she gave her precious daughter and companion out in marriage and the home environment has become lonelier or less interesting. A woman who loved travelling while young is likely to evaluate her quality of life in terms of her inability to travel frequently, as she advances in age. Therefore, some of the symptoms may be due to natural life events that occur in every home. So, it is a complex situation and every woman is considered by doctors, as unique and treated on merit. The approach is for you to be appraised by your gynecologist, who will determine whether estrogen is appropriate for you or not. In any event, remember that estrogen cannot solve all your problems, as explained previously.

### 42. Is estrogen administered alone or with other drugs?

In young women, the body produces estrogen from the ovary and progesterone from the corpus luteum. The effects of these two hormones on the lining of the womb lead to the regular, cyclical bleeding experienced before menopause finally sets in. In the absence of progesterone, estrogen given alone may cause the inner lining of the womb to grow or to become abnormally thick. Some doctors believe that this abnormal thickness may lead to cancer of the lining of the womb, in some women. For this reason, progesterone or progestogen is prescribed with estrogen for about 2 weeks in a month. This is given to women whose wombs are still intact, in order to prevent thickening of the lining of the womb.

### 43. What are the side effects of hormone replacement therapy?

The common side effects or complaints of estrogen are:
- Leg cramps - this is the most common complaint and about 21% of women on estrogen replacement, suffer from side effects. The pain is usually worse while in bed and disappears or reduces with time
- Breast tenderness - this may be felt as pain, discomfort, or feeling of tightness in the breasts
- Retention of fluid - is also a fairly common problem. This may appear as fullness in some parts of the body
- Nausea
- Vaginal discharge - some women on estrogen replacement experience increased vaginal discharge
- Irritation of the eyes

### 44. What are the most common problems that make women discontinue HRT?

There are three most common problems that are notorious in frustrating women to discontinue HRT. These are:
- Breakthrough bleeding
- Bloating
- Fear of breast cancer

### 45. What are the alternatives to HRT?

Where a woman is much troubled by the estrogen and progestogen combination, synthetic steroids may be prescribed by the doctor. A good example is Tibolone which has estrogen, progesterone, and androgenic properties. Tibolone causes a remarkable reduction in the distressing symptoms of menopause in many women. It is also effective in preventing bone loss but it may be worthwhile to discuss available alternatives with the doctor.

### 46. Is there any new effective drug on the horizon?

Yes. Many women should benefit from the new class of drugs called selective estrogen receptor modulators (SERM). With SERM, the risks of withdrawal bleeding, spurious post-menopausal bleeding due to HRT and breast cancer are most unlikely.

**47. Does HRT increase blood pressure?**

No. There is no clear evidence to suggest that HRT increases blood pressure in menopausal women. However, at that age, blood pressure may increase due to old age and other diseases of old age.

**48. Does HRT benefit the heart in any way?**

Yes. HRT reduces the risk of heart attacks and other cardiovascular diseases. Protection against cardiovascular disease is an important benefit for 2 reasons:
- Cardiovascular disease is the cause of death in over 40% of women in the USA, Europe and other countries of the civilized world
- There is an increase of incidences of cardiovascular disease in women after menopause

So, HRT may prevent cardiovascular disease.

**49. Who are those that should not take HRT?**

To determine whether HRT is suitable or not, doctors usually interview each woman extensively. This is followed by physical examinations and appropriate investigations. It is after taking these steps that the doctor is able to take a decision. The type of HRT, the dose and timing or whether HRT is contra indicated are then determined. There are women who should never be given HRT, while some can be given HRT in modified prescriptions, under very strict supervision by the doctor.
- Those that should not be given HRT at all include women that fall under the categories listed below:
  - Suspected endometrial cancer
  - Suspected breast cancer
  - Previous or confirmed cases of thrombo-embolism
  - Active liver disease
  - Uncontrolled hypertension
- Those women who may be given HRT under modified prescription and strict doctors supervision, include those who have the following:
  - Chronic liver disease
  - Benign breast disease
  - Uterine fibroids
  - Endometrial polyp
  - Unconfirmed thrombo-embolism
  - History of migraine

It is good to avoid HRT if these women are also on drugs used for the treatment of epilepsy.

**50. What are the other means of relieving menopausal symptoms apart from HRT?**

There are a few alternatives to hormone replacement therapy. However, their effects are controversial. Some women profess their efficacies, while the experiences of other women suggest that there are no benefits. Some of the alternative methods include the use of the following:

- Primrose
- Soy bean diets
- Garlic medications
- Black cohosh plant (herb)
- Other numerous herbal preparations

Also, there are various supplements which lay claims to their abilities to reduce hot flashes and other menopausal problems. They come in both orthodox packages and herbal preparations. Their claims of benefits are also controversial. Before embarking on any of these alternative treatments, the doctor's advice and guidance is important. There is the potential danger that untested or scientifically unproven medications, may turn out to be harmful or even toxic to health in the long run.

**51. Are there self-help measures out there that may be beneficial?**

Some women have tried out many alternative remedies in the effort to secure solutions to their symptoms. Their testimonies and claims are as diverse. Generally speaking, at menopause, the following tips may be useful:

- Food: You need to take good food and eat right. At the age of menopause, the purpose of food is to nourish you; you are not eating in order to grow anymore, so you need to cut down on the quantity of food at each meal. However, ensure that the food is balanced in terms of quality. Light breakfast, little quantities of food for lunch and dinner are good. You should avoid heavy foods as much as you can. The digestive system at old age is slow and less active. Plenty of vegetables and fruits will help in moving the bowels, and ensure that you feel light. Try and eat fruits daily. If you make a timetable of your diet and adhere to it, you are more likely to get better results. There are many vitamins supplements that are available, but it is better to ask for your doctor's advice, to ensure you get the right one
- Rest: You need to rest adequately and relax as much as possible. Rest is like a tonic that allows the cells of the body to recover faster from stress. Rest also slows down the aging process. Sleeping is a universal way to rest all parts of your body, including the mind and brain
- Exercise: Indulge in regular but non strenuous exercises. The emphasis is that you make it routine. It should not be stressful. Exercise tones up your aging body and improves blood supply to the brain and other parts of the body. Daily walking, light jogging, and stretching are all good. It is useful to remember that any exercise that

leaves you breathless is too much and may harm you. Also, note that work and exercise are two different things
- Set realistic Goals: At your age, you should set only goals that you consider realistic. If your goals are too ambitious, and not achievable, the failures will add to your worries. Let peace of mind be one of your goals!
- Drugs: There are drugs that can help to take care of some of your complaints. These include hormonal drugs, but they must be prescribed by your doctor. It is easy to abuse drugs at this period because you are desperately looking for solutions that may fix the problems. You are more inclined to try out many drugs in the hope of finding one or two that can help ease your complaints. It is important to resist this tendency. Ask your doctor for his or her advice
- Make friends: Get the best out of your situation; after all, you cannot change it. Make friends and keep in high spirits. Avoid staying alone as much as you can. Engage in discussions and other things that make you feel more fulfilled and happy

These tips should make life more meaningful for you. Always remember that many women are experiencing what you are passing through, so you are not alone.

## 52. Why is menopause difficult to deal with?

In many situations, the age of 51 years and beyond represents the period when most women experience menopause. This time also coincides with the period when other important life events begin to happen at the home front and family. These events, include:
- Children leaving home or being married off
- Retirement from official work place, making life more redundant and boring
- Divorce or death of a husband
- Poor financial status and less or no spendable income
- Other diseases and situations that are more common in old age are:
  - Diabetes
  - Hypertension
  - Cancers
  - General weakness and more frequent common illnesses
  - Worries over children and other family members

## 53. What is stress incontinence?

Stress incontinence is a condition whereby a woman involuntarily leaks urine when the pressure in her tummy is increased. This means that she cannot control urination on her own like other adult women. So, she may expel urine from the urinary pipe when she coughs, laughs or sneezes, etc.

**54. What are the conditions responsible for urinary incontinence?**

The majority of cases of urinary incontinence are due to:

- Stress incontinence - in this condition the woman will leak urine when she engages in activities that cause the abdominal pressure to increase, thus forcing urine to leak from the bladder. Such activities include coughing, laughing, and sneezing. This is why it is called stress incontinence
- Urge incontinence - A normal adult has the ability to hold urine for a reasonable length of time. In urge incontinence, the woman feels a compelling urge to urinate. She does not have control over when and where the urge will come and once the urge comes, she must rush to urinate quickly. This is why it is called urge incontinence
- Incontinence due to fistula - This may also be due to direct communication between the urinary bladder or urethra and the vagina. This type of hole is called a fistula. Fistula may occur following a difficult childbirth. This situation is more common in teenage pregnancy because the birth canal may be too narrow to allow the passage of the baby. Fistula is also common in many developing countries where the external female genital tract and vagina are cut or circumcised according to local cultures or traditions

**55. What about elderly women who leak urine uncontrollably?**

Yes, some elderly women leak urine involuntarily. This is common when they laugh, sneeze, shout, jump, or other situations where the abdominal pressure or force is increased. Since elderly women lack the hormone called estrogen, they suffer from weakness and loss of tone in the muscles of the bladder and urethra. Aging in these muscles also contributes to the problem. The weakness results in improper function of the bladder and urethra and leakage of urine. This is one reason why even old women should engage in appropriate exercises and keep fit.

**56. Do young women leak urine too?**

Yes, but this tends to happen almost exclusively in the poor or less developed countries, where teenage pregnancy and circumcision are common. The most common type in young women and girls is vesico-vaginal fistula (VVF), one of the most unfortunate consequences of teenage or underage pregnancy. With VVF, there is a hole between the bladder (which contains urine) and the vagina.

**57. How common is VVF in developing countries?**

Leakage of urine especially due to VVF is very common in many developing countries. The burden of this disease is most common in sub-Saharan Africa, following difficult child birth in teenagers. For example, it is estimated that up to 800,000 cases of VVF occur every year in Nigeria. This is typical of other developing countries too. The young girls so afflicted, suffer great social stigma, depression, and rejection. They are regarded as out-casts in their own localities and they are rejected and avoided by family and friends.

### 58. Is there no treatment for VVF?

VVF and other types of urinary incontinence are quite treatable. There are many centers in many developing countries dedicated to the treatment of VVF. One big challenge is that most of the patients are so downcast that they are afraid to come out for treatment. Health education and campaigns should be done to address the issue of reluctance, to assess treatment in developing countries.

### 59. Can ordinary infection cause urinary incontinence?

Yes. Urinary tract infection can cause incontinence. There are also tropical infestations by parasites that cause incontinence.

### 60. Can injury during sexual intercourse result in leakage of urine in women?

Yes. Injuries during sexual intercourse can occur in adolescents in teenage marriages. This is because of the immaturity and lack of strength of the tissues of the vagina and bladder against the aggressive thrusts of the penis of their full grown adult partners or husbands.

### 61. Is it possible for a woman to leak urine during sexual intercourse?

Yes, some women leak urine involuntarily during sexual intercourse. This problem is also suspected to be due to the over activity of the urinary bladder muscle, otherwise known as detrusor muscles. In some women, this leakage may be common or recurrent and is embarrassing. It is advisable for women who experience this problem to see a gynecologist and where necessary a urologist. The services of a psychologist may also be beneficial in some cases.

### 62. How can VVF and other incontinences be prevented?

Since most VVF cases are due to difficult childbirth or prolonged obstructed labor, health education, improved socio-economic conditions in poor communities, curtailing harmful traditional practices and family planning awareness are important aspects of the prevention of VVF. Pregnancy should be by choice and not by force. Teenage pregnancy should be discouraged. Those unfortunate women who have been afflicted with this condition should be accorded dignity and encouraged to seek treatment at dedicated medical facilities.

### 63. Why do some adults still wet their beds?

Many cases of bedwetting are due to malfunctioning or over activity of the muscles of the urinary bladder. In medical parlance, this is called Idiopathic Detrusor Muscle over activity (IDO).Other conditions that can cause bedwetting include urinary tract infection, infections of the urinary bladder muscles, bladder stones, too much fluid intake at night and drugs, e.g. diuretics.

### 30. Can women also leak stool involuntarily?

Yes, some women continuously leak stool or feces. This may be due to difficult child birth resulting in injury and a hole between the rectum and the vagina This condition is called Recto-vaginal fistula (RVF). Some cases of RVFs are due to penetrating injuries which can occur, sequel to scarifications on the back wall of the vagina. This type of scarification or cut is commonly practiced by some herbalists for the treatment of barrenness in many developing countries. Leakage of stool constitutes a serious social embarrassment and stigma. These women usually confine themselves indoors to reduce social interaction and mingling with other women in order to curtail their shame.

### 64. Is there any treatment for Recto-vaginal fistula?

Yes, `both VVF and RVF are treatable. The difficulty has been that many sufferers do not declare their conditions or seek treatment on time. There are dedicated hospitals that cater for these problems in many developing counties where these problems are rampant.

### 65. What are the treatment modalities for womb prolapse?

There are palliative and surgical methods of treatment for womb prolapse. The choice of treatment depends on the degree or severity of the condition. The appropriate treatment is determined by the doctor.

### 66. What is the relationship between menopause and women who have had their wombs removed through operation?

For reasons which are not totally understood, women who have had their wombs removed through surgery usually experience the problems associated with menopause earlier than others, even if the ovaries are intact. Surgical removal of the womb is called hysterectomy in medical parlance. This information is important for women who are planning to have hysterectomy.

# DEAR DOCTOR:

**67.  As I get closer to menopause, what challenges should I expect?**

Every aspect is important and may impact your life in different ways. For example, the following could occur:
- Vaginal dryness will cause pain during sexual intercourse and if not carefully handled may lead to sexual disharmony, especially if your husband is not aware of your feelings or complaints
- Because of loss of self-confidence, many women result into trying out several remedies to improve their libido, look younger, and become a "sweet sixteen" once more
- Even though there are remedies for some of the symptoms, menopause is a biological process which every woman who is old enough will eventually attain

**68.  Doctor, since I stopped menstruating, I no longer feel like a woman. What is happening to me?**

This kind of feeling may be experienced by a few women after menopause, so it is not unusual. This is more of a psychological problem and is mainly because of the absence of menstruation. Some women feel that they are no longer qualified to be called women, simply because they have stopped menstruating. This view may be rooted in the socio-cultural beliefs in communities where menstruation and child bearing are regarded as proofs of true womanhood. This notion of low self-esteem or self-worth may also be experienced by women who feel profoundly unhappy because of the gradual loss of youthful glamour, ugly bodily changes, and other problems of menopause. At the height of such notions, the woman may look down on herself and greatly discount her value. This perception of low self-esteem is perhaps more common in the early period, just after attaining menopause and should improve with time. At this time, the services of a psychologist may be beneficial.

**69.  I am 42 years old. My womb was removed 3 years ago due to excessive bleeding during child birth. Now I feel hot and sweat a lot. Doctor, what is happening to me? Could it be menopause?**

Yes, it is possible that you are experiencing symptoms of menopause even though your womb has been removed. Doctors have noticed that women who have had their wombs removed experience symptoms of menopause 2 – 5 years earlier than usual. This type of situation may be confusing, since you automatically stopped menstruating after your operation. This type of menopause is called occult menopause.

**70. Doctor, is it still appropriate to have sexual intercourse considering the fact that I am no longer menstruating?**

Absolutely yes. It is normal to enjoy sexual intercourse after menopause. Women in some parts of the world, for cultural reasons believe that it is a dirty habit to have sexual intercourse after menopause, since the monthly menstrual flow cannot flush out the seminal fluid deposited by their partners anymore. Other women believe that sexual intercourse may result in illnesses. There is no truth in all these. Semen is not dirt and does not cause illness. It is safe and normal to have sexual intercourse after menopause.

**71. Is it possible for me to be pregnant even after menopause?**

Yes, but it has to be through in-vitro fertilization (IVF). When you attain menopause, you do not have good quality eggs and do not ovulate any more. If your womb is intact and healthy, you may still achieve pregnancy through IVF but another woman will have to donate her eggs for this purpose. Egg donation is commonly utilized in IVF procedures, for women who do not have good eggs in their ovaries because of age or other medical reasons.

**72. How many ways can I take my estrogen prescription? Is there any preferred route?**

Estrogen hormone replacements can be achieved by using estrogen in different ways. The main routes are:
- By mouth as tablets
- On the skin as gel or patches
- Under the skin as subcutaneous implants
- Through the vagina as cream, vaginal pessary or tablets

The various forms of estrogen and routes of usage have advantages and disadvantages. Therefore, estrogen replacement should only be prescribed by a doctor. He will determine the type that is best for you, as well as the dose and route. It is wrong for you to administer such drugs on yourself just because it works perfectly for your friend. You are a different woman.

**73. Doctor, I am on combined estrogen and progestogen HRT. I noticed a remarkable weight gain soon after my family doctor added progestogen. Should I stop HRT because I continue to gain weight despite eating much less?**

It is quite possible that your weight gain is due to progestogen. The well-known side effects of progestogen in women include:
- Weight gain or bloating
- Mood change to severe mood swings
- Irritability
- Breast pain

Sometimes, these symptoms may discourage some women from taking the drugs. It is advisable that you complain to your doctor. He may be able to make some adjustments on the dose and combination or prescribe an alternative that will be less troublesome.

**74. I am 52 years old and a mother of 5 children. For over one year now, I can feel and touch something coming out of my vagina. The doctor told me it is my womb. Please, how can this be?**

Your doctor is most probably right. This condition is called womb prolapse. Normally, the womb is kept in its natural position in the pelvis by the support of strong ligaments and tissues which surround it. This is why it does not come down or get displaced. With advancing age or menopause, the ligaments and tissues become weak and lack the strength to support the womb as usual. Therefore, the womb may gradually descend through the vagina, especially when the pressure in the tummy and pelvis are increased. The abdominal pressure may be increased when you cough, sneeze, or bear down during defecation; especially if you are constipated. The ligaments may also be weakened due to repeated episodes of difficult childbirths and habitual lifting of heavy objects among others. The complaints of women with womb prolapse depend on how serious the condition is. Like you, the complaints by many women is that of feeling or touching something bulky in the vagina, which becomes more pronounced when they cough, sneeze, bear down, or strain. There may be back pain especially while in the standing position. There are medical and surgical treatments for womb prolapse. You should consult your gynecologist who will examine you and decide the type of treatment suitable for you.

**75. Doctor, what do you think has caused the collapse of my womb?**

Womb prolapse usually occurs when the support of the womb becomes weak. There are some conditions that may increase your risk of developing womb prolapse and if you already have it, they may make it worse. These conditions include:

- Medical conditions like
  - Chronic cough,
  - Chronic constipation and
  - Tumors in the abdomen
- Surgical operations around the womb
- Obstetric conditions like
  - Difficult childbirth
  - Obstructed labor
  - Instrumental deliveries
- Lifestyles, occupation, and others:
  - Obesity,
  - Lifting of heavy
  - Old age
  - Menopause

**76. Doctor, my friend started HRT but had to discontinue 3 months after because it was so stressful? How am I sure that I will be able to cope?**

It is not unusual for some women to experience aggravated symptoms at the initial period of starting HRT. These are called 'start-up' effects and are due to the side effects of the drugs. "Start-up" effects usually last for about 3 months. The complaints include:

- Increased appetite
- Weight gain
- Breast pain and tenderness
- Increased nipple sensitivity
- Leg pain or pain in the calf muscle

It is usual practice for doctors to tell you of the likelihood of experiencing any of these problems before starting HRT. In most cases, good relief from these symptoms can be expected after 3 months. It should be possible for you to cope with the usual problems with little perseverance.

**77. Sometimes, urine stains my underwear when I laugh or shout. I am 60 years old. One of my friends has the same complaint. Doctor, what could be responsible?**

Increased frequency of urination, pain during urination, urgency, and poor control of urination which doctors call incontinence, may happen due to menopause. This is due to the effect of lack of estrogen on the muscles of the urinary bladder. Estrogen deficiency makes the muscles of the urinary bladder to be weak and lax. Because of the weakness of the bladder muscle, when you laugh, shout, or sneeze, spurts of urine may escape through the urine pipe. This condition is called stress incontinence. You should see your doctor for evaluation. It is also important for the doctor to exclude other causes of such symptoms, especially infections of the urinary tract.

# CHAPTER 21
# Miscellaneous

BODY ODOR • MOUTH ODOR • SKIN BLEACHING

*"The Secretary of Hygiene or Physical Culture will be far more important in the cabinet of the President of the United States in the year 2035, than the Secretary of War"*
– NIKOLA TESLA

## BODY ODOR

**1.    What is body odor?**

Generally, each individual has a unique smell or odor. In most cases, people smell good in their own unique ways. This is the reason why some domestic animals would most certainly recognize the approach of a familiar person, even in the dark or while still out of their view. Human beings and some animals have highly sensitive organs of smell and can perceive and recognize odor easily. This is why animals like dogs can easily detect drugs like cocaine, heroin, etc. However, the term body odor is used when a person exudes an unpleasant or offensive smell. Few people suffer from this distressing social problem.

**2.    When does normal body odor generally begin in life?**

In human beings, body odor does not usually appear before puberty unless it is caused by some identifiable diseases or conditions. In females, puberty is attained at about the age of 13 years. At this time, a young adolescent girl, develops a characteristic body odor, which is one of the hallmarks of physiological maturity.

**3. What is the role of sweat glands in body odor?**

There are 2 types of sweat glands:
- Apocrine glands: These are sweat glands found in certain parts of the body where they also make secretions. They are the odor producing glands and are important with respect to body odor. Apocrine glands are found in the pubic area, armpit, breast, and ear. They are the cause of the pungent smells in the armpit, pubic area, nose, ear wax, etc.
- Eccrine or skin glands: These are found under the skin. Their main function is to regulate skin temperature and cool the body. The sweat from eccrine glands contains a lot of salt which makes it difficult for bacteria to breakdown protein

**4. What is the cause of body odor?**

Body odor occurs mostly when bacteria that live on our skin breakdown the proteins in our sweat into acids. The smell of the acids is responsible for the offensive odors, so although sweat has no odor, the protein it contains is broken down into "smelly acids."

**5. What are the major acids produced when bacteria break down proteins in sweat?**

The type of acid produced depends on the type of protein in the sweat. However, the two most common acids are:
- Propionic acid: This is produced by the action of propionic bacteria on sweat. Propionic bacteria are present in the ducts of our sebaceous glands. Propionic acid has a pungent, chocking, and irritating smell.
- Butanoic acid: This is produced when the bacteria called staphylococcus epidermidis which live on our skin break down protein in our sweat.

**6. Where is body odor more likely to be perceived?**

Body odor is common in places that are hairy, wet, enclosed, and rich in apocrine glands. Such places like the armpit, groin, pubic part, ear, belly button, anus, foot, etc., are therefore more likely to smell more often.

**7. How is body odor sustained?**

Using the armpit as an example, the hair entraps the perspiration or sweat together with the bacteria it contains. The wet environment allows the bacteria to multiply very rapidly. These bacteria then break down the protein in the sweat into acids. The salts and protein in the sweat form white crusts, which stick on the hairs and perpetuate the odor. The same process happens in the groin, pubic region, under the breast and ear.

## 8. Is it abnormal to sweat?

No. Sweating has a very important role in our daily living and well-being. It serves 2 very important functions. Firstly, it allows us to excrete some undesirable waste products from the body. Secondly, when sweat evaporates or dries from our skin, the heat of evaporation is taken from our body and this leads to reduction in temperature. That is, the body cools down. This type of temperature regulation is important, for example, during physical exercise or hot weather and serves to cool our body.

## 9. What is the relationship between excessive sweating and body odor?

Individuals who sweat excessively may not necessarily have body odor. This is because sweat from the skin contains high amounts of salt. You will notice this salty nature if you taste your sweat. High amount of salt makes it difficult or harder for bacteria to break down protein in sweat. So, if there is good hygiene, excessive sweating should not result in body odor.

## 10. Which habits are associated with the increased occurrence of body odor?

These include:

- Diet – consumption of foods like curry, spicy foods, ginger, garlic, etc., make sweat more pungent. Also, red meat may predispose some individuals to rapid development of body odor
- Obesity – This predisposes to increased sweating. The various thick and overlapping skin folds promote dirt in the hidden areas like the armpit, undersurface of the breasts, groin, etc. Obesity also makes these places inaccessible to proper washing or cleaning
- Clothing – Heat or sweat promoting fabrics like nylon and synthetic fabrics, aid rapid bacteria multiplication and reduction of ventilation
- Life style – Some practices, e.g. spraying perfume (other than deodorant) on the armpit, will result in further chemical breakdown of sweat and stronger, more offensive odors. Of course, there are typical body odors associated with habitual lifestyle issues like cigarette smoking, etc.
- Hair hygiene – Inadequate or poor attention to the hair in females, increases the risk of hair diseases like dandruff and other fungal infections
- Fasting – During periods of fasting, some individuals neglect their health. Some do not bathe, clean their mouth, or keep their dresses clean
- Diseases and ill health – May reduce the level and quality of hygiene. Some systemic illnesses like liver diseases, kidney failure, or complication of diabetes, may be associated with body odor

## 11. Which occupations and lifestyles influence body odor?

Some occupations are associated with distinct body odor. The putrid, fish-like body odor that fishmongers exude is unmistakable. Bakers also have characteristic body odor; that of freshly baked bread, even though more tolerable than fishy odors. Chronic alcoholics exude typical ammonia – like, alcoholic mouth and body odors, even when they are not actually drunk. It does appear as if their body is saturated with 'stale alcohol'. Occupational or lifestyle body odors are more common in men. This type of body odors can be reduced through frequent bathing and avoidance of direct skin contact with fish or bread e.g. by wearing gloves or other protective body gears. This is one situation where a strong smelling perfume may make some difference and increase social acceptance. When alcohol consumption is discontinued or an alcoholic is rehabilitated, it takes some time for the odor to disappear completely. Good personal and general oral hygiene surely accelerates the return to normal odor, in alcoholics. Other lifestyle-associated odors that are also common include the use of habitual substances like cigarettes and marijuana. These substances are associated with characteristically strong odors that are perhaps more socially acceptable, especially cigarettes. However, the danger is that a smoker never smokes alone, those around the smoker automatically smoke when they inhale the same air. Fortunately, fewer women smoke and much less so, than men. But then, it is probably more socially acceptable for a man, for example, to smell of cigarettes than for a woman to exude the characteristic suffocating odor of cigarette. The only sure way to abolish odors from any habit forming substance is to stop it.

## 12. Why is body odor more common in obese women?

There are reasons why obesity may promote body odor, especially in women who are severely overweight. Because of the body form, women, are generally more prone to infections of the genital tract than men. This demands that women do more to keep their body clean and hygienic. When a woman is severely obese, her ability to clean her body properly is hindered. Because she is overweight, she has fat pads in many areas of her body. The fat pads create crevices and make areas around the exterior of the genital tracts especially the vagina, anus, thighs, groin, undersurfaces of the breasts, armpits, etc., very difficult to clean. Also, obese women are more likely to sweat more than usual; this, combined with the difficulty in washing and cleaning their bodies properly, promote body odor.

# MOUTH ODOR

### 13. What is mouth odor?
When oral hygiene is good and an individual is healthy, the mouth should not have any distinct odor. A person is said to have mouth odor, if while she talks or coughs, a bad or foul smelling odor comes out from the mouth, as perceived by people around him or her. In medical language, mouth odor is called halitosis.

### 14. How common is mouth odor?
Mouth odor is common in people with poor oral hygiene. In general, about 25% of people have mouth odor, but the extent or severity varies from one person to another.

### 15. Why does the mouth smell?
The main reason why the mouth smells is due to the actions of bacteria. Commonly when we eat, some food particles are left in the mouth. These food particles usually settle at the back and surface of the tongue, the bases of the teeth and in between the teeth, under the gum and at back of the mouth. Bacteria in the mouth and throat break down the food particles, especially the protein elements. The odor of these broken-down proteins is what is perceived as mouth odor.

### 16. Why is oral hygiene extremely important?
Proper oral hygiene is very important in the prevention and reduction of mouth odor. Doctors advise that the teeth should be brushed and cleaned at least 2 times per day. It is good practice to brush the teeth and clean the mouth after meals and last thing before going to bed. Cleaning of the teeth should be done with an appropriate toothbrush and paste. The tooth brush should be applied in an up-and-down direction. Brushing the teeth horizontally is not effective. In some parts of the world, it usual practice with natives to use chewing sticks to clean the teeth and mouth generally. The use of chewing sticks is historical and predates the modern way of using tooth brush and paste in many cultures. However, doctors believe that the use of chewing sticks is inferior to the use of a tooth brush and paste. Mouth odor, dental plaques, and other dental diseases are very common among such natives who use chewing sticks.

### 17. How best can we care for our tongues?
It is desirable to brush the tongue at least once every night after super. The surface of the tongue has small projections that stick in tiny food particles eaten at meals. This is the reason why the tongue is discolored after meals

or drinks. Unless the tongue is gently cleaned regularly, tiny remnants and particles of different meals pile up on the tongue. These form a robust mixture that becomes a fertile ground for bacteria multiplication. This situation sets the stage for the decay of such food mixtures. The warmth in the mouth cavity, actions of protein-splitting bacteria, and the presence of digestive enzymes in the mouth result in putrid mouth odor. So, cleaning the tongue is an important integral part of good oral hygiene. Try and gently apply the brush over your tongue before bed at night. After brushing, inspect the tooth brush and you will be surprised at the discoloration and amount of dirt on the brush. Such is the importance of cleaning the tongue.

### 18. What is the relationship between mouth odor and sugary beverages?

Consumption of sugary, starchy or sweet food stuffs, chewing gums, chocolates, candies, etc., accelerate the formation of dental plaques and holes in the teeth. It is also associated with increased occurrences of mouth infections and ulcers. All these conditions are known to cause or aggravate mouth odor.

### 19. Is it true that meat causes mouth odor?

Yes. Those who indulge in consuming plenty of meat per meal are prone to mouth odor, typical of stale meat. This is very common in communities where meat consumption is part of the staple diet or menu. The smell of meat is typical, but chicken smells differently from red meat, etc. However, the possibility of mouth odor is ever present. This is because meat particles commonly lodge in the spaces between the teeth and between the gum and the teeth. These particles are usually left overnight or for a considerate length of time depending on the degree of oral hygiene. The leftover meat particles are stale and exude typical odors which could be easily perceived by other people when you talk. Unfortunately, you are less likely to smell your own mouth odor.

### 20. Why are people more likely to have mouth odor when they are fasting?

Normally, when people talk, the saliva and the air in the mouth escape. This happens each time we talk, sing, or laugh and ensures that there is no stagnation in our mouth. So, normal talking, laughing, etc., help to evacuate droplets of our saliva, gases from our throat and mouth, and even fresh odor from the remnants of food particles. Such particles may be in between the teeth, on the tongue or and the gum as frequently as possible. For this reason, people with normal oral hygiene do not exude mouth odors. However, when people fast, they are usually weak, less active, and talk much less. Many people also sleep more often and for longer periods during fasting. Therefore, the mouth is closed most of the time, giving ample time for saliva and gases from the throat to accumulate in the mouth. Gases from broken down protein particles by bacteria, stay longer and the odor gets more intense, so there is poor turn-over of waste products in the form of gases and stale digested food droplets from the mouth. The odor is also fouled by stale saliva because of stagnation. Therefore, mouth odor is more common during fasting. This is also the reason why mouth odors are more common in the mornings after a long night sleep, even in those who are not fasting.

### 21. Why is mouth odor more common during pregnancy?

Mouth odor may be present in a woman early in pregnancy, when many women produce saliva excessively. Welling-up of saliva is one of the symptoms of pregnancy but when it is not disposed of through spitting and allowed to accumulate in the mouth, the breath exudes a typical ptyalin-saliva odor, which is quite irritating. The odor is much worse early in the morning when the woman wakes up. Such mouth odor normally disappears before the 18$^{th}$ week of pregnancy because at this time, production of saliva is very much reduced and the woman is better adjusted to pregnancy.

### 22. How does old age affect mouth odor?

At old age, women are less active and more careless with their health generally. Also, the teeth have suffered much from wear and tear. They are old, fewer, weak, and many are poorly aligned. The mouth has also suffered from diseases which are usually more common in old people. Some old people are physically not capable of taking good care of themselves anymore. Some even forget basic care such as caring for the mouth. Poor oral hygiene and aging, are responsible for the increased occurrence of mouth odor in old people.

### 23. Are people with mouth odor always aware that their mouths smell?

At the initial stage, it is possible for people with mouth odor to perceive it because it has just started, like a new scent, and the nose can smell it easily. However, if the odor persists for a considerable length of time, in a matter of days, the ability of the nose to smell it gradually disappears, so the person cannot perceive the odor anymore. This is one of the antisocial problems of chronic or longstanding mouth odor. While people around are facing away and avoiding the bad odor oozing from the mouth, the person is also trying to talk more directly and draw closer. This is because the speaker is not aware that the mouth odor is the reason why people move away during conversations.

## 24. Can mouth odor increase the risk of depression?

Next time you come across somebody with mouth odor, never assume that he or she knows that she actually has mouth odor. Many of such people do not know, except they are lucky to have been told by someone else. Most of those who are aware that they have mouth odor are too conscious of the fact, to the extent that they would rather isolate themselves from people and gatherings, than be avoided. Some would only talk sparingly to people who they trust and who can tolerate them. Unless active steps are taken to seek medical help, chronic mouth odor can lead to withdrawal and psychological illnesses including depression.

## 25. What is the best way to reduce mouth odor?

The single most important way to prevent or reduce mouth odor is good oral hygiene. The self-help measures include:

- Brush your teeth: Brushing the teeth at least 2 times per day. The second should be at bed time. It is also good practice to brush the teeth after meals. It is important to clean the inside surfaces of the teeth and the spaces in between them. The surfaces of the tongue, the gum, and back of the throat should also be cleaned gently with the brush
- Dental flossing: This is a highly effective way to keep the spaces in between the teeth and gum clear and clean. Flossing removes leftover fragments of meat, fruits and foods. It is desirable to floss each time before you brush your teeth, after each meal. This translates to 1-3 times per day. Flossing after dinner is highly recommended.
- Avoid smelly items: eating highly smelly foods like garlic, ginger, and onions and drinking smelly beverages. It may not be totally bad to consume these items in your meals but eating them habitually is not recommended. While consumption of sugary and sweet food items may not cause mouth odor directly, they increase the possibility of dental plaques and holes in the teeth, which are causes of mouth odor
- Dental checkup: It is necessary to have a dental checkup at least twice a year. This is a big step in preventing dental diseases, aside from treating already established problems. When you are actively suffering from mouth infection or dental diseases, it is compulsory that you see the dentist
- Fasting period: Take special care of the condition of your mouth during periods of fasting. You may still need to converse, even when you are in a sober mood
- Pregnancy: Pregnant women are more likely to experience welling up of saliva. Accumulation of saliva has its own characteristic odor which is strong and irritating. Many pregnant women experience this condition. One of the ways to reduce mouth odor during pregnancy,

is to avoid things that aggravate or increase salivation. This may include avoiding some type of foods, smells of food, perfumes, etc. Fortunately, people do not run away or avoid pregnant women just because of mouth odor

- Illness: Take care when you have a cough! If the origin of your cough is an infection, you are more likely to have mouth odor, especially if you bring out phlegm. This is the truth, even though it is commonly disregarded perhaps because a cough is a common ailment. This type of cough does not include those due to conditions like asthma, that are not as a result of infections

### 26. Is there any medical treatment for mouth odor?

Some mouth odors are caused by diseases of the mouth, throat and wind pipe, liver and chronic digestion problems. Many are due to poor oral hygiene, holes in the tooth or dental caries, plaques, and highly spicy foods like garlic and ginger. Consultation with the doctor is necessary. Many times, solutions to mouth odor may entail visits to the dentist to take care of dental problems, followed by regular checkups. For odors caused by foods, stoppage of such consumptions may be the only solution. There are suggestions in the soft-sell media that foods like garlic, ginger, onions, etc., are helpful in many diseases and conditions including hypertension, diabetes and obesity. However, most of the claims have not been proved conclusively. Many people who take such foods believe in their efficacy, and it is sometimes difficult to convince them to stop or modify their consumption.

## SKIN BLEACHING

### 27. What is responsible for skin coloration?

Skin color is due to the effect of a pigment in the skin called melanin, which is produced by a type of cell in the body called melanocytes. The degree of pigmentation in an individual is proportional to the amount or concentration of melanin in the skin. This means that dark colored individuals have high concentrations of melanin, while fair complexioned individuals have lower concentrations of melanin. Melanin concentration in an individual is partly genetic or familial. That is, if one or both parents are dark, their offspring is more likely to be dark, but if they are fair in complexion, their offspring is more likely to be fair. However, environmental conditions also have great influence on the skin appearance and color. For example, people who live in hot climates, where the heat is great usually appear dark in color. This may be as a result of burning sunshine, as in many parts of Africa and Asia. In a country like India, there are fair skinned as well as dark skinned people. The dark skinned Indians are those that live mainly in the hot regions of the country. Even in some African countries like Nigeria, those who live in the northern parts nearer the Sahara Desert, are usually darker. Another factor is long-term exposure to sources of heat in occupations that expose workers to heat. Long term exposure to heat radiation from charcoal fire, firewood, locomotives, etc., can gradually make the skin darker.

### 28. What does skin bleaching mean?
Skin bleaching is an intentional act of applying substances on the skin, for the purpose of changing its color from black or dark to 'white'. Skin bleaching is more common in the Black African race and Asians. Whether it is bleaching clothes or skin, the intention is the same, to make it lighter.

### 29. What is the difference between skin bleaching and toning?
The differences are subtle. Both are done to achieve lighter complexions. However, the word bleaching connotes a stronger intention or desire, to change the skin color more dramatically. This may include lightening of dark spots, marks, scars and achieving a light skin from an originally highly pigmented, dark skin. Skin toning suggests an intention to achieve a lighter and more even skin that appears 'flawless'. Therefore, dark complexioned individuals tend to bleach, while fair complexioned persons tend to tone their skins.

### 30. Why do people bleach their skins?
The overriding reason for skin bleaching is beauty. Many people believe that making their skin lighter makes them more beautiful, and they will therefore do their utmost to achieve this, using all manner of local creams and soaps. Psychologically, they are not satisfied with the color or degree of pigmentation of their skin. As legitimate as it sounds, it appears that most people do not know the consequences of bleaching or if they do, they just don't care.

### 31. What parts of the skin are affected during bleaching?
The skin has two main layers. The topmost layer is called the epidermis while the deeper layer is the dermis. The epidermis is the layer that is mostly affected during bleaching. With intensive skin bleaching, the superficial aspects of the dermis may also be involved in some areas of the skin.

### 32. In what ways do bleaching creams work?
Melanin is responsible for skin coloration. Most bleaching creams work by reducing the amount of melanin pigments in the skin.

### 33. What are the main chemicals used for bleaching?

Bleaching is most commonly achieved by the application of chemicals or bleaching creams on the skin. Bleaching creams come in different formulations and varieties. In the past, most bleaching creams commonly contain one of the following as its major components:
- Hydroquinone
- Mercury
- Topical steroids
- Retinoic acid, Vitamin A or Retin A

### 34. Are there no natural skin lighteners that are free of chemicals?

Whether a skin lightener is produced by a combination of chemicals in the factory or extracted directly from a plant, they are all chemicals. However, those extracted directly may be considered to be more 'natural'. There are many skin lightening creams which contain natural ingredients. Such natural ingredients include:
- Vitamin A: as retinoic acid - This works by reducing the amount of melanin pigment in the skin. The skin becomes lighter in color. The retinoids also improve the thickness of the epidermis
- Arbutin: a plant extract
- Kojic acid: an extract from fungus

Some women feel more comfortable using natural bleaching agents than those produced by chemical combinations in the laboratory.

### 35. Is mercury commonly used as a bleaching cream?

Because of serious health hazards, mercury was banned as a cosmetic ingredient in the USA, Europe, and many other countries. Unfortunately, about 25% of bleaching creams available in Asia and Africa still contain mercury. Mercury is available as a cosmetic ingredient in soaps, creams, or gels in many parts of Africa and other places where there are poor regulations. There are varieties of local skin mixtures, concoctions, and creams made from locally available chemicals, most of which are caustic to the skin. In sub-Saharan Africa, many ladies formulate their own bleaching creams by mixing or grinding together different soaps, powders and chemicals, to make "potent" bleaching creams. The native black soap is a popular component of bleaching creams in many African communities.

### 36. What are the bad effects of mercury?

Mercury is a heavy metal. It has very stubborn itching and irritating effects when it comes in contact with the skin. More importantly, mercury is one of the deadliest poisons ever known and should not be allowed to get into the mouth or applied on the skin. The liver and the kidneys are the two important organs in the body that function to degrade and subsequently remove poisonous substances from the body. Because of these, the effects of mercury poisoning are more common in the liver and kidneys, resulting in liver and kidney failure.

**37.     What are the features of mercury poisoning?**

The disastrous effects of skin bleaching using mercury include:
- Kidney failure
- Liver failure
- Brain damage
- Mental illness
- Other diseases of the nerves in the body

**38.     What should be done before bleaching creams are applied to the skin?**

The most important thing is to seek the advice of a doctor, to know if a particular cream is good or not. People who are sick or have diseases that may get worse should not use bleaching creams. People with systemic illnesses like diabetes and extensive skin infections are at higher risks of more serious infections with bleaching creams. So, the doctor's advice is important. Here are some key points that you should always observe before applying any cream:
- Read the manufacturer's instructions carefully and be sure to understand the information on what the ingredients are and how to apply the cream.
- ALWAYS EXCLUDE MERCURY! Be sure that your cream does not contain mercury in any form. Some manufacturers may use some confusing names to denote mercury. So beware!
- If the cream contains hydroquinone, be sure it is not more than 2%
- Search through the list of ingredients to ensure you don't react to any one on the list.
- If the list contains the names of major ingredients without stating their respective amounts, it is an indication that the cream cannot be trusted. It may contain dangerous ingredients in high amounts. DON'T USE IT!
- Follow the manufacturer's instructions or directions on how to use the cream. AVOID mixing different creams together with the intention of getting a more potent cream with faster bleaching action.
- Check the dates of manufacture and the expiry. It is assumed that before deciding on the cream, it has been given prior approval by the regulatory authority such as the FDA in the USA. However, this needs to be double checked. Manufacturers usually state contraindications to drugs, creams, etc in the package. These are conditions where the uses of such medications are forbidden. You must read through the list to see if any applies to you.

- If you are not sure of the type of cream that is best for you or the genuineness of the information in the insert, consult your doctor before you get started.
- Lastly, if after applying the cream, you notice or feel any adverse reaction or sensation, immediately wash the skin with water and proceed to see your doctor without delay

### 39. Apart from using bleaching creams, are there other safer methods of skin lightening?

No method is completely safe. Every method has its own side effects or complications but then, the problems of some alternative methods of skin lightening are relatively less. The main alternative method is called skin resurfacing. In skin resurfacing, the top layer of the skin is removed through operation. This creates an intentional wound. The wound heals from below and a new skin is grown from the deeper layer of the skin or dermis. The new skin is higher in collagen activity, more elastic, and more 'youthful'. Skin resurfacing can be achieved through:
- Laser treatment
- Skin surface restoration-chemical peels
- Dermabrasion

Skin resurfacing is a procedure that must be prescribed and performed by skin specialists or other trained and certified skincare health providers. Skin resurfacing is not suitable for everybody, so the advice of the dermatologist is paramount.

### 40. What is laser resurfacing?

Laser resurfacing is a procedure that uses laser beams to remove the upper layer of the skin (epidermis) and the upper part of the deep layer. The wound created by the laser action, heals with thickening of the epidermis. Collagen activities are increased which makes the skin look younger. Previously dark spots become more evenly toned while skin wrinkles are greatly reduced.

### 41. What is a chemical peel?

Chemical peels are mostly acids. They are applied on the skin to destroy or remove the top layer of the skin. New skin grows from the deeper layer or dermis. Acids are dangerous on the skin but the effect depends on the particular acid used, its strength, or concentration.

### 42. What about dermabrasion?

This procedure also reduces wrinkles and removes dark spots on the skin. However, it is cruder and less friendly than laser resurfacing, as the surface of the skin or epidermis is mechanically scraped off to create a wound.

**43. Generally speaking, what are the complications that may arise as a result of skin bleaching?**

There are specific problems that may develop as a result of bleaching. In many instances, this largely depends on the type of cream or method used. Generally, people who bleach may have one or a combination of the following:
- Irritation
- Skin discoloration
- Infection
- Thinning of the skin
- Poor wound healing
- Duodenal and stomach ulcers
- Skin ulcers
- Hair damage and boils
- Inappropriate exfoliation - scales
- Premature aging of the skin
- Allergic reactions

**44. What is the effect of bleaching on injury and wound healing?**

A bleached skin is much more prone to injury or trauma. Wound healing is also much slower than in normal, healthy skin. With bleached skin, infections spread more easily and faster. For example, wounds from burns are more severely infected and much more difficult to treat.

**45. Does skin bleaching cause body odor?**

Skin bleaching may cause body odor, depending on the type of cream involved. Body odor due to bleaching is more common in women who mix or grind together various soaps and creams, hoping to achieve faster results. Initially, the body odor is similar to that of the cream. In the long run, the cream mixes with sweat and gets embedded under the skin. This produces a bad, pungent, and repulsive odor which may be unique to the individual woman. Such an odor may be perceived from a distance. In some instances, even the woman's clothing may exude the odor. If the odor is linked to the use of bleaching creams and it becomes persistent or constantly present, there is a high probability of skin damage and other unpleasant consequences.

**46. Can the color of bleached skin be permanent?**

No, skin bleaching is not permanent. Melanin is responsible for skin pigmentation or coloration. The color of the skin depends on the concentration of melanin. Most bleaching creams can only reduce the effect of melanin for as long as they are applied. Thus, once the cream is stopped, pigmentation by melanin is restored and the skin color gradually changes to its original form. The mistake made by women who bleach is to assume that the lightening effect of bleaching creams and soaps are permanent. In most cases, the skin color is reversed to what it was originally, soon after the cream is stopped. In addition, it takes a long time before bleached skin can regain its original shade of coloration and beauty. The usual picture after discontinuing a cream is a darker skin that looks dry, discolored, inferior and much older.

### 47. How does intense sunshine make the skin darker?
Prolonged exposure to severe heat from the sun causes sun burns. Such heat destroys the skin's surface including the melanin pigment. As part of the natural repair mechanism of the body, the cells produce more melanin. The increased concentration of melanin results in a darker skin.

### 48. How does old age affect skin color?
It is normal for the skin to become darker with advancing age. This effect is more noticeable in the exposed parts of the body, especially the face. It is also more pronounced in dark skinned people. The skin also becomes wrinkled, thinner and loses it elasticity, after the age of 60 years in many individuals. In individuals that indulge in skin bleaching, because of the destruction of the upper layer of the skin, these adverse effects of aging take place earlier than 60 years and are more severe.

### 49. Why is the face usually darker than the rest of the body in most women?
The concentration and effect of melanin varies in different parts of the body. In some individuals, melanin pigment is more highly concentrated in the face than other parts of the body. In such persons, the face usually appears remarkably darker than other parts of the body. Secondly, the face is the only part of the body that is perennially not protected or covered by clothing. This exposes the face to adverse effects from the environment. These include dust, fumes and hot radiation from the sun. The result of all these include bumps on the face, pimples and darker facial skin. However, parts of the body that are covered by clothing are protected from such adverse effects especially intense sunshine. Consequently, these parts appear lighter than the face and other parts of the body that are usually exposed.

### 50. Can skin bleaching lead to cancer?
Yes. One of the worst consequences of skin bleaching is the increased incidence of cancers, especially cancer of the skin. Both hydroquinone and mercury which are common in bleaching creams and soaps are capable of causing cancer of the skin. Mercury is poisonous and in addition, can damage many organs in the body. It is notorious for causing kidney damage which usually results in kidney failure.

**51.    Does bleaching have any medical use or advantage?**

There is no important medical benefit derivable from bleaching. In a few instances, doctors may prescribe appropriate creams to be applied on old, black scars or dark marks for cosmetic reasons, especially if the scars are conspicuous and the woman is worried. The purpose is to lighten the color of the scars and make them blend more with the surrounding skin. This makes the scar more socially acceptable and less embarrassing to the woman. However, this treatment is only appropriate if it is prescribed and supervised by the doctor.

## DEAR DOCTOR:

**52.    What can I do to prevent body odor?**

Ideally, self-help measures should be started early in childhood, so that they become established practices before puberty. Briefly they are:

- Keep dry – all places that perspire should be kept clean and dry. The hair in the armpit should be shaved or kept clean by regular washing and mopping. If the hair is to be unshaven, then it must be clean and dry
- Perfumes- Do not spray perfumes on the cloth in the armpit area. This will produce a strong offensive odor when it mixes with sweat in the armpit. Perfumes are meant to be sprayed on the skin; not the dress. Clothes soaked with sweat in the armpit, for example, will take in a lot of sweat crusts and ensure the sustenance of the horrible odor, apart from staining the dress
- Avoid tight fitting nylon or synthetic fabrics. They retain heat and promote sweating
- Avoid spicy foods, garlic, red meat, etc.
- Avoid obesity through regular exercise and dieting
- Bathe with antibacterial soaps when necessary. Warm water is better because it kills bacteria
- If you are fasting, do not neglect your health. Do not forget to bathe regularly, clean your mouth, and be cheerful
- Wash your feet at least once daily preferably in warm water. Wear clean socks once a day and clean your shoes. Allow the shoes to ventilate at the end of each day. This is more important for men and ladies who wear covered shoes
- Deodorants and antiperspirants may help, but must be used correctly

**53.    Doctor, I take garlic regularly and have been accused of mouth odor many times. Please, what can I do to cure this?**

Garlic is one of the items that have strong characteristic odors. Other examples are ginger and onion. The odor of garlic can be strong and long lasting, especially if you chew them like many women do. The odor is not socially friendly and is not acceptable to many people. It can make people avoid staying around you or engaging in conversation with you. People take garlic for different suspected and unproven medicinal beliefs. You should seek your doctor's advice to see if there are alternatives to raw garlic that can be prescribed for the same ailment or benefits. Surely, the only way to abolish the odor is to stop eating garlic completely. This is the cure.

### 54. How can I tell someone that he or she has mouth odor?

Tell them and let them know in a most private and friendly manner. Many people with mouth odor do not know. If you tell them in a way that shows you care, they will be most grateful. Some may also ask for your advice. If you do not have any advice that may be useful to them, tell them to see a doctor as soon as they can. It is a wrong attitude to announce their plight derisively, cover your face or nose, or deliberately face away. Remember that if you don't make an effort to bring it to their attention, you will, in a way contribute to the sustenance of their mouth odor. In every case, the appropriateness of the circumstance should guide your action.

### 55. How can I sustain the lightening effect of my cream and make it more permanent?

Almost all bleaching or skin lightening creams have user instructions from the various manufacturers. The creams need to be used according to manufacturer's instructions. They also need to be kept and stored properly, even though most are usually kept at room temperature. To achieve a longer lasting effect, the creams need to be used regularly and continuously, for as long as you want the effect to last. When skin lightening creams are discontinued, the skin gradually returns to its previous color. So, for you to enjoy the new color, you need to continue applying the cream. The other important thing to do is to protect your skin as much as possible from the direct rays of hot sunshine and other sources of heat. This can be achieved through the use of sun screens or sun blocks, sun shielding creams, umbrellas, etc.

### 56. I am pregnant; can I continue to use my bleaching cream?

Generally, it is not appropriate to use any drug that is not prescribed for you during pregnancy. Drugs in this sense include tablets, capsules, injections, creams, etc. Many drugs are not safe during pregnancy. They may cause problems for you, the baby in the womb, or both of you. The effects on the baby include:

- Congenital deformities
- Damage to organs like the kidneys, liver, heart, and brain

- Bleeding in pregnancy, abortion, premature labor and delivery
- Small baby and low birth weight
- Death of the baby in the womb or after birth

Because of these potential problems, it is better to stop using bleaching creams as soon as pregnancy has been confirmed. If you think that your cream is probably safe, you should confirm with the manufacturers and also seek the advice of your doctor before continuing with it

**57. Since I am not swallowing the creams, how does the cream that I apply on my skin affect my growing baby?**

The skin covers the exterior of the body. It has little holes or pores on its surface through which substances pass into the inside of the body. Indeed, the skin is like a 'net'. Liquids and creams pass through easily. Therefore, the cream applied on the skin surface nourishes the skin from inside. In the same manner, your bleaching cream will enter through the holes in the skin, enters your blood stream, and is carried around your body. It eventually gets to your baby through the placenta. So, creams that contain harmful substances such as mercury may eventually get to your kidneys and those of your baby.

**58. I have been using bleaching cream for about 5 years and there is no evidence of cancer. Does this mean it is safe?**

No. It is a fact that skin bleaching can result in cancer of the skin. However, this may develop slowly and after a variable period of time. It may take years for cancer and other diseases to manifest. Therefore, you should carefully consider the risk of such diseases like cancer against the cosmetic benefits of bleaching.

**59. Doctor, I have a liver problem. Since it was diagnosed, my skin seems to have turned darker. Why is this so and how can I cure this?**

The skin is the general gateway to the body. The skin quality and color tend to reflect the situation of our general health. In some disease conditions, the skin commonly manifests with different types of rashes, itchiness, pimples, and change in color. This is the situation in liver diseases. The skin may also change color or become darker, due to other diseases including heart and kidney failures. Skin changes may also be due to systemic infections like tuberculosis, chronic weight loss, long standing skin infections and chronic skin ulcers, etc. When the diseases are cured, the skin discoloration may be reduced or improved but not totally reversed. Dark spots or coloration caused by conditions like chronic leg ulcers may be difficult to reverse completely.

www.ingramcontent.com/pod-product-compliance
Lightning Source LLC
Chambersburg PA
CBHW061502180526
45171CB00001B/5